GERIATRIC PHARMACOLOGY AND THERAPEUTICS

GERIATRIC PHARMACOLOGY AND THERAPEUTICS

EDITED BY

J.C. Brocklehurst

MD, MSc, FRCP
Professor of Geriatric Medicine
University of Manchester

BLACKWELL SCIENTIFIC PUBLICATIONS
OXFORD LONDON EDINBURGH
BOSTON PALO ALTO MELBOURNE

Editorial offices:
Osney Mead, Oxford, OX2 0EL
8 John Street, London, WC1N 2ES
23 Ainslie Place, Edinburgh, EH3 6AJ
52 Beacon Street, Boston
Massachusetts 02108, USA
706 Cowper Street, Palo Alto
California 94301, USA
107 Barry Street, Carlton
Victoria 3053, Australia

First published 1984

Set, printed and bound by
Butler and Tanner Ltd,
Frome and London

DISTRIBUTORS

USA
Blackwell Mosby Book Distributors
11830 Westline Industrial Drive
St Louis, Missouri 63141

Canada
Blackwell Mosby Book Distributors
120 Melford Drive, Scarborough
Ontario M1B 2X4

Australia
Blackwell Scientific Book Distributors
31 Advantage Road, Highett
Victoria 3190

British Library
Cataloguing in Publication Data

Geriatric pharmacology and therapeutics.
1. Geriatric pharmacology
I. Brocklehurst, J.C.
615.5′8′0880565 RC953.7

ISBN 0-632-01303-6

Contents

List of Contributors

J.C. Brocklehurst
MD, MSc, FRCP
Professor of Geriatric Medicine, University of Manchester, University Hospital of South Manchester, Manchester, England

C.M. Castleden
MD, MB ChB, FRCP
Consultant in Geriatric Medicine, Leicester General Hospital, Gwendolen Road, Leicester, England

W. Davison
MA, MB ChB, FRCP
Senior Consultant Physician, Department of Geriatric Medicine, Addenbrooke's Hospital, Cambridge, England

D.E. Hyams
MB BS, FRCP
Senior Director, Medical Operations, Merck Sharp and Dohme Research Laboratories, Rahway, New Jersey, USA

M.D.W. Lye
MD, MB ChB, MRCP
Professor of Geriatric Medicine, University of Liverpool, P.O. Box 147, Liverpool, England

J.E.F. Pohl
BSc, MB BS, FRCP
Consultant Physician, Department of Medicine, Leicester General Hospital, Gwendolen Road, Leicester, England

D. Robertson
MB BS, FRCP(C), FACP, FRCP(Ed)
Professor and Head, Division of Geriatric Medicine, University of Saskatchewan, Saskatoon, Canada

Preface

It is now well recognized that medicine in old age, while sharing most of the problems which arise in the practice of medicine in younger people, has a whole additional range of problems of its own. These arise because of the background of aging, the accumulation of pathology and the altered drug effects that occur in old people. The combination of all these factors affects not only the presentation of many diseases in the elderly but also the way in which old people react to a therapeutic regimen.

While this book does not attempt to rewrite the whole field of pharmacology and therapeutics, it does aim to deal with all those aspects of medical treatment in old people which have their own special problems and which differ in their nature and presentation from treatment at younger ages. In highlighting the differences in pharmacology and therapeutics in old age a necessary preliminary is to consider something of the processes of aging itself and how they affect pharmacodynamics and pharmacokinetics. Subsequently we consider the implications of an aging society: both as to its effect on the prescribing habits of physicians (and the nation's drug bill) and also regarding the problems that old people have in personally managing their own medications.

Geriatric Pharmacology and Therapeutics is written by a group of authors, most of whom are also involved in teaching geriatric medicine to medical students. The book has been written primarily for family practitioners but it will also be of use and interest to geriatricians and internists.

This book is intended for an international readership and a small number of drugs discussed are not available in North America. In each chapter the drugs discussed are listed in tables and any not available in North America are indicated.

J.C. Brocklehurst
University of Manchester

Chapter One
A General Introduction to Aging

W. DAVISON

Old and young, we are all on our last cruise
Robert Louis Stevenson (1850–94)

OVERVIEW

Aging is an essential characteristic of living things setting a limit to the potential life span of the species, even under best conditions. Some possible basic biological mechanisms and the functional consequences of aging in the human are outlined. The key role of an intact central nervous system in the fight for survival is emphasized. Attention is drawn to the possibility that much morbidity and mortality (more especially in the male) is due to an unhealthy life style.

Some social characteristics of the elderly are looked at and the changing demography is considered, especially the impact on health and welfare agencies. Lastly, there is a look at the elderly at home, their life satisfaction and health. It is hoped that this chapter will help the family practitioner view his ailing elderly patient in perspective, both biologically and sociologically.

AGING: A FUNDAMENTAL BIOLOGICAL PROCESS

What is aging?

Aging comprises those fundamental changes not due to disease occurring in individuals after maturity, which are more or less common to all members of the species and which increase the probability of death. The relative uniformity of the process of senescence and the consequent inevitability of death, is an unpalatable fact that each man's philosophy of life must embrace. Aging inevitably results in death and the increasing probability of imminent death with advancing years after puberty was expressed mathematically more than 150 years ago by Benjamin Gompertz. He showed that this probability doubles every 8 years over the age of 35. In the developed world people are least liable to die in the years just before puberty, thereafter the risk of imminent death increases exponentially (Finch & Hayflick 1977, p. 513). Aging is the increasing inability to resist death.

Aging as an evolutionary adaptation

Death by aging is essential for the vigour and the survival of the species. It helps to keep down total population size and those who die make way for youth. Without death, life as we know it would be impossible. With these processes of death and birth comes the possibility of change in the species by genetic mutation. The more favoured mutants are more likely to survive and procreate; the less favoured mutants more likely to succumb. Presumably the different species-specific life spans have evolved to confer on each species the maximum vigour and survival potential for living in its own environment in a particular epoch; for example, in *homo sapiens* the long postmenopause may have evolved to allow more intellectual development (which provides the hallmark for our species). The long postmenopause allowed the longer-lived members to act (before books and computers) as vital repositories of knowledge, i.e. as data banks. Thus older people earned their postreproductive lives by conferring considerable survival advantage on the young. This crucial role has been eroded in modern society.

Table 1.1 Possible molecular mechanisms of aging.

Biological clock
Error hypothesis
Hayflick limit
Accumulation of waste
Cross-linkage of proteins

The biological clock

The predictable rate of aging in each species suggests some kind of biological clock mechanism programmed genetically to run for a set time before allowing death to occur. A mechanism of this sort seems essential to allow natural growth and development; for example, the early death of tissues between the digits on the hands and feet of the human fetus (morpho-genetic death), and (in another species) the death of the tail and gills of the tadpole to allow the normal metamorphosis to a frog to take place (phylogenetic death). Controlled death and regeneration is as important within individuals as it is for the development and survival of the species as a whole.

The error hypothesis

It has been suggested that aging may be due to an accumulation of errors in the molecular content of the cells of the body. DNA and RNA provide the key control mechanisms for protein synthesis but they can be damaged by mutagens such as radiation, free radicals (e.g. superoxide) and drugs. There is a continuous turnover of enzymes, hormones and neurotransmitters and at each stage in the biochemical processes there is the possibility of error. If errors accumulate beyond a certain level, the cells or tissues will become incompetent and may die; for example, if the brain cells deteriorate chemically then even if the cells themselves survive, ultimately the brain as a whole would cease to function satisfactorily, homeostatic controls would fail and death would ensue. If dysfunctioning cells in any tissue are allowed to survive and proliferate, death of the whole organism will eventually occur as in many malignant diseases.

The rate at which errors accumulate depends partly on the rate of error production and partly on the rate of error removal and this applies at both the molecular and the cellular level. In cell division normally the replication of DNA is a highly accurate and reliable process so that the daughter cells have all the proper constituents, viz. chromosomes, RNA and proteins. However, damage to the genetic material may produce coding errors and result in faulty cell proteins.

The Hayflick limit

In the first half of this century it was commonly believed that certain vertebrate cell types such as the fibroblast could grow in culture indefinitely. The work of Carrel and later Ebling suggested this. However, in the mid 1960s Hayflick and others observed that some 40–50 doublings was the upper limit for cells grown from human fetal tissue. This 'Hayflick limit', as it has come to be called, is now generally accepted as the ultimate life span of genetically normal human fibroblasts in culture.

Accumulation of intra- and extra-cellular waste

Some cells are actively dividing and replacing themselves throughout life. These cells are all 'young' even though the whole organism is 'old'. This is true of the cells of the blood, gastrointestinal mucosa and outer layers of the skin. Other cells have to last literally for a lifetime. If they die before death of the whole organism, they are not replaced. Examples of these postmitotic cells are heart muscle cells and neurones. Throughout life they gradually accumulate lipids, lysosomes and lipofuscin. Opinion is divided as to whether these accumulations are deleterious with respect to normal aging.

One of the most constant biological features of aging is the increasing quantity of lipofuscin or 'wear and tear pigment' found in many tissues. Its origin and effects are not known but production from lysosomes is a probability. Formation of lipofuscin can be inhibited by antioxidants and its removal from neurones can be achieved by centrophenoxine in the experimental animal. The benefits which might accrue from preventing the formation or affecting the removal of lipofuscin from the human brain are none too clear but some clinical reports are encouraging. There is also extracellular accumulation of other substances, such as amyloid which may have adverse effects on cell or organ function.

Aging of connective tissue

Connective tissue aging may contribute to the failure of the more metabolically active tissues as well as causing many of the other manifestations of old age, including thinning and fragility of the skin, loss of elasticity of blood vessels and stiffening of heart muscles and joints. Collagen is the main connective tissue protein. Its stiffening with age is due to chemical cross-linkage of adjacent parts of macromolecules with resultant altered physical properties. Similar changes occur in elastin and other proteins of the interstitial tissues. Lathyrogens such as beta-aminopropionitrile (BAPN) and penicillamine have been shown to inhibit cross-linkage in collagen.

Immune system failure

The immune system (IS) functions less effectively in older animals than in the young, and some parts of it (e.g. thymus) atrophy comparatively early in life. Normally the IS protects the body against invasion by bacteria, viruses and fungi and also prevents accumulation of the body's own unwanted cells. Cells which are not acceptable because they are effete, foreign to the host or malignant are identified and destroyed. If the IS fails in this task, it may allow alien cells to invade, or may fail to recognize 'self' cells and proceed to destroy them as if they too were alien (autoimmunity).

General failure of the IS would help to explain the susceptibility to infection and the increased incidence of autoimmune diseases and some malignancies with age. There is an inverse relationship between the overall incidence of cancer and the activity of the IS and this is seen most clearly in the aged. Experimental attempts to combat these problems have used immunosuppressive drugs to prevent or suppress autoimmune reactions. In some cases, immune cells are infused from a healthy young donor to counteract the immunodeficiency of the elderly recipient. The results are not encouraging. Existing immunosuppressants (e.g. azathioprine and cyclophosphamide) are much too toxic and non-specific in their effects to use as general life-extending agents. Also the use of IS cell homografts is beset by formidable technical problems of immunological match and mismatch. One suggestion is to use IS cell autografts which were removed in the full bloom of youth and stored in a tissue bank, as is done with sperms, for use when required in old age!

WHAT DOES BIOLOGICAL RESEARCH TELL US?

Despite the mass of research into biological and especially molecular aspects of aging there is no evidence yet to suggest that we can influence the rate of human aging. We can, however, affect the incidence of disease and thus maximize activity and prolong life. Medical practice must focus on the promotion of good health and the identification and effective treatment of disease. The retardation of aging is not yet on the medical agenda despite many claims to the contrary (Finch & Hayflick 1977).

Functional consequences of aging

Age changes comprise a decline in efficiency, a loss of homeostasis, a weakening or damage to structure and an eventual breakdown in health. Death is the outcome. Primary aging, although an inherent process, is also influenced to a greater or lesser degree by the social and physical environment. It must be distinguished from secondary aging which refers to the effects of trauma and disease.

The general appearance and behaviour of an individual will give a good indication of his age. Careful camouflage by clothes, cosmetics (even cosmetic surgery) and 'acting young' may for a time give an impression of extended youth but soon the truth will out! Greying of the hair, frontal balding, wrinkling of the skin and puffiness under the eyes are all manifestations of middle-age. By the age of 50 years half the population have at least half their body hair grey, irrespective of their sex or early hair colour. Also over 60% of this age group have bitemporal recession and some vertical thinning. Failing vision (presbyopia), slowing of dark adaptation and decline in hearing (presbycusis) also develop. There is need for improved illumination to allow adequate vision and also need to provide good contrasts in the environment to give clear visual signals. Taste and smell sensitivity also decline.

Even in the absence of disease, changes take place which affect pharmacokinetics (Finch & Hayflick 1977, Chapter 8). The lean body mass (LBM) consisting of brain, heart, lungs, liver, kidney and other organs together with the voluntary muscle mass (which is maximal at age 20–30 years) decreases and body fat increases. By age 80 years about half of the striated muscle cells have been lost and replaced in this way. This reduction in LBM can be demonstrated by the 15–20% drop in exchangeable potassium per kilogram body weight between age 20 and 75 years. Thus despite continued physical exercise there is a decline in both strength and stamina. The loss of stamina is noticeable in both work and leisure by the age of 40 years and is well established by 60. It is more marked in sedentary males than in manual workers and females. Total respiratory capacity (including arterial oxygen saturation), glomerular filtration rate and tubular functions are all reduced. There is loss of one-third of the nephrons and the mean value of glomerular filtration rate in healthy 80-year-olds is only half of that of young people. Even in the presence of a normal blood urea a big drop in renal function must be assumed. The importance of this lies in the liability to overt renal failure during illness and the reduced ability to excrete drugs via the kidney, even in the absence of disease known to affect renal function.

Basal metabolism is very high in childhood, drops rapidly from before puberty to the mid-twenties and continues to decline, albeit more slowly, for the rest of life. To avoid obesity it is necessary to reduce calorie intake in keeping with these changes—say by 5% in each decade from 40 to 60 years and by 10% in each decade from 60 to 80 years (Trémolières & Geissler-Brun 1975). That is to say the 60-year-old needs 10% less energy from food than at 40. The 'ideal' body weight (i.e. that which confers the lowest mortality in statistical studies) is 15% below the average weight in the USA. If the body weight is 30–50% above the mean in middle age the mortality risk doubles.

Table 1.2 Some functional consequences of aging.

Loss of vigour and mobility
Altered pharmacokinetics
Failing special senses
Liability to fall and fracture
Failing thermoregulation
Failing intellect

Aging of the nervous system

Differential aging occurs in all body systems. Nevertheless in terms of self-care the role of the central nervous system (CNS) is paramount. Evidence of this abounds in everyday medical practice; when the intellect goes, self-care is no longer feasible.

Brain weight decreases with age, more especially very late in life, so that the brain weight of the 80-year-old is found to be some 10% less than that of the 30-year-old. Progressive neuronal fallout has long been accepted as the most plausible explanation of loss of both brain volume and intellect. Certainly some neuronal loss occurs but it is less general than previously believed, being much more marked in certain areas of the brain than in others (Birren & Sloane 1980, p. 75). Some brain shrinkage may be due to loss of stroma rather than neurons. Characteristic histopathological and neurochemical changes also occur with aging but will not be detailed here. However, let it be noted that malfunction of brain cells rather than simply neuronal fallout may be the main problem affecting the aging brain; for example, defects occur in central neurotransmitter synthesis of acetylcholine, dopamine and other catecholamines as well as γ-aminobutyric acid. Aging brings increased forgetfulness, difficulty in acquiring and assessing new information and concepts, as well as slowing of sensorimotor responses. Psychic energy or drive (conation) is lost so that the speed and agility of the mind diminishes with increasing years. There is a narrowing of interest and although 'crystallized' intellect performs well enough into great age (which is adequate for high court judges and clergymen!), 'fluid' intellect falls off markedly; most elderly people do not exhibit a quick grasp of complex new data, nor can they analyse it rapidly. Thus they are less adept in newly developing mathematical sciences. Despite these changes, high level intellect can be maintained by various adaptive strategies, including the use of experience, a slower pace and a smaller volume of work.

Sleep requirements change throughout life and older people sleep less well. Older women spend more time in bed and sleep longer and wake less often in the night than do men. Men take longer to go to sleep and their sleep is more broken. Most older people adjust satisfactorily to these changes but the more neurotic individuals with unresolved anxiety, characteristically complain of broken sleep and many find difficulty in coping without sleeping tablets. As a result there is an age-related increase in the consumption of hypnotics.

There are well-established, age-related declines in thermoregulatory functions; for example, elderly people often show reduced ability to discriminate between skin temperature differences as wide apart as 5 °C—there is diminished sweat response to heating and impaired shivering response to cooling. These changes, together with intellectual failure and impaired mobility, put elderly patients at risk of hypothermia in cold weather. Thus in a survey of over 1000 elderly people living at home in the first quarter of 1972 in England it was found that 10% had borderline hypothermia with a deep body temperature of less than 35.5 °C. Also in 75% of the homes in this survey the ambient temperature was at or below the minimum generally accepted housing standard temperature (18.3 °C). Impaired thermoregulatory responses were found to be very common. Detailed tests, on a subsample of the survey showed impaired thermoregulation of some degree in 50% of subjects. Further tests a few years later showed that the disorder was progressive (Exton-Smith & Evans 1977, p. 41). Coping with a very warm or a very cold environment becomes more difficult with increasing age. Rapid temperature swings are particularly stressful and produce a sharp increase in morbidity and mortality.

Loss of postural stability is another decline in CNS function. Women are twice as liable to fall as men. The risk of falling increases linearly with age; in one study, 30% of women in the 65–69 years age group reported falls, compared with more than 50% of the women aged 85 and over. In the very old (aged 75 years and over) tripping, giddiness and drop attacks are all important causes followed by loss of balance. Tests of control of sway in the upright posture show a progressive decline with age after maturity (age 30–40 years) and again the phenomenon is much more marked in women at all ages (Exton-Smith & Evans 1977, p. 47). Visual failure and inadequate illumination and lack of colour contrasts in the environment increase the chance of falling.

Falls are incapacitating in themselves but also they put the victim at risk of additional hazards, especially hypothermia and fractures. Not surprisingly there is an age-related increase in fractures. After the age of 60 years the incidence of femoral neck fracture doubles every 5 years in women and every 7 years in men. Thus for the female population the cumulative risk of sustaining a fractured upper femur is 25% by the age of 90 years. Apart from a liability to fall, the other major causative factor in the occurrence of fractures is the age-related decrease in quantity and quality of bone (Exton-Smith & Evans 1977, p. 51). Much evidence exists to show that loss of bone with age is a universal phenomenon but postmenopausal oestrogen deficiency causes accelerated loss and puts the female especially at risk (Stevenson & Whitehead 1982). Poor nutrition, inferior skeletal status in earlier years, lack of physical exercise and the effects of disease, including osteomalacia, are all implicated in addition to aging *per se*.

From what has been said it is clear that health in old age is determined by a multiplicity of factors of which aging is but one. Inheritance, early growth and development, education, life style, environment and the impact of disease are also important in the crucible of life. An understanding of the relative contributions of these multiple factors offers hope of a greatly enhanced quality of life for old people, even without being able to comprehend, let alone modify the aging process itself.

Demographic and social trends

How old can you become?

It is well known that people are living longer and there are more old people now than ever before. However, there are no well-documented cases of people in the USA or UK living to age 120 years or more, suggesting that age 120 or thereabouts is the theoretical maximum life expectancy for human beings. The few who approach this maximum represent the biological elite. Nowadays people are achieving a bigger tranche of the theoretical maximum life span, and the average life expectancy at birth has risen by 20 years this century.

However, people are not living all that much longer from the standpoint of the middle-aged and elderly. Thus the life expectancy for an infant born

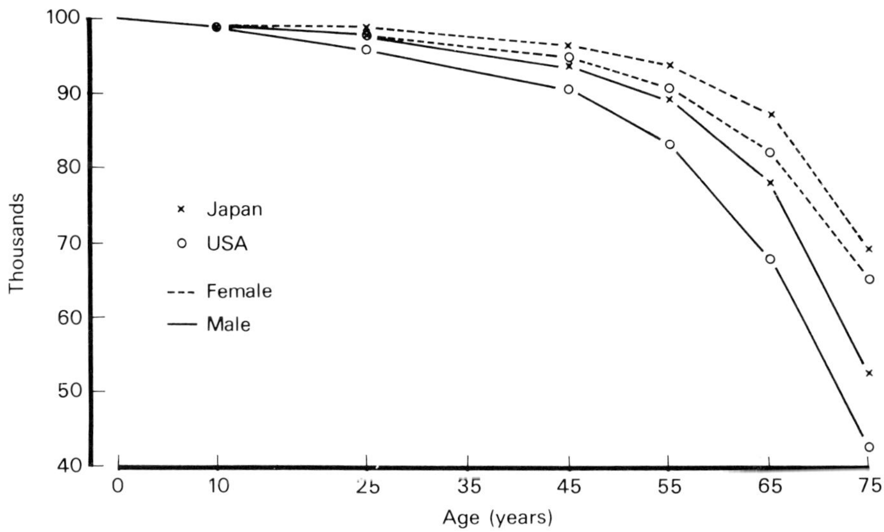

Fig. 1.1 Numbers surviving out of 100 000 born alive (WHO 1978).

in the USA today is very much better than for one born in 1900 but the life expectancy for the average 40-year-old male has improved little over the same period, certainly not by more than 3 or 4 years. Middle-aged females have done rather better by gaining an extra 8 or 9 years since 1900. In 1975 the average expectation of life of white females was over 77 years and for white males almost 70 years. For non-whites, male and female, the expectancy was 6 or 7 years less.

Males die earlier

Contemporary male mortality rates in middle age in the USA are 60% higher than those for women. Why should this be? The longer life span of the female is seen in species other than man and so the possibility exists that this is a fundamental biological phenomenon not responsive to external influences. However, there is evidence that human male behaviour patterns largely determine this excess mortality in middle age. More than half the excess male deaths in middle age are attributable to ischaemic heart disease with its possible aetiological factors including diet, lack of exercise, cigarette smoking and a persistently intense aggressive competitive life style. About a third of the excess is due to deaths from road traffic accidents, cirrhosis of the liver, respiratory tract cancer, bronchitis and emphysema. Virtually no heavy drinkers (i.e. consuming more than 100 g alcohol per 24 h) survive into old age (Trémolières & Geissler-Brun 1975).

An overall improvement in these mortality rates must come from a change of life style and there is evidence in western countries that this message is being accepted and acted upon, more especially in the middle (professional) classes. The dramatic fall in cigarette smoking amongst the middle classes, and physicians in particular, and the worldwide interest in regular and strenuous physical exercise to promote positive health are examples of this. Mortality rates are still declining in the middle-aged and in the elderly. The current life expectancy of the average 65-year-old American is 16 years or more. If cancer and cardiovascular deaths were eliminated, it would add about 10 years to the average total life expectancy.

The elderly

The elderly are usually regarded as those aged 65 and over, to provide a social and legislative frame of reference. Different countries have different statutory retirement ages. In the USA for retirement and state-facilitated pension purposes the age of 65 is used for both sexes, whereas in the UK the retirement ages for men and women differ, being 65 and 60 respectively. In France the retirement age is 60 years for both sexes and in Norway 70 years. However, those so defined do not constitute a homogeneous group and in addition to frailities attributable to aging, many have multiple chronic disabling conditions and often social problems. Despite this the majority can cope at home even when living alone, although the ability to do so falls off rapidly in extreme old age.

These somewhat arbitrary cut-off points represent thresholds beyond which most people will engage in little or no paid employment. Thus income levels drop dramatically but this loss is abated by pensions and possibly a lump cash payment on retirement. There are no dependant children, and for the relatively affluent the house mortgage is paid off and of course there is a drop in income tax and many other factors. Furthermore those fortunate and prudent people in work prior to the official retirement age will have provided for their own retirement by moving to a more convenient house with less expensive overheads. Consumer durables and clothes will have been renewed and so forth.

However, the relative prosperity of many of the newly retired is a far cry from the penury of some of those who have been retired for many years and whose resources have so dwindled that they have insufficient income to make ends meet. Special attention must be given to the needs of these extremely old, frail and economically impoverished people.

Utilization of health and welfare resources

The proportion of elderly people with severe dependency increases markedly with age, yet less than 5% of the elderly are in institutional care on a long-term basis (mainly nursing homes in the USA and in the UK divided almost equally between Local Authority residential care homes and the hospitals). In British hospitals rather more than one-third of all elderly people are in the geriatric service, about one-third in the acute services and just under one-third in mental hospitals. The very old, however, are concentrated in the geriatric services which provide for two-thirds of those aged 75 years and over in hospital.

Table 1.3 Elderly in institutions in England and Wales 1976 (Hospital In-patient Enquiry, England and Wales 1974 and 1976).

Accommodation	No. approx.	% approx.
Geriatric service	51 240	0.73
Acute services	48 590	0.69
Psychiatric services	44 970	0.64
Local Authority homes	123 470	1.75
Voluntary and private homes	25 820	0.37
Total in institutions	294 090	4.17
Population aged 65 +	7 054 800	100.00

* HIPE = Hospital in-patient enquiry for England and Wales. See references.

The rapid expansion of specialist geriatric services in the UK has helped the hospitals to cope with the rising tide of elderly, sick people. Additionally the throughput of elderly people in the general services is considerable, especially in internal medicine, orthopaedics and ophthalmology. In these services more than half the bed days may be given over to older folk. In the UK and USA and other countries utilization of the institutional resource increases rapidly with age. The rate of admission to hospital of the over 75s in the UK runs at 20% of the age group population per annum (see Table 1.4) which is 3 times the admission rate of the age group 15–45 years, excluding maternity and psychiatry.

Hospital utilization is related to age and inversely related to income

Table 1.4 Hospital discharges expressed as a percentage of the age group population and showing duration of stay in days (all departments excluding psychiatry and maternity) (Hospital In-patient Enquiry, England and Wales 1974).

		Duration of stay	
Age group	Discharge rate	Median	Mean
14–44	6.9	4.1	7.1
45–64	8.7	8.2	12.8
65–74	13.4	11.4	20.8
75+	20.7	14.5	41.2

both with respect to rate of admission and duration of stay. Multiple factors contribute to this.

Long-term care utilization also mounts rapidly with age and 90% of all nursing home provision in the USA is taken up by residents aged 65 years and over (see Table 1.5). In the UK the equivalent provision for the elderly is on a much less lavish scale. For planning purposes an aggregate figure of less than 40 places per 1000 aged 65 years and over has been aimed at, apportioned 25 residential care, 10 geriatrics and 3.5 psychiatric hospital care. In both countries psychiatric services for the elderly are grossly deficient. Psychiatric morbidity rates rise rapidly with age but referrals to psychiatric out-patient clinics and admissions to mental hospitals are low in this most vulnerable client group. Also dental care is poorly taken up by the elderly, probably due to a combination of low expectations and financial

Table 1.5 Nursing home utilization by the elderly in the USA 1974.

Total use by elderly =	44 places/1000 pop. aged 65+
	12 residents/1000 aged 65–74
	59 residents/1000 aged 75–84
	237 residents/1000 aged 85+

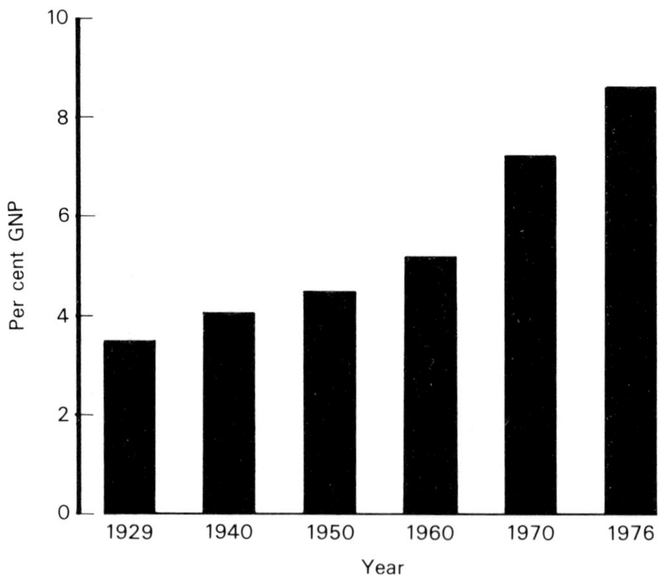

Fig. 1.2 National Health Expenditure USA (per cent of Gross National Product) (DHEW Publication No. 77–1232 1976–77).

barriers, yet dental disease is common and good care should aid health, appearance, comfort, nutrition and social interaction.

Since people aged 64 years and over have high illness rates and often chronic disability and weak social support they make heavy demands on health and welfare services. The financial implications of this pose pressing political problems. In 1976 the American per capita expenditures for personal health care were $249 for those aged less than 19 years, $547 for those aged 19–64 years and $1520 for the elderly. Not only does the total cost rise with age but also the proportion of that cost coming from the public funds rises even faster. Thus for the youngest group only 26% of expenditure on health came from the public funds whereas for the elderly the figure was 68% (DHEW Publication No. (HRA) 77–1232 1976–77). The current intense interest in the elderly by health and welfare authorities, in large measure, stems from the relatively sharp increase in charges on the public purse by this age group together with the promise of much further expenditure due to changing demography (see Table 1.6). The escalation of general health and welfare costs is faster than the prevailing growth in the economy even after allowing for inflation. Changes in quality and quantity of care account for less than one-half of the increased costs in the past few years.

Table 1.6 National health expenditure (USA) as approximate percentage of gross national product (GNP) and per capita (DHEW Publication No. 77–1232 1976–77).

Year	% of GNP	Per capita expenditure
1929	3.5	$29
1940	4.1	$29
1950	4.5	$78
1960	5.2	$147
1970	7.2	$334
1976	8.6	$638

In an attempt to curb health and welfare expenditure less reliance will need to be placed on further increases in hospital and nursing home care. Hospitals and nursing homes have long been the major expense in health care and in recent years they have gradually increased their share of the total budget due to increased staffing (the staff:patient ratio has doubled in 30 years) and the burgeoning of medical technology; for example, the use of increasingly sophisticated diagnostic techniques and other developments in fields such as cardiology including open heart surgery, renal dialysis, organ transplantation and joint replacement.

There is a particular and urgent need to plan appropriately for health care of the older age groups. Good geriatric care should be readily accessible to allow elderly people to live their lives to the full. In a developed country the virtual elimination of death in younger age groups is a benefit to be enjoyed; but old age must not become a nightmare experience, burdensome to the individual and to society. However, health care provisions must always be cost effective if there is to be a genuine intention to provide a service of value to all in need and not simply to a select few. The falling death rates in the elderly over the past 15 years will mean that the proportion of elderly people aged 65–74 years will decrease and those aged 75+ will increase (see Table 1.7). This increase in the numbers of aged, rather than simply elderly is the nub of the problem and is a trend likely to continue to the end of the century.

Table 1.7 Proportion of the elderly aged 75 years and over, USA 1977 data.

Year	% aged 75+	
1900	less than	30
1970	almost	40
2000	estimated	45

Projected numbers of the aged are based on current mortality rates, and will be underestimated if the mortality rates amongst older people continue to decline.

Health of the elderly at home

Increasing emphasis in medical practice must be on the old (i.e. those aged 75 years and more) who are living at home. Although life is a continuum, different age groups do have discernible characteristics of a medical and social nature. These distinctions are clear to elderly people themselves and have been revealed time and again in the community surveys. Physical and mental old age usually does not bear too hard on people until well after retirement. By the age of 75 most old people will have sustained a moderate decline in general health, in the ability to cope and in social activity. After the middle 80s these trends accelerate and there is a sharp fall off in social contacts outside of the home and in self-care capability. However, even at these great ages, people can retain their independence and manage to live on their own with very little outside help.

An Age Concern, England survey (Abrams 1978) of elderly people aged 75 years and over from 4 different urban areas and excluding all those in institutional care, showed that almost half (47%) were living alone and of those living alone 85% were women. Three-quarters of all elderly widows were living alone. Of the over 75s 30% had never had children and at the time of the survey 38% of respondents had no living offspring.

The biggest single factor giving a satisfactory life in old age appeared to be good interpersonal relationships with neighbours and friends. Good health and happy family links ranked second; sufficient money was subordinate to these other social factors, even though it is important (over 40% said they needed a modest extra amount of money each week to spend, especially on heating, food and clothing). Happiness is not immediately susceptible to improvement by more State cash benefits, but rather by the exercise of social skills by people as they grow older and also by health and welfare agencies encouraging and supporting families, friends and neighbours who care for the elderly. Peace, solitude and sunshine were not highly rated as important ingredients of a happy life in old age. The early development of good interpersonal relationships and their maintenance throughout life is the best way to a satisfactory life in old age. Preparation for retirement should start early.

Second only to good interpersonal relationships and help from family and friends, good health is a key factor in a happy life. In the Age Concern, England survey (Abrams 1978) only 39% of the over 65s said that they enjoyed good health 'to a great extent' and this was the lowest attainment score recorded for any of the specified bases for a happy old age about which they were questioned. Clearly, medical care has a large part to play in determining the quality of life of elderly people.

In the over 75s only 10% said they had no physical (medical) problems or disabilities. The most widespread ailments on self-assessment were: arthritis or rheumatism (60%), difficulty in walking and unsteadiness on the feet (50%), forgetfulness (44%) and poor eyesight (42%). Overall these disabilities accounted for one-third of all declared ill health. Another 7 common ailments were deafness, backache, breathlessness on slight exertion, swelling of the feet, giddiness, indigestion and persistent fatigue. A much lower prevalence was noted with respect to long spells of mental depression (14%), urinary incontinence or poor bladder control (11%), trouble with teeth and gums (6%) and difficulty in passing water (5%). Generally there was a much higher incidence of disability in women, even after allowing for age differences. In the age group over 75 years the average woman is only about 2 years older than the average man. The higher morbidity of these aged women was especially marked with respect to the rheumatic diseases, backache and unsteadiness on the feet. There were no ailments reported in this survey which were significantly more frequent in men than in women.

REFERENCES AND FURTHER READING

Abrams M. (1978) *Beyond Three-score and Ten.* Age Concern, London.

Birren J.E. & Sloane R.B. (1980) *Handbook of Mental Health and Aging.* Prentice-Hall, New Jersey.

Exton-Smith A.N. & Evans J.G. (Eds) (1977) *Care of the Elderly*. Grune and Stratton Inc., New York.

Finch C.E. & Hayflick L. (Eds) (1977) *Handbook of the Biology of Aging*. Van Nostrand Rheinhold, New York.

DHEW Publication No. (HRA) 77–1232 (1976–77) US Department of Health, Education and Welfare.

Hospital In-patient Enquiry, England and Wales (1974) and (1976) HMSO, London.

Stevenson J.C. & Whitehead M.I. (1982) Postmenopausal osteoporosis. *British medical Journal* **285**, 585–8.

Trémolières J. & Geissler-Brun C. (1975) Nutrition and metabolism. In von Hahn H.P. (Ed.) *Practical Geriatrics*. S. Karger, Basle.

WHO (World Health Organization) (1978) *Annual Statistics*, Vol. 1, Table II.

Chapter Two
Principles of Geriatric Therapeutics

W. DAVISON

I do not wish two diseases, one nature made and one man made.
Napoleon I (1769–1821)

OVERVIEW

Medical and social problems of the elderly indicate that the cornerstone of medical care for this age group is Family Practice. In geriatrics (as in paediatrics and psychiatry) a positive, enabling approach to care is required, promoting family health and welfare and minimizing dependency on outside agencies.

Because of known gross underreporting of illness by the elderly, sociomedical screening plus active medical intervention is indicated. Vague non-specific presentation of illness in old age challenges the doctor's diagnostic skills. The value of compassion, kindness and commonsense when dealing with people in trouble is stressed. The need for prudent, frugal prescribing, planned procrastination and placebos is discussed.

THE MEDICAL APPROACH TO OLD AGE

Aging and death are inevitable. Prolonged ill-health prior to death is common but not inevitable. Currently, the rising tide of elderly sick people poses the threat that it will swamp the health and social service organizations. The 'silent epidemic' of brain failure (mostly senile dementia) alone is likely to overwhelm the mental health and welfare services.

These massive and daunting problems demand an equally large and active response. A great deal can be achieved by the elderly themselves, by younger people preparing for old age, by care practitioners of all types and by health and welfare authorities, to ease the burdens of an aging population. Practical strategies include the adoption of a healthier life-style but in addition, resources must be diverted from younger to older members of society. Medical and social care for the elderly requires a more positive organizational basis. There is plenty of evidence that elderly people do not approach health and welfare services as and when they require them. Often the elderly person is unaware that his disability is due to disease, he may ascribe it simply to old age and, even if disease is considered likely, a lack of therapeutic potential may be assumed.

If medical intervention is to be practised in a positive way, it is vital that those intervening have a good overall grasp of the problems of aging from a biological, social and medical standpoint. Intervention must be well thought out both in terms of the old person's needs and that which society should and can afford to give. Otherwise doctors allocate too much to individual patients and then complain about the lack of total resource. This applies to medicines, domiciliary care services, specialist investigations and especially to sojourns in hospital.

The practitioner should be aware of his own self-interest in the doctor–patient interaction because it is virtually impossible (and probably undesirable) to exclude the profit motive from medical activity. The 'profit' may be money, the promotion of self-esteem, the luxury of giving, or all three; but it is a force to be reckoned with nevertheless. A balance must be struck between altruism, commerce and self-satisfaction so that the needs of the patient, physician and society are all met.

Medical care is increasingly a matter of dealing with medical and social problems of the very young, the very old and the lower social classes. In the more affluent nations most people avoid serious ill-health throughout childhood, adolescence and middle-age and so the main burden falls on the old.

Family medicine

The essential principle of family medicine is that the family and not the individual is regarded as the unit. Patterns of ill-health exist throughout the family and not just in the patient who comes (or who is sent or brought) to see the doctor. There is a fundamental concept of family homeostasis (and disequilibrium). Every change in one person causes changes in other closely related persons and in the family as a whole (Huygen 1978). In a family crisis there is great stress, all members suffer and as a result perceived ill-health increases. When a family member does well, all members feel the better for it.

The origins of disease in families are usually complex but can often be unravelled with persistence and patience. In geriatrics it is not uncommon for the patient to be pushed forward as 'the problem'—a sort of scapegoat for stress in the family. Alternatively, the elderly person may actually volunteer to enact this role in order to help the family or to atone for previous, real or imaginary, mismanagement of family affairs.

It is important to assess the ability of the family to cope with the burdens of sickness and everyday life. But how can these things be measured? It is usually not just the stress itself which is the problem but the family reaction to it. Fortunately most illness is dealt with perfectly satisfactorily by families and only the minority of illness comes to the primary-care physician. The doctor must not take over the caring role from the family. The doctor's role is to enable the patient and the family to cope with their own problems using, as far as possible, their own resources.

In the UK the speciality of general practice is generally responsible for primary care and there are more than twice as many general medical practitioners (GPs) or family physicians as there are medically qualified consultants (established, hospital-based specialists). In the USA primary care is shared among many specialists with only a minority of the work undertaken by a family practitioner. However, there is a revival of interest in primary care and these physicians are increasing in number. This is a welcome reversal of the 50-year-old trend towards specialization and it could lead to improved medical care for elderly people.

Table 2.1 The flight from primary care: physicians in USA (DHEW Publication No. (HRA) 77-1232 1976-77).

Year	% in general practice	% in specialities
1930	80	20
1970	20	80

UNDER-REPORTING OF ILLNESS

It is well known that there is gross under-reporting of illness in the elderly even when financial and physical barriers between patient and doctor are non-existent. Unless the family practitioner actively seeks illness in his older clients, much (possibly most) illness will go undiagnosed and untreated. This would be a pity because much illness and disability can be helped (if not actually cured!) by simple means. Even chronic progressive incurable disease is worth diagnosing because the well-informed doctor is then better placed to give appropriate advice to both patient and relatives.

It is not uncommon for sick elderly persons to be supported by younger members of the family and indeed this is as it should be. However, it is important that the needs of the young supporters are not overlooked. This would be unfair to the young and ultimately to the old person also. If the family is left struggling with an insupportable burden, sooner or later a sociomedical crisis develops and the old person will be admitted to institutional care, never to return home. The family will have been so exhausted by their unrelieved toil that they refuse utterly to take on the burden of care ever again. This reaction is wholly reasonable and understandable in the circumstances, yet earlier attention to the family's needs might have prevented or greatly delayed the total dereliction. Timing is important but generally in the face of scarcity of resources doctors act too late rather than too early.

Early intervention, together with a frugal well-focused use of resources, is the recommended approach. Where the family practitioner has the back-up of hospital-based geriatric services headed by a specialist in geriatric medicine, this specialist should be consulted early rather than late.

Sociomedical screening

Depending on the manpower available and the personal interest of the practitioners, screening of elderly people in the practice can be done by the physician or some other person. 'Physician extenders' are increasingly used for this purpose, especially the nurse practitioner or the health visitor. All the over 75s should be visited systematically each year or every two years and asked to agree to a health check. Most old people will be delighted that someone is taking a special interest in them. Those patients who demur are often those most in need of evaluation and extra care should be taken not to let them slip through the net, although at the same time avoiding unnecessary confrontation. The recently bereaved, the housebound, those lately discharged from hospital and those who normally live alone should be regarded as high-risk cases. The health visitor conducts an uncomplicated structured interview, assesses the overall home situation and the doctor makes a simple physical and mental examination, preferably in his office or surgery where the facilities are good and help is readily available. Attention must be given to the eyes, ears, mouth and feet. Disorders in these parts of the body are exceedingly common and can often be relieved by treatment. The clinical examination by the doctor is supplemented when indicated, by biochemical, haematological, radiological and other investigations or by referral to a specialist.

Yield from screening programme

Screening in this way will reveal many medical and social problems previously unknown to the primary-care team; for example, foot troubles, deafness, visual impairment, urinary tract disorders, thyroid under- or over-activity, anaemia, osteomalacia, mental depression and dementia. A basic mental test questionnaire should be used routinely to access mental function because the earlier stages of intellectual failure are easily underestimated. A series of straightforward questions demanding precise simple answers will quickly disclose impaired mental function.

Other problems are usually 'known' to the physician yet the patient would benefit by the review of his current medical and social status, including drug use, family attitudes and the financial aspects of ill-health. These 'known cases' will be patients suffering from long-term illness. Virtually all will be on long-term treatment and scrutiny of the drug schedule will often allow a dramatic reduction in drug consumption, to the patient's benefit (Tulloch 1981, Bruce 1982).

DEPRIVATION, DISEASE AND DIAGNOSIS

Social and financial deprivation

In addition to the medical and nursing components of the screening programme, it is important to assess the financial and social aspects because financial and social deprivation so often precipitate the demand for medical attention. The plight of the chronically poor worsens with retirement and at a higher income level we have a group of 'new poor'. That is to say, people whose resources were adequate at retirement but who have suffered more than most from the ravages of inflation.

Poverty, social isolation and illness go together and compound the old person's problems. Most State aid schemes have concentrated on relief of poverty, which, though costly in financial terms, is the easiest type of aid to give. Relief from social deprivation is much more complicated and difficult to achieve because, in essence, people need the affection of other people. Regrettably, many of the people most in need are not at all attractive to others. So although we are enjoined by religious and moral philosophy to 'love one another', this in practice often proves to be impossible.

The range of services and types of financial help available will vary from place to place and the members of the primary-care team need to know what is available and how to secure it for the patient's benefit.

THE MEDICAL CONSULTATION

The basis of the medical consultation is that the patient brings his problem to the physician and asks the physician to solve it, viz:

Patient: 'Here is my pain, ulcer, broken leg, mental depression, or whatever. Please relieve, heal, repair or cure it'.

Physician: 'You do this—take the tablets, avoid eating salt or let me do this—special blood tests, X-ray, surgical operation and all will be well'.

This simple medical model works in many medical and surgical diseases, for example, pernicious anaemia, scurvy or myxoedema and in acute appendicitis or a case of a broken leg. Indeed medicine works so well in these and many other examples that patients and physicians tend to be baffled and frustrated that it does not work in the vast majority of medical transactions, not even in something as banal as the common cold.

Irrespective of the age of the patient, good therapeutics rests on a scientific foundation but is brought into action by the professional skill and humanity of the doctor. He is himself a powerful therapeutic agent that 'works' (i.e. ameliorates disease to the obvious satisfaction of the patient) even when the evidence that 'it works' would fail to convince the impartial scientific observer. Thus the credibility of medicine stands despite the impotence of the profession in the face of most diseases. Kindness and commonsense are great therapeutic gifts. Illness is a social as well as a physical phenomenon and the patient's self-assessment of his health is at least as important to his functional ability as is the doctor's assessment. Therapeutic listening is valuable to allow the patient and the family to express their emotional feelings and to explain their attitudes to the physical and social problems. The physician must allow time for careful explanation of drug regimens and, if necessary, he should supply written or printed instructions.

PRESENTATION OF DISEASE IN OLD AGE

The old person who is taken ill often presents one or more non-specific declines in function. The physician is informed that the old lady is 'confused and has gone off her feet'. This simply means that she is unwell and it is the doctor's job to make a full assessment to find out what is wrong and how best to attempt to put it right. Just to prescribe a tranquillizer or a vestibular sedative or a tonic is both too little and also too much medicine. There is often a temptation to use too little diagnosis and too much drug treatment in geriatric practice. The patient may have multiple long-term illnesses, may be on long-term drug treatment and yet previously was able to manage the tasks of daily living. The inability to cope can be precipitated by some minor upset such as an intercurrent infection, an error in medications, psychosocial stress or even a shift in the ambient temperature. Disease and disability may masquerade as old age and senility. Furthermore, the interplay of psychosocial factors is often much more relevant than the physician is inclined to admit. Mental confusion, postural instability, incontinence and immobility all occur much more readily in the elderly than in the young and a lack of appreciation or possibly a courageous indifference to pain and a weak reaction of the body to infection are more commonly seen in this age group. The patient with arthritis may be immobile due to apathy, anxiety, overbearing relatives, unsteadiness on the feet or failing vision rather than to the joint disease *per se*. Diagnosis of all components of the disease is essential and the intellectual challenge can be formidable.

Diagnosis is the keystone of treatment

The keystone of medical treatment is accurate diagnosis but diagnosis can be difficult because patients present with an inadequate history, multiple pathology and polypharmacy. Additionally there can be confusion in the elicitation and interpretation of physical signs. However, it has to be admitted that the inadequate diagnosis is often due to distraction of the physician by the great age of the patient. It is often helpful to ignore the patient's age until the diagnosis has been made. In management and prognosis age assumes much greater relevance.

DRUG TREATMENT FOR THE ELDERLY PATIENT

The elderly are a major target for the drug prescriber. A large percentage take drugs and multiple drug treatment is common. In England around 80% of the over 75s are on regular drug treatment (mostly long-term repeats) and more than one-third take 3 or 4 different medicines each day. The most frequently used preparations are analgesics, psychotropics and genitourinary and heart drugs (cardiac glycosides and diuretics). Much drug use is unnecessary and some is frankly hazardous.

By way of illustration, in a large English town it was found that 15% of the patients referred to the hospital geriatric out-patient clinic were long-term consumers of barbiturates, 41% were taking other hypnotics and only 8% were not taking hypnotics (Macdonald & Macdonald 1977). The referring doctors mentioned giddiness or falls as a reason for referral in 84% of those on barbiturates and in only 24% of those not taking these drugs. Another study suggested that over 10% of admissions to UK geriatric units were precipitated by inappropriate drug treatment (Williamson & Chopin 1980). Gross overprescribing of oral iron is well documented in Sweden where the *per capita* consumption is three times that of Germany and the UK and five times that of France. For some reason, doctors in all these countries prescribe iron more readily to older people so that iron consumption rises as a function of age; yet the iron requirement of most elderly people is very small. Most old people taking iron do so without a clear indication. Indeed it would appear that 70% of elderly people taking iron in Sweden do so unnecessarily (Reizenstein *et al.* 1979).

These and many other reports suggest widespread iatrogenic misuse of drugs by the elderly. Adverse reactions to drugs are three or four times higher than those recorded for patients of pre-retirement age. It is ironic that drugs should be subject to such stringent premarket testings and post-market monitoring when they are used in such a haphazard fashion. The next big advance in geriatric therapeutics should be the better use of currently available drugs rather than the development of new and more potent remedies (see Table 2.2).

Procrastination in prescribing

Procrastination in prescribing need not be just a passive lack of action by a physician who cannot act decisively. It can be a positive act of putting off for a clearly defined reason. Used in this way, procrastination is valuable

Table 2.2 Guidelines for prescribing for the elderly.

Have precise diagnosis and clear objectives
Be expert with a small range of drugs
Use generally lower doses of toxic drugs
Prune the drug list regularly
Print instructions for patient and helpers

(Thomson 1979). Putting off doing something (i.e. prescribing a drug) is a particularly useful device in geriatric practice. However, to be well done it usually requires doing something else as a means of gaining time. Common indications for deferring prescribing exist when dealing with viral upper respiratory tract infections, when it is necessary to allow overtreated stasis ulcers to settle, when time is needed to confirm a diagnosis and quite often when the patient is obviously dying. Methods of delay include a definite agreement with patient and relatives that a period of 'observation' is indicated, that it is necessary to wait for the results of a test (e.g. throat swab or chest X-ray) and possibly the use of a placebo. As with all medical practice it is of fundamental importance that the patient's confidence is maintained.

Placebos

Placebos have a role in medical practice but their use is complicated by the emotional reactions they evoke in many patients, doctors and nurses. Most physicians and nurses do not understand placebo reactions. The extent to which patients react to placebos has been greatly underestimated, so much so that a positive response to a placebo (e.g. relief of pain or insomnia) may be taken as proof that the symptoms were not genuine in the first place (Goodwin *et al.* 1979)! Thus the use of placebo in procrastination may relieve the symptoms but it may also erroneously relieve the physician of his duty to make a proper diagnosis. Yet 30–40% of patients distressed by pain in hospital would respond as well to placebo injections as to 10 mg of morphine. Unfortunately it is patients thought to be malingering, rather than those who might benefit, who are given placebos by doctors and nurses. Sometimes it is the nurse who provides the major impetus for placebo use. In fact the use of placebos as a weapon in the conflict between 'difficult' patients and hospital staff is common practice. The overdemanding 'difficult' patient is much less likely to respond to placebo than the compliant 'good' patient. Nevertheless, the chances are that the 'good' patient will receive the morphia (as a reward) and the 'difficult' patient will be given the sterile water injection (as retribution)! The essence of a placebo is that it should do no harm. Ascorbic acid is often used, but many knowledgeable patients will recognize it—and trust may then be put in jeopardy.

On no account should benzodiazepines, antidepressants or phenothiazines ever be used as placebos. Placebos should have no demonstrable pharmacological activity. The tonics and bitters are almost certainly the best.

Minimum drug schedules

A central tenet of geriatric pharmacology is the use of minimum drug schedules. This is necessary because as the number of preparations used increases, the incidence of adverse drug reaction increases exponentially and also the degree of patient compliance or adherence to the drug schedule falls. Additionally, each drug taken represents a pharmacological burden on the body's economy, and, in most health care systems, it also represents a drain on the patient's financial resources. Lastly, it is easier for the physician to retain some semblance of control over what is happening when fewer drugs are prescribed. Once-daily drug regimens are ideal if drugs are to be used at all. With better knowledge of pharmacokinetics and with the use of some longer acting preparations it will be found that more and more drugs can be given on a once-daily basis; for example, with some antibiotics, anticonvulsants, antidepressants, antirheumatics, diuretics, digoxin and various hormones.

PHYSICIAN HEAL THYSELF

It seems probable that many drugs are prescribed as much to relieve the anxiety or embarrassment of the doctor as to resolve a disease process in the patient. This occurs because the orthodox medical model puts the onus on the physician to produce a cure for, or at least to relieve by physical means, the patient's disease. However, many forms of distress cannot be removed by drug treatment. Feelings of anxiety, loneliness, lack of purpose, rejection by family, and the like, are mostly matters best tackled along social rather than medical lines. Certainly, psychosedative drugs can dull the mind, induce an artificial state of sleep and so put a barrier between the patient and his problems. However, the psychosocial difficulties remain and the long-term use of drug treatment creates additional hazards. Helping the patient to face up to the realities of life, and mobilizing social support, would be a better answer to many of these cries for help.

REFERENCES AND FURTHER READING

Bruce S.A. (1982) Regular prescribing in a residential home for elderly women. *British medical Journal* **284,** 1235–7.

Coni N.K., Davison W. & Webster S. (1980) *Lecture Notes on Geriatrics*, 2nd Edition. Blackwell Scientific Publications.

DHEW Publication No. (HRA) 77-1232 (1976-77) US Department of Health, Education and Welfare.

Goodwin J.S., Goodwin J.M. & Vogel A.V. (1979) Knowledge and use of placebos by house officers and nurses. *Annals of internal medicine* **91,** 106-10.

Huygen F.J.A. (1978) *Family medicine—the medical life history of families.* Dekker & van de Vegt, Nijmegen.

Macdonald J.B. & Macdonald E.T. (1977) Nocturnal femoral fracture and continuing widespread use of barbiturate hypnotics. *British medical Journal* **2,** 483.

March G. & Kaim-Caudal P. (1976) *Team Care in General Practice.* Croom Helm, London.

Reizenstein P., Ljunggren G., Smedby B., Agenäs I. & Penchomsky M. (1979) Overprescribing iron tablets to elderly people in Sweden. *British medical Journal* **2,** 962-3.

Thomson G.H. (1979) Prescribing procrastination. *Journal of Royal College of General Practitioners* **29,** 550-2.

Tulloch A.J. (1981) Repeat prescribing for elderly patients. *British medical Journal* **282,** 1432-1.

Williamson J. & Chopin J.M. (1980) Adverse reactions to prescribed drugs in the elderly: a multi-centre investigation. *Age and Ageing* **9,** 73-80.

Chapter Three
Practicalities of Drug Treatment

W. DAVISON

Life is very sweet brother, who would wish to die!
George Borrow (1803–81)

OVERVIEW

A large proportion of the work in family practice relates to the medical care of the elderly. Medical input is required across the whole range of illness at home, in skilled nursing homes and in residential homes, as well as in hospital. This chapter considers the practicalities of drug treatment in ambulatory, long-term and terminal care, looking especially at prescribing practice, review of total drug schedule, management of repeat prescriptions, the vexed question of compliance and the use of suitable containers.

GENERAL

Prescribing habits

It is important for the physician to review his prescribing habits from time to time, preferably in collaboration with colleagues. The principles of good prescribing are simple enough (see Chapter 2) yet self-audit often shows multiple errors in the family doctor's prescribing habits (Shaw & Opit 1976, Tulloch 1981, Bruce 1982). The common errors include: prescribing drugs which are really not necessary, prescribing too many doses in the day, persistence with treatment long after the indication for it ceased and the use of unnecessarily hazardous drugs. Elderly patients living at home mostly manage their drugs as well as younger people but a sizeable minority will have difficulty on account of forgetfulness, lack of rapport with the doctor or mental confusion. With rational, economical prescribing and supervision by an interested relative serious dangers will be averted. Many errors of drug taking by elderly people (mostly omissions) are not harmful and indeed some are beneficial! Inspection of the vast drug hoards in many patients' homes provides indirect evidence of both non-adherence and gross overprescribing.

No drug should be prescribed unless it can be expected to do good, is unlikely to do harm, and unless equally good results cannot be obtained by safer means. These self-evident rules are often broken in the medical care of the elderly. Self-medication, using over-the-counter medicines or pills from the family hoard, is quite common. Perhaps a quarter or a third of patients indulge in this. In general the self-prescribed medicines are laxatives, analgesics, tonics and cough remedies. Drug-dependency cases are a problem. Patients who have been on barbiturates and other hypnotics or anxiolytics for years swear that they cannot do without them. With determination and persuasion by the physician most can be weaned off and so remove the long-term risk of adverse effects.

Record keeping

A high standard of practice records is an essential prerequisite for good prescribing. The problem-orientated format of recording is strongly recommended (Weed 1971). Each case also needs a drugs record sheet or card showing the names of all the drugs in use with start dates, doses, frequencies

DRUG RECORD SHEET

Surname	First Names	Date of Birth
Johnson	Frederick W	19.1.01

Sensitivities (known / suspected)	Response	Date
Penicillin	Rash and wheeze	Jan '75
Aspirin	Urticaria	Oct. '80

Special precautions

Prostatism, glaucoma

Serial	DRUG	DOSE	QNTY	STARTED	STOPPED
1.	Digoxin tabs	125 microgr × 1	30	15 Jan '80	16 Feb
2.	Furosemide tabs	40 mg × 1	30	15 Jan '80	16 Feb
3.	Bendrofluazide tabs	5 mg × 2	60	17 Feb '80	
4.	Propranolol tabs	40 mg × 3	90	17 Feb '80	

Fig. 3.1 Patient's drug record sheet.

and stop dates (see Fig. 3.1); also information regarding known drug sensitivities. This card should be consulted and written up prior to every prescription. Failure to do this exposes the patient to unnecessary hazards.

Return home from hospital

Traditional hospital and nursing home care is over-protective. Institutions should adopt a more enabling approach to care and this is so especially in the run-up to discharge. As the acute episode subsides, the patient must take more and more responsibility for himself including the handling of his own drugs (Crome *et al.* 1980).

As soon as possible the drug schedule should be stripped to its bare essentials, in preparation for discharge. At this point the patient should be given a supply of his medication clearly labelled and in the form and packaging to be used at home. He should be instructed in drug use, given a set of written instructions and allowed to cope on his own but with unobtrusive observation and supervision to assess competence and to iron out any difficulties. If despite all this the patient cannot manage, the control of his drugs must be lodged with an appropriate relative or friend. Once-daily dosage is used whenever practicable, as for example with digoxin, diuretics and thyroxine. Doses should be linked to some regular event of the day, such as rising, eating or retiring. A fixed daily routine is easiest to follow.

Contact with the patient at home or by a visit to the surgery is necessary soon after he leaves hospital. This usually occurs within a week or ten days when the family practitioner receives the hospital discharge summary. In a sizeable minority, contact is not made until much later and even then possibly just because things have gone wrong. Early contact can be conveniently made on a home visit by the practice nurse. During the visit she can check all aspects of patient management including the medicines.

Drug management in residential homes

Residential care homes for the elderly and nursing homes with no pharmacy service pose particular problems which have not yet been resolved. In the hospital or skilled nursing facility the nurse administering the drug should work directly from the patient's prescription card. The prescription is both the instruction to the pharmacist and to the nurse. No transcription, with its possible errors, is required.

In the residential home and lesser-grade nursing home, the prescription goes to the pharmacy (off site) for dispensing and is retained there. The doctor should maintain a drug list for each patient in the home but usually this is done by a member of staff, possibly with no pharmaceutical training. The list is compiled from the container labels and is thus transcribed twice from the prescription. Difficulties arise because of this, since the staff are not trained in the use of medicines and because usually there is a less good flow of information between doctor and staff in this type of care home than in a hospital or a skilled nursing home. Special individual packaging of drugs using blister packs or foil strips will overcome some of the problems.

Terminal care

In Western countries, three quarters of all deaths occur in people aged 65 and over and except in sudden death the doctor is almost always involved. Good care for the dying is very important but it is often neglected. Inadequate medical management can leave the patient and his relatives acutely anxious, frustrated, resentful or suffering intolerable distress. A more thoughtful, compassionate but positive approach to the dying patient is indicated.

Drugs can be used to provide relief from distress but without undue mental clouding. It is usually better to attack the physical problems first and the mental and emotional problems later. Relief from pain, breathlessness, abdominal distention or cough can allay anxiety, restlessness and insomnia. Early use of hypnotics, sedatives and tranquillizers while leaving the physical problems unresolved, will probably make things worse rather than better.

'Don't use a sledge-hammer to crack a nut' is a well-known aphorism which is valid in geriatric therapeutics. This applies to the relief of pain in the dying patient. The severity of the pain is not necessarily great simply because the patient is dying. It may be tolerable with simple reassurance and a mild analgesic but if it really is severe then sufficient analgesia must be provided to give consistent and enduring relief. Physicians working in primary care have many opportunities to help dying patients. They should be prepared to do it well.

Limited aim prescribing

Multiple pathology is the rule in geriatric medicine; multiple symptoms and signs invite multiple drug treatments but there are real limitations on what drugs can be expected to do. Drugs are not the answer to all our patients' problems. Often social stress is the main problem even though the patient's complaints are of bodily illness. Social help or counselling rather than drugs is indicated in these cases. Also, there are limits to the patient's ability to handle multiple drugs from both the compliance and from the pharmacological standpoints. The good safe prescriber works with a strictly limited number of well-tried and trusted remedies. He aims to use these drugs sparingly and with consummate skill. Too often doctors aim to treat 'everything' and because of the numerous drugs involved they not infrequently become muddled, as do the patients. Consequently, at best, time and money are not well spent and at worst, the outcome can prove to be disastrous.

New drugs

The doctor must resist the temptation to try out each and every new drug. He should allow time for the first flush of enthusiasm to abate before coming to his own reasoned decision. He also needs time to become familiar with the basic pharmacology, indications, contraindications and possible adverse reactions of the newcomer. This is especially important in geriatric practice because of the generally reduced tolerance to side-effects (see Chapter 5).

If a new drug is to be accepted into the prudent prescriber's formulary then generally some other remedy must be discarded to make way for the newcomer. Failure to do this will result in prescribing too great a number of different preparations to be manageable. The new drug should be able to offer clear advantages based not only on comparative cost and effectiveness but also on simplicity of regimen (the fewer tablets and doses the better), speed of onset and duration of action and acceptability to the patient. Bioavailability and penetration into body spaces such as bone, CSF or joints together with specificity for the selected target organ are also important.

Repeat prescriptions

Some 80% of people aged 75 years and over in the UK are on regularly prescribed drug treatment and 25–30% of them additionally self-medicate. Two-thirds of regular drug users take 1–3 drugs and one-third takes 4–6 drugs daily (Law & Chalmers 1976, Skegg *et al.* 1977). Among the most commonly prescribed repeats for the elderly are drugs for the heart and blood pressure, analgesics, oral hypoglycaemics, hypnotics and psychotropics. Over a third of the females in this age group are on long-term psychotropic drugs.

Most prescriptions written for elderly people in general practice are for repeat medication (Murdoch 1980) and probably the majority are issued without the patient being seen by the doctor. Repeats are granted without discussion and there seem to be no generally accepted arrangements for good medical control of the patient's drug treatment. There are obvious dangers in prescribing thus, as for example when a rather toxic drug, intended for relatively short-term use is taken by the patient for very long periods of time. Thus corticosteroids given to damp down a flare-up of rheumatoid arthritis, digoxin given to treat heart failure precipitated by a chest infection or a hypnotic given to tide over a particularly stressful life episode may be continued indefinitely, sometimes with disastrous effects.

FAMILY PRACTICE POLICIES FOR REPEAT PRESCRIPTIONS

Long-term repeat prescriptions fall into a number of well-defined groups each with a different degree of justification for the chronic repeat.

Continuous long-term treatment is indicated in patients with, for example, diabetes, hypothyroidism and pernicious anaemia. Medical review would be justified at up to yearly intervals, for these, depending on the stability of the case. Most elderly diabetics should be seen more frequently than the patients with hypothyroidism, who, in turn, should be seen more often than the case of pernicious anaemia. Adding another drug to the patient's schedule may upset a previously stable drug regimen necessitating more frequent review.

Intermittent long-term treatment is used for patients with chronic bronchitis, congestive heart failure and indigestion where the illness fluctuates and requires variations in drug treatment. Some patients can cope with these changes themselves, for example, by taking a course of antibiotics to damp down an acute exacerbation of chronic bronchitis or by taking an extra dose or two of diuretic when oedema increases in the case of heart failure. The actual frequency of medical review would be indicated by the stability of the case, perhaps within the range of 2 to 6 months.

No repeat without medical consultation is a group which should include most new cases, patients with less stable illness and possibly all those on psychotropic drugs including antidepressants, anxiolytics and hypnotics. The aim is to keep the schedule of these drugs to a minimum and to maintain a high degree of patient–doctor interaction because of the serious nature of the illnesses and the tendency to develop drug dependence or other adverse effects. Antidepressant drugs have a fairly low therapeutic index (i.e. low safety margin between therapeutic and toxic blood levels) and a toxic confusional state may result from high peak serum drug levels. Sudden cessation of certain drugs, including hypnotics, sedatives, antidepressants and antiparkinsonian drugs is hazardous. Attempts should be made to wean patients off the anxiolytics and hypnotics because chronic repeat prescribing is not usually in the patient's long-term interest.

Prescribing policies need to be worked out by the physician for many other drugs including antibiotics, laxatives, antidiarrhoeals, anti-inflammatory drugs and analgesics as well as topical preparations, especially steroid creams and ointments. Dermatitis medicamentosa is common in elderly patients due to the widespread use of inappropriate topical medication. Topical steroids, antibiotics and antihistamine preparations are common offenders.

Control of repeat prescriptions

As indicated, each family practice needs some general policy regarding repeat prescriptions (see Table 3.1). As a basis, the likely medical review interval for the more common disorders for which drugs are prescribed should be agreed by the partners, written down and made known to all who work in the practice. Experience has shown that primary care physicians work to much longer review intervals than they themselves would regard as desirable. The reason for the discrepancy is not lack of time (as most aver) but lack of an administrative mechanism to limit the repeats without further medical consultation. Inadequate record keeping is at the heart of the problem (Ho-Yen 1979). Good medical records giving the date, diagnosis and prescription, followed by instructions regarding repeats and medical review are needed. Without this, control over prescribing is lost and the potential to monitor the patient's progress is also, in large degree, lost. When patients attend for medical review, it is a good plan to have them bring *all* their medications with them, including those which are self-prescribed. This helps greatly to visualize the total drug burden and to review the complexity of the drug doses and timings.

Table 3.1 Guidelines for control of repeat prescriptions.

Practice policy for common disorders
Good records with details of drugs
Repeat prescription card
Repeat prescription register

Some physicians go further and each patient carries his own medication card with information about the drugs, including dates, doses and the number of repeats allowed before medical consultation. A possible layout is shown in Fig. 3.2. This acts as a guide to the patient, the practice receptionist and the pharmacist. No repeat prescriptions are issued without production of the card which is then suitably endorsed with the date of the repeat. Use of the card does not remove the necessity for good record keeping in the normal medical folder and there would be a serious disadvantage if the two records were discrepant in any particular. Also the prescription card is open to falsification to some degree by the patient or another. An alternative system involves keeping a separate practice repeat prescription register which must be consulted and endorsed by the

DOCTOR :

PATIENT :

Number of repeats allowed				↓	Dates of repeats					
Date	Drug	Dose	Frequency		1	2	3	4	5	6

No repeat prescription without this card

Fig. 3.2 Layout for repeat prescription card.

receptionist or clerk before the repeat prescription mechanism is initiated or the patient is referred for medical review (Ho-Yen 1979).

COMPLIANCE

The majority of patients intend to take the drugs as ordered but may then forget or modify the regimen to suit themselves, depending largely on their own perception of the relative importance of the various medicines. If they feel upset by a drug or believe they would manage just as well without, they give up the treatment altogether. Alternatively, if drugs cause dependence (psychological or physical) patients will go to great lengths to secure further supplies. It is impossible to be sure that a patient is adhering to the medical prescription although doctors frequently delude themselves that they can easily recognize the likely compliers and the non-compliers (Haynes *et al.* 1979). A combined approach using interview, tablet counts and reference to the prescription record cards will reveal the degree of compliance (Wandless *et al.* 1979).

Old people probably manage their medications every bit as well as younger people but the drug burden is greater. An American study showed some lack of compliance to occur in 40–50% of elderly patients living at home. Mostly these were cases of intentional drug underuse because the patients did not believe the drugs were necessary in the doses prescribed (Cooper *et al.* 1982). A British study showed that deviations of 10% or more occurred with half of prescriptions and women especially were non-compliant (Wandless *et al.* 1979).

Table 3.2 Factors decreasing compliance.

Multiple drugs
Complicated regimen
New prescription
Disability, especially mental
Lack of symptoms
Lack of supervision
Abhorrent medication

Compliance tends to be least good with first prescriptions. Antibiotics, because they are given in short courses and on a three or four times a day schedule, are often not taken as prescribed. However antirheumatics, used long-term, are not taken as prescribed either, possibly because of adverse effects. Three or four different preparations is about the maximum that most sensible old people can manage for themselves. Larger numbers make for confusion in pill-taking as well as increasing considerably the risk of an adverse drug reaction. Of all the factors studied in relation to compliance, the number of drugs to be taken and their frequency give the best indication. Few drugs (ideally one) to be taken once daily gives best compliance. The age of the patient is of little relevance, training patients in drug handling helps, brief simply written instructions help, as does clear labelling plus the use of a daily drug reminder tick chart or calender. Most of all, rational, frugal prescribing aids compliance. Additionally, good rapport (as perceived by the patient) between physician and patient improves compliance.

Table 3.3 Factors increasing compliance.

Few drugs
Simple regimen
Written instructions
Chronic drug taking
Memory cues
Clear (typed) labels
Special packaging
Supervision
Pleasurable, addictive medicines!

Memory aids

Errors of omission and timing are the most frequent errors in pill-taking. Even intelligent, well-motivated people of good education may fail in pill-taking because of absent mindedness, and having forgotten to take the pill, are unaware of the omission.

Where the intention to comply exists, simple memory aids such as written instructions, check lists or calendars are helpful. Some memory aids are merely common sense cueing strategems involving placement of pills or reminders in suitable places to be encountered at a suitable time.

When away from home it is not always possible to arrange suitable cues to the act of pill-taking. Certainly it is a great deal less easy than at home and some more active reminder is required. A drug list or diary is of no avail if the patient fails to consult it. These are passive memory aids because the patient has to trigger off the activity. An *active* memory aid is required when one is mentally occupied (see Table 3.4).

Table 3.4 Effective memory aids.

Temporal proximity to action
Active rather than passive
Specific to action required
Portability, simplicity, reliability

However, if the patient carries his pills and his drug list and also wears an alarm wrist watch with two alarm settings he is equipped to achieve the hitherto unachievable! That is he can comply with a four times in the day drug schedule. He takes his first dose while attending to his morning toilet, the second when the first alarm goes, the third dose when the second alarm goes and the fourth dose at bed time.

An alarm wrist watch has much to commend it as an external memory aid. It is readily portable and is normally carried around throughout the waking day. Most importantly the alarm gives a temporally proximate cue. Despite the high tone of these alarm watches they are audible to most active 'young' elderly for whom this memory aid is most suited. Provided the alarm is used to cue pill-taking only, it will serve as a convenient, appropriately timed, reminder. More elaborate micro-electronic memory aids, which may be helpful to the pill-taker are available, and others are being developed, but they are beyond the scope of this book. None has yet proved its worth in the matters discussed here.

From time to time the doctor or aide should check on the elderly patient's medication at home, partly to monitor by query and pill counting the degree of compliance with respect to the drugs prescribed, and partly to remove unwanted medicines from the home or at least to advise on their destruction. Old drugs are unreliable, some become toxic and all present a hazard to children. Some patients might object to these drug scavenging forays. However, when the reasons are explained most will surrender the unwanted hoard without further ado.

Presentation of medicines

At the present time most (95%) of the medicines consumed by the elderly are in tablet or capsule form. These have the merits of accurate dosage, longer shelf-life, small volume and great convenience in carriage and swallowing especially when away from home. Liquid preparations for administration by mouth can be easier to swallow but problems may exist because of an unacceptable taste or difficulty in using a measuring spoon (e.g. on account of tremor or poor visual acuity) and hence messiness and erratic dosage. The broad-based plastic measuring beaker is less of a problem for the tremulous, provided that the dose is not too critical.

The standard screw-top bottle, especially one with a sizeable diameter to the cap, has stood the test of time and is manageable by the vast majority of elderly people. For those with weak, stiff or deformed hands the wing-top variant can be helpful (see Fig. 3.3). Because of the dangers of unauthorized pill-taking to small children a variety of child-resistant containers (CRC) has been developed (see Fig. 3.4). Some elderly people, with stiff fingers, and poor eyesight have difficulty with them. Next to the screw top the simple snap top is the easiest to use.

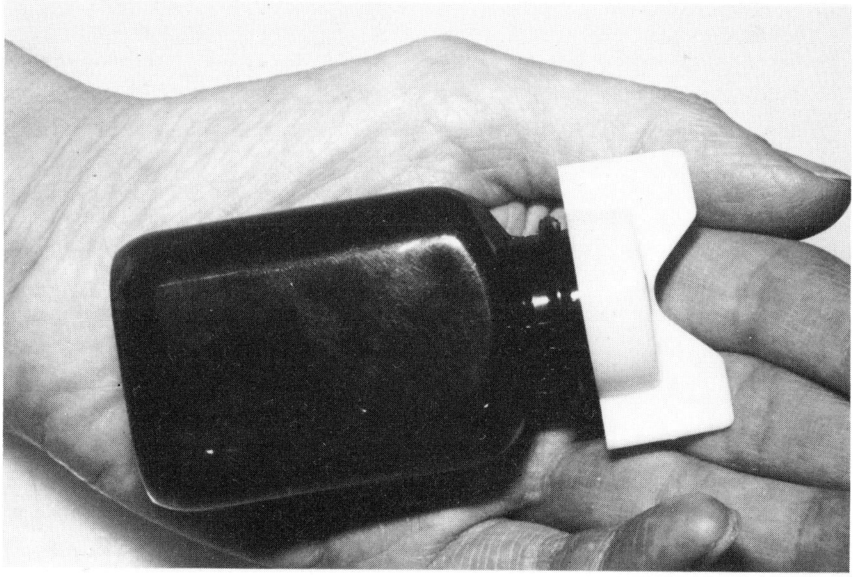

Fig. 3.3 Winged screw cap bottle.

Opening reclosable child-resistant containers

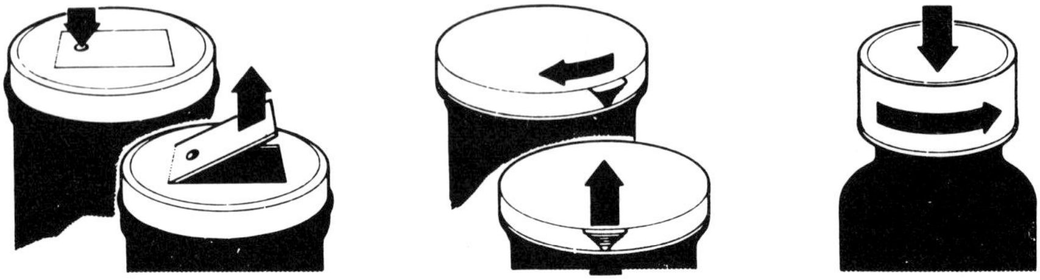

Pop-Lok (solids only) **Snap-Safe** (solids only) **Clic-Loc** (solids or liquids)

Fig. 3.4 Child-resistant closures.

Bubble packs and strips are increasingly popular, both for routine merchandizing and more recently for individual patient prescriptions, especially in institutions. The pharmacist puts the desired number of pills into each blister and then the whole sheet is sealed using a special press. Appropriate labelling can be done before or after sealing depending on the circumstances. Every blister (pill or cluster of pills) is labelled. Many nursing homes (long-term care homes) now use this 'unit system' with individual sheets or strips of plastic bubbles made up for each patient.

More flexibility is gained by using a multidose container which can be filled by the patient or a helper to cover the needs of a day or even a week. The 'Mediset' or 'Dosett' is such a container (see Fig. 3.5). This signal-red

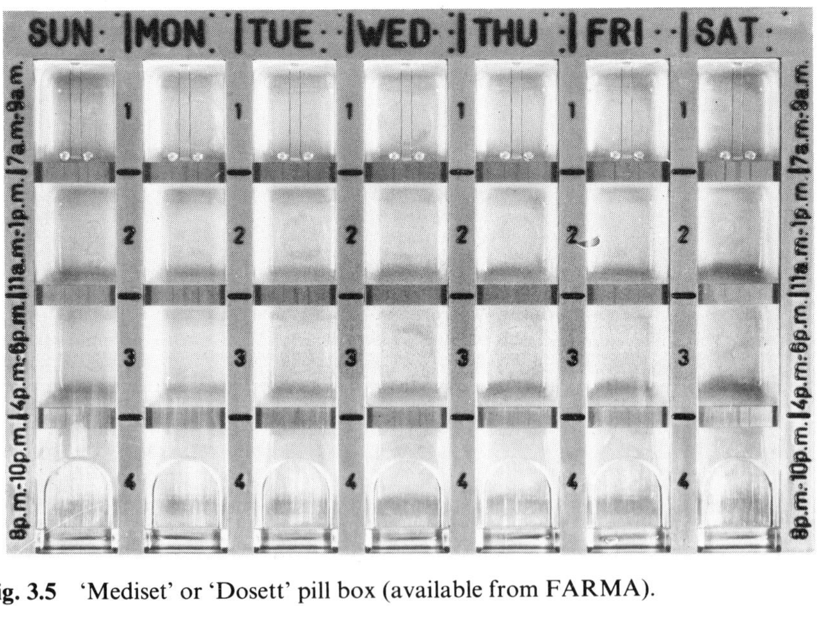

Fig. 3.5 'Mediset' or 'Dosett' pill box (available from FARMA).

coloured box holds a week's supply of pills with 4 separate compartments for each day. labelled 1 to 4 and with times. All lettering on the front is in raised characters to allow the box to be operated by those with very poor visual acuity, relying on touch. Each day's supply has a single transparent slide cover with a series of stops. Pulling to the first stop opens compartment 1 (also labelled 7 a.m–9 a.m.), pulling the slide open to the second stop then opens compartment 2 (also labelled 11 a.m.–1 p.m.), and so on. A certain amount of care is required to pull open the drawer just the requisite amount. On the back of the container there is provision for a drug list to be displayed covered by a plastic window (see Fig. 3.6). This allows the patient or helper to check that what is in the box tallies with the drug list.

Prescription for MR. JOHN JAMES

Medicine	Dosage	Number of tablets 7 a.m. 9 a.m.	11 a.m. 1 p.m.	4 p.m. 6 p.m.	8 p.m. 10 p.m.	Doctor
Thyroxine 0.1 mg.	Two tablets each morning	2				[illegible]
Bendrofluazide 10 mg.	One tablet each morning	1				[illegible]
Quinidine Sulphate 200 mg.	One tablet four times daily	1	1	1	1	[illegible]

Keep the DOSETT away from children!

Fig. 3.6 Drug list on reverse of 'Dosett'.

With all these systems there is the advantage of the patient having to do less 'work' (thinking) and of being able to see at a glance what he has taken and what he has not, which reminds him of his compliance or non-compliance and thereby provides a cue for him to take his pill. Even though the container has to be refilled weekly by the patient or helper this container should reduce the 'need to remember' burden in everyday life throughout the week. The Dosett is somewhat bulky to carry but there is another type of container available where the whole week's supply is in a plastic wallet but each day's supply case may be removed and carried separately. It has been estimated that at least three-quarters of all long-term pill-takers use some aid even if it is just a row of three egg cups on the kitchen table!

Those with a special interest in geriatric pharmacology and therapeutics need no reminding that there is little merit in pressing for higher levels of compliance when the drugs prescribed, in the doses set by the doctor, are so often ill-suited to the patient's real needs. The chapters which follow hope to go some way to repair this major defect in the medical care of the elderly.

REFERENCES AND FURTHER READING

Atkinson L., Gibson I. & Andrews J. (1977) The difficulties of old people taking drugs. *Age and Ageing* **6,** 144–50.

Atkinson L., Gibson I. & Andrews J. (1978) An investigation into the ability of elderly patients continuing to take prescribed drugs after discharge from hospital and recommendations concerning improving the situation. *Gerontology* **24,** 225–34.

Bjorn J. & Cross H.D. (1970) *Problem Orientated Private Practice.* Modern Hospital Press, Chicago.

Bruce S.A. (1982) Regular prescribing in a residential home for elderly women. *British medical Journal* **284,** 1235–7.

Cooper J.K., Love D.W. & Raffoul P.R. (1982) Intentional prescription non-adherence (noncompliance) by the elderly. *Journal of the American Geriatrics Society* **30,** 329–33.

Crome P., Akehurst M. & Keet J. (1980) Drug compliance in elderly hospital in-patients. Trial of the Dosett box. *Practitioner* **224,** 782–5.

Eidenberg L. (1979) 'A friend, not an apple, a day will help keep the doctor away'. *American Journal of Medicine* **66,** 551–3.

Haynes, R.B., Taylor D.W. & Sackett D.L. (Eds) (1979) *Compliance in Health Care.* Based on McMaster Workshop/Symposium on compliance with therapeutic regimens. John Hopkin's University Press, Baltimore.

Ho-Yen R. (1979) A study of repeat prescription cards in a general practice. *Journal of the Royal College of General Practitioners* **29,** 473–7.

Law R. & Chalmers C. (1976) Medicines and elderly people: a general practice survey. *British medical Journal* **1,** 565–8.

Matin Eric W. (1971) *Hazards of Medication.* J.B. Lippincott, Philadelphia.

Murdoch J.C. (1980) The epidemiology of prescribing in an urban general practice. *Journal of the Royal College of General Practitioners* **30,** 393–602.

Shaw S.M. & Opit L.J. (1976) Need for supervision in the elderly receiving long-term prescribed medication. *British medical Journal* **1,** 505–7.

Skegg D.C.G., Doll R. & Perry J. (1977) Use of medicines in general practice. *British medical Journal* **1,** 1561–3.

Tulloch A.J. (1981) Repeat prescribing for elderly patients. *British medical Journal* **282,** 1672–5.

Wandless I., Mucklow J.C., Smith A. & Prudham D. (1979) Compliance with prescribed medicines: a study of elderly patients in the community. *Journal of the Royal College of General Practitioners* **29,** 391–6.

Weed L.L. (1971) *Medical Records. Medicine, Education and Patient Care,* (*The Problem Orientated Record as a Basic Tool*). Year Book Medical Publications, Chicago.

Chapter Four
Drug Handling in Old Age

D. ROBERTSON

> Faulty diagnosis naturally gives rise to faulty treatment, but even when a correct diagnosis is made the aged are frequently improperly treated through our ignorance of the action of drugs and other therapeutic agents upon the senile organism. Assimilation is slow, cumulative action is frequent and the secondary action of drugs is often more pronounced than the primary effect ... ask yourself if you have any other rule for diminishing dose in old age than a rough guess.
>
> *I. L. Nascher*
> 'Geriatrics'. Medical Record, New York.
> April 20, 1912

OVERVIEW

Most drugs prescribed for the older patient are administered orally, absorbed into the portal blood from the upper gastrointestinal tract and distributed throughout the body via the circulation. Drug in plasma exists in two forms, 'bound' and 'free'. Free drug leaves the plasma and enters the tissues where it binds to cellular receptors and exerts its effect through changes in cell permeability or metabolism. In general, the magnitude of drug effect depends on the number of receptors and the concentration of available or 'free' drug to which they are exposed.

With advancing age and in the presence of a number of age-related diseases there are changes in the way in which drugs are handled by the body. Changes in body composition and in drug disposition by renal excretion and hepatic metabolism result in a higher plasma level of free drug than would be the case if the same dose was administered to a younger individual. There is evidence that some tissues and organs, such as the central nervous system, are more sensitive to drugs.

PHARMACOKINETICS AND PHARMACODYNAMICS IN OLD AGE

The World Health Organization defines a drug as 'any substance or product that is used or intended to be used to modify or explore physiological systems or pathological states for the benefit of the recipient.' Few drugs, whether naturally occurring or synthetic, have exclusively beneficial effects. Most drugs exhibit a spectrum of effects: some beneficial some inconsequential and some deleterious or frankly dangerous.

When the physician makes therapeutic decisions on behalf of his patients, his choice between available therapeutic agents is influenced by the diagnosis, the likely outcome with and without intervention and the anticipated effects of treatment. Whether a proposed therapy is surgical, physical, psychological or pharmacological, the practitioner makes an individualized risk-benefit assessment weighing the expected benefits of treatment against possible adverse effects with the 'benefit of the recipient' in mind. In order to plan appropriate pharmacological treatment of the elderly, the prescriber must be aware of the effects that aging and age-related diseases exert on the way drugs are handled by the older person.

In the healthy older person there are age-related changes in both *pharmacokinetics*—drug absorption, distribution and elimination—and in *pharmacodynamics*—the biological and therapeutic effect of the drug. In general, the changes in pharmacokinetics and pharmacodynamics which occur in normal aging and in many of the disease states commonly encountered in the elderly result in an exaggeration of the expected therapeutic effect or the appearance of unwanted drug actions.

Therapeutic effect occurs when active drug reaches the target organ, diffuses through the extracellular fluid and binds to cellular receptors. Drug action at a cellular level usually results from stimulation or inhibition of enzymes or from alterations in membrane permeability. The magnitude of drug action depends on the concentration of free drug at the receptor site and the sensitivity of the target tissue, which is largely determined by the number of available receptors.

The relationship between drug in free and bound form in the plasma and drug in the extracellular fluid is shown in Fig. 4.1. With the exception of topically applied preparations and drugs injected directly into body cavities, most drugs reach their site of action via the circulation. Access to the circulatory system may be by direct intravenous injection or, more commonly, by absorption from another site such as the upper gastrointestinal

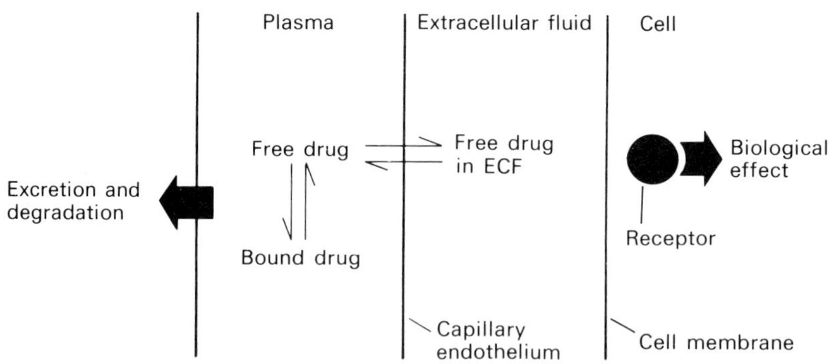

Fig. 4.1 The relationship between drugs in body compartments.

tract or the rectum. Because of the convenience of oral administration, approximately 80% of all drugs and almost all of the drugs used by the elderly living at home are administered orally. The ways in which normal aging, disease states and concurrent pharmacological therapy affect drug absorption will first be considered.

Drug absorption

For drug absorption to occur in the upper gastrointestinal tract the drug must be presented to the absorptive area in an appropriate physical and chemical state. It must remain in contact with the absorptive area for an appropriate length of time, and blood flow to the absorptive site must be adequate. Although some absorption of acidic drugs or drugs in solution may occur in the stomach, most drug absorption occurs by passive diffusion through the small intestinal mucosa.

Normal age changes in gastrointestinal structure and function include reduced mucosal surface area, reduced splanchnic blood flow and reduced gastric acid secretion. Age-related decrease in splanchnic blood flow and morphological changes in the small intestinal mucosa could theoretically impair drug absorption in the older patient, although in studies of drug absorption in young and old subjects no differences were found in the absorption of many drugs including acetaminophen (Divoll *et al.* 1982) and acetylsalicylic acid (Castleden *et al.* 1977b; see Fig. 4.2). Theoretically, diminished gastric acid production and the reduced volume of gastric secretion found in many elderly persons may impair absorption of tetracycline which is best absorbed at an acid pH. Conversely achlorhydria may improve the absorption of other drugs, such as Penicillin G, which are degraded by exposure to stomach acid.

While most drugs are absorbed by simple diffusion and the rate of absorption appears to be unaffected by aging, absorption of substances which are actively transported across the small intestinal epithelium or absorbed by facilitated diffusion is reduced. Active transport of glucose, galactose, and 3-0 methyl D glucose declines with advancing age and absorption of iron, calcium, and thiamine is diminished in older individuals.

Since most drug absorption occurs in the upper small intestine, the speed with which gastric contents are released into the duodenum will influence drug absorption. Any condition which accelerates the delivery of the drug in a suitable form to the intestine will lead to an earlier and a higher peak plasma level.

Gastric emptying in the older person is probably completed within 4 hours, though it may be affected by position, emotion, pain, and the nature and pH of gastric contents. The reported effects of aging on gastric emptying are conflicting. However, altered gastrointestinal anatomy and drugs in common use in the elderly may shorten or prolong gastric emptying time.

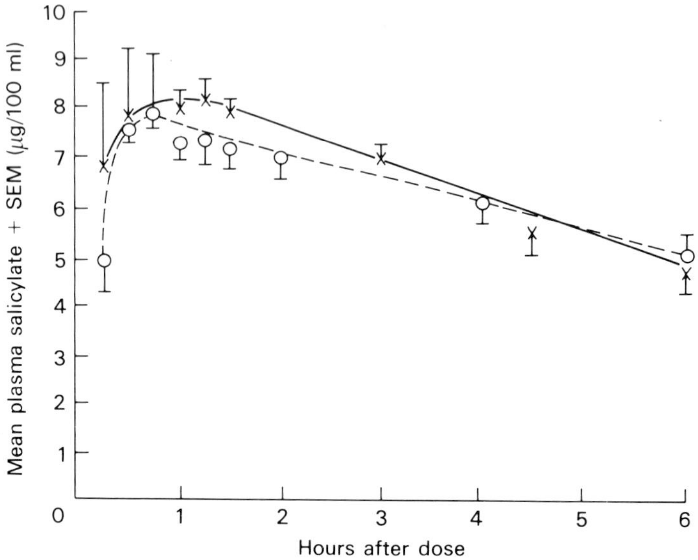

Fig. 4.2 Plasma salicylate concentrations after an oral dose of 900 mg soluble aspirin to young (x–x) and old (0–0) subjects. (Redrawn from Castleden *et al.* (1977b) by kind permission of the authors and the editor of *Age and Ageing*.)

Following gastrectomy or gastroenterostomy, bypass of the normal delay produced by the pyloric sphincter leads to earlier drug absorption; a similar effect may be produced medically by administration of metoclopramide. Administration of metoclopramide (Maxeran, Reglan) concurrently with paracetamol (Nimmo *et al.* 1973) or with tetracycline, lithium carbonate, or levodopa (Parsons 1976) accelerates drug absorption. Reduced drug absorption may occur with the administration of anticholinergic agents which delay gastric emptying. Propantheline and other drugs with anticholinergic activity given together with paracetamol or sulfamethizole lead to reduced absorption (Nimmo *et al.* 1973, Parsons 1976). This effect is of considerable therapeutic importance since many drugs prescribed for the elderly, such as antidepressants, antihistamines and antipsychotics, have anticholinergic activity.

The results of concurrent administration of digoxin with drugs which either accelerate or delay gastric emptying yield paradoxical changes in digoxin absorption. Whereas metoclopramide improves absorption of some drugs, when digoxin and metaclopramide are administered together digoxin absorption is diminished. Presumably accelerated gastric emptying and intestinal motility caused by metoclopramide allows the ingested digoxin to be transported beyond the site where it is optimally absorbed (Manninen *et al.* 1973) since these changes are seen only when digoxin is administered in tablet form and not when liquid preparations are used.

Absorption studies using single drugs administered in the fasting state may not accurately reflect the clinical situation where several drugs may be taken simultaneously, often with food. It is well known that absorption of the fat-soluble vitamins A, D, E and K is reduced when mineral oil is administered, and that insoluble complexes may form between tetracycline and foods containing magnesium, calcium, iron and aluminum. Other interactions reducing absorption include binding of digoxin, salicylates and indomethacin with antacids and binding of oral anticoagulants, thyroid preparations and cardiac glycosides with cholestyramine in the gastrointestinal tract.

The elderly patient receiving drug therapy may have disease states which affect absorption. Pain from any cause or emotional upset may delay gastric emptying; metabolic and endocrine disorders, such as hypercalcemia, hypokalemia or diabetes, slow intestinal transit; and neoplastic infiltration of the intestine or mucosal edema in fluid retaining states may impair absorption. In summary while aging does not affect drug absorption from the gastrointestinal tract greatly, disease, drugs or foods may interfere with absorption.

After an ingested drug diffuses through the intestinal mucosa it enters the portal venous system where several processes commence almost simultaneously; it is bound in a reversible fashion to plasma protein, and in the case of some drugs also to erythrocytes and during the first pass through the liver, drug extraction and metabolism occurs. The amount of extraction and metabolism during the first pass through the liver varies from drug to drug and is quite significant for drugs such as nitroglycerine, propranolol and lidocaine. On reaching the systemic circuit, drugs circulate throughout the body and are available either to enter the tissues to exert a therapeutic effect or to be disposed of by excretion through the kidneys and bile, or by metabolism in the liver and elsewhere.

These several processes occur simultaneously and independently in a dynamic system but for convenience, the effects of aging upon drug binding, distribution and elimination will be considered separately.

Drug binding

Drugs transported in the plasma exist in two forms; 'free' and 'bound'. Free drug in the plasma is that fraction which is available to diffuse into the tissues and also is subject to renal excretion and to enzymatic degradation. For a given drug the ratio between 'bound' and 'free' drug is remarkably constant and a state of equilibrium exists between the free drug and the drug which is bound to albumin or in some cases to erythrocytes. As the free drug enters the tissues the bound drug acts as a mobile reservoir from which drug is released thus preventing major fluctuation in the amount of free drug available to the tissues. The interrelationship of free and bound drug in the tissue and plasma was shown in Fig. 4.1.

Since the most important blood component for drug binding is albumin, changes in serum albumin concentration may be expected to affect drug binding. There is a slight decline in serum albumin in healthy old age and a greater reduction in many older patients. Greenblatt (1979) found a lower serum albumin in older hospitalized patient: in 11 090 subjects, 4538 of whom were over 60 years of age, significant differences in serum albumin were found between the young and the old. Subjects were patients in whom diseases associated with altered serum protein levels had been excluded.

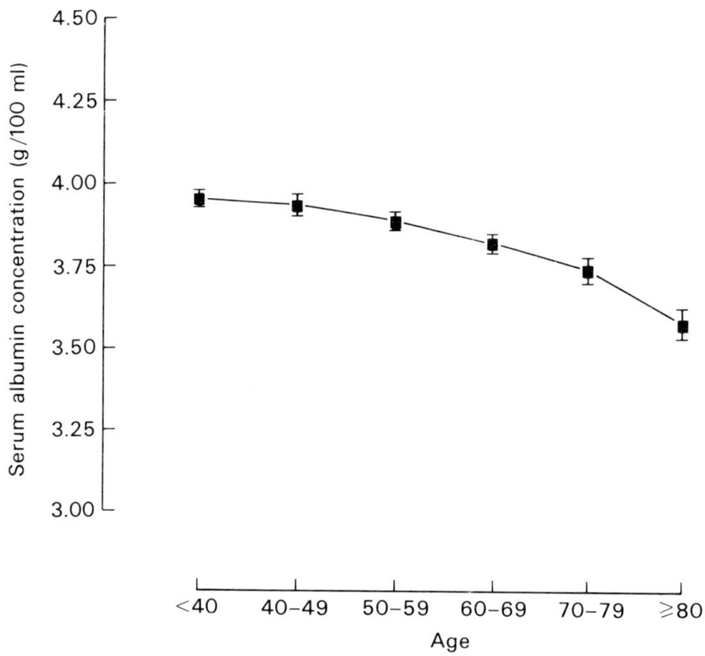

Fig. 4.3 Mean (±SE) serum albumin concentrations in 11 090 hospitalized medical patients by age. (Redrawn from Greenblatt (1979) by kind permission of the author and the editor of the *Journal of the American Geriatrics Society*.)

The result of a lower serum albumin level, whether it occurs in healthy old age or as a consequence of disease, is a reduction in the number of drug binding sites. The higher level of free drug in the plasma leads to enhanced therapeutic effect. The effect of reduced serum albumin levels on highly protein-bound drugs is illustrated in Fig. 4.4.

Interactions between highly protein-bound drugs may occur as a result of competition for binding sites (see Fig. 4.5); for example, when sulfonamides or salicylates are administered together with oral hypoglycemic

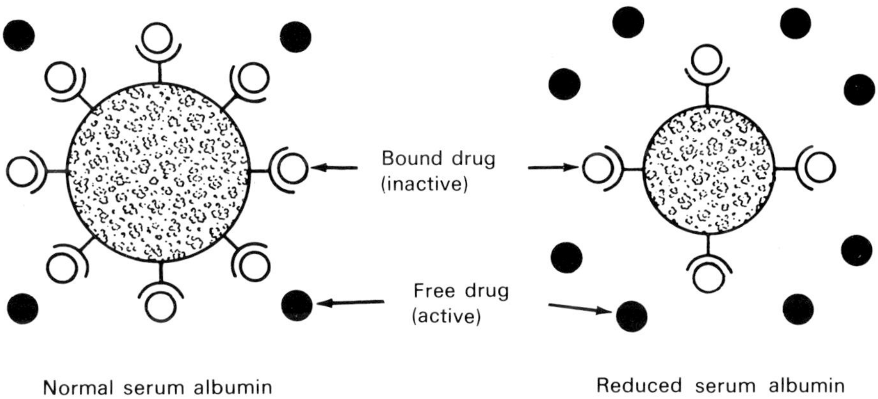

Fig. 4.4 The effect of reduced serum albumin on protein binding of drugs.

agents the hypoglycemic agent may be displaced from its binding sites and profound hypoglycemia may occur. Displacement of oral anticoagulants from protein binding sites occurs when chloral hydrate, clofibrate, nalidixic acid, or phenylbutazone are administered (see Case Study 1). The increased risk of hemorrhage in patients receiving oral anticoagulants and acetylsalicylic acid results not from protein displacement but from the effect of ASA on platelet function and the gastric mucosa. A full account of drug interaction with oral anticoagulants will be found in reviews by Koch-Weser and Sellers (1971a, b).

Case Study 1

Mr L. McK., a 72-year-old retired office worker, enjoyed good health until he suffered a myocardial infarction. Two months

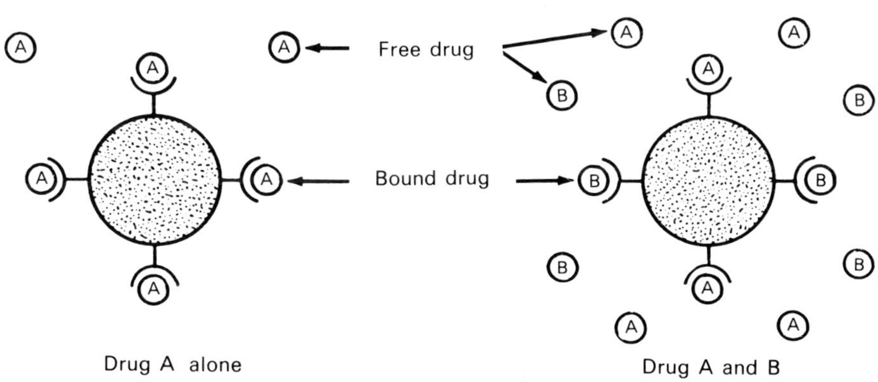

Fig. 4.5 Drug displacement from protein binding sites.

after the myocardial infarction he experienced a sudden onset of right hemiplegia and expressive dysphasia. Cerebral embolism of mural thrombus from the left ventricle was diagnosed and long-term anticoagulant therapy with warfarin was instituted. He was stabilized on a small dose of warfarin and satisfactory control was achieved.

Following discharge from hospital he attended the outpatient department for physical therapy. After therapy he developed pain in his right shoulder and for several days he took several of his wife's 'arthritis pills'. One week later he experienced a rectal bleed and fell to the floor. This resulted in tissue injury and an extensive hematoma of his right buttock and thigh.

When reviewed by his physician the one-stage prothrombin time was 68, (control 14). The 'arthritis pill' which he had taken intermittently over the preceding week was phenylbutazone.

Case Study 1 illustrates the problem which may result from concurrent therapy with two or more drugs which are highly protein bound. Although competition for protein binding sites between two or more highly protein-bound drugs may occur at any age, it is an everyday clinical consideration when dealing with older patients who may be receiving several drugs.

A number of the drugs commonly prescribed for the elderly are highly protein bound. Warfarin, for example, is 99% protein bound and tolbutamide is 96% protein bound. These drugs may be contrasted with digoxin of which 80% is free in the plasma and only 20% protein bound. Highly protein-bound drugs may be displaced from their binding sites and into the plasma by other highly protein-bound drugs which bind more avidly to the binding sites. When, for example, warfarin, 99% of which is in the bound form, is administered concurrently with drugs such as phenylbutazone and chloral hydrate, warfarin is displaced with potentially disastrous clinical consequences.

Outpatient anticoagulant therapy in elderly patients is potentially hazardous. Hypertension, renal impairment, female sex, mental confusion, poor compliance and concurrent drug therapy increase the risk of adverse drug reaction.

Drugs may be bound to other blood constituents, notably erythrocytes. Changes in erythrocyte binding have been described for meperidine (Demerol, Pethidine) as for chlormethiazole (Heminevrin). However, age changes in erythrocyte binding are minimal compared with those caused by changes in serum albumin levels or compared with drug displacement from protein binding sites.

Drug distribution

After the initial phase of intravascular distribution and binding to albumin, and in some cases to erythrocytes, drugs are distributed throughout the body. Differences in cardiac output and blood flow to various tissues affect the speed with which equilibration is achieved so that well-perfused organs, such as the brain, heart and muscles achieve equilibration rapidly whereas in less well-perfused areas, such as adipose tissue, the process may take several hours.

There is considerable variation between drugs in their pattern of distribution to different tissues and compartments of the body. Some drugs, such as digoxin, may have a low serum level yet they are bound avidly by skeletal muscle, cardiac muscle and brain. The apparent volume of distribution (V_d), calculated from the plasma concentration, after equilibrium, following an intravenous injection of a known quantity of drug, is the volume of fluid into which the drug *appears* to distribute with a concentration equal to that in plasma. The V_d of drugs which are taken up avidly by body tissues, such as digoxin, may greatly exceed actual body water. Compounds such as the dye Evans Blue do not enter tissues to any appreciable extent and have a V_d of around 3 litres, the same as plasma volume.

With advancing age the proportion of body water, intracellular water and lean body mass decreases and the proportion of body fat increases. This is reflected in an age-related decrease in the apparent volume of distribution of drugs such as ethanol and acetaminophen and an increased volume of distribution of highly lipid-soluble drugs such as lidocaine and diazepam. In the case of diazepam the mean volume of distribution is twice as great in the 80-year-old as it is in the 20-year-old. It is the alteration in $\mathrm{V_d}$ rather than an impaired hepatic metabolism which increases the biological half-life of benzodiazepines in the older patient. Case Study 2 describes the consequences of the injudicious administration of benzodiazepines to an elderly woman who developed adverse drug reaction due to the accumulation of benzodiazepines and their metabolites.

Case Study 2

Mrs L.S., a recently widowed 70-year-old woman, left her home and moved into an apartment in a senior citizens' highrise building. Since she could no longer travel to visit her former physician she consulted a new physician and on her first visit complained of weakness, tiredness, abdominal pains, occipital headache and insomnia. Flurazepam 15–30 mg q.d.s. was prescribed. Dissatisfied with this treatment, she consulted another physician who prescribed diazepam 5–10 mg t.i.d.

Several days later she was observed staggering in the apartment building in a state of undress, and when returned to her apartment she collapsed to the floor. She was taken to the emergency department of a hospital where she became agitated and noisy. She received diazepam 10 mg i.m., was examined and returned home. Later that day she was referred to a geriatrician as a 'social problem' because of recurrent falls and failure of self-care.

Physical examination revealed multiple bruises, ataxic gait and slurred speech. She was admitted to hospital where all drugs were discontinued. Over the next 10 days her gait, speech and mental function improved and she was discharged home.

Drug elimination

The effect of a drug is terminated either by its elimination from the body in unchanged form or by its biotransformation into pharmacologically inactive or less active metabolites which are subsequently excreted. Biotransformation occurs predominantly in the liver, although some metabolic degradation may occur in many organs including the lungs, kidneys and the gastrointestinal tract. Most drugs and their metabolites are excreted in the urine, although in some circumstances drug excretion in bile, sweat and expired gases may be important. The rate at which drugs are eliminated may be expressed either as the elimination half-life ($T_{\frac{1}{2}}$) or as total body clearance. Elimination half-life is the time (in minutes or hours) taken for the plasma concentration in the post-absorptive, post-distributive phase to fall by 50%. Total body clearance is a better measure of drug disposal since it is not influenced by changes in the apparent volume of distribution which have already been described in the elderly. Total body clearance is expressed as a hypothetical volume of blood cleared of drug in unit time. It is the sum of hepatic metabolism, net biliary and renal excretion and elimination and metabolism at other sites.

Hepatic metabolism

First pass effect

Oral administration of glyceryl trinitrate is ineffective in relieving angina pectoris whereas sublingual administration is used widely to prevent or relieve anginal pain. The difference in efficacy is explained by 'the first pass effect'. This refers to the extraction and metabolism of a drug from the plasma during its first hepatic circulation. Some drugs, such as glyceryl trinitrate, are almost completely metabolized during their first pass through the liver, and must, therefore, be given by a route which bypasses the liver, such as percutaneously or sublingually. Other drugs, such as propranolol and lidocaine, are extensively but not completely metabolized during the first pass through the liver, thus there is a considerable difference between comparably effective oral and intravenous doses.

Hepatic metabolism, whether during the first pass or subsequently, occurs in the hepatocyte. Active, highly lipid-soluble drugs are converted to less soluble and usually less active forms prior to renal or biliary excretion. Hepatic metabolic reactions may be divided into two phases although not all drugs undergo both types of reaction. In *Phase 1* metabolism drugs undergo oxidation, reduction or hydrolysis. The resulting compound is usually inactive or less active than the parent compound. However, in some circumstances the product of hepatic degradation is metabolically active, as is the case with diazepam which is metabolized to desmethyl diazepam, which is itself pharmacologically active and has a long biological half-life. *Phase 2* reductions include conjugation, reduction and acetylation and usually render drugs or their metabolites more soluble by conjugation with glucuronic acid, sulfate, glycine, or acetate.

Hepatic enzyme activity

Hepatic drug metabolism occurs mainly in the smooth endoplasmic reticulum of the hepatocytes. However, non-microsomal biotransformation does contribute to the degradation of many drugs in common use. Within the smooth endoplasmic reticulum a series of mixed-function oxidases, collectivelely known as the Cytochrome P450 system, has been studied intensively. The rate of degradation of drugs metabolized by this system may be used as a measure of hepatic enzyme activity.

Antipyrine (Phenazone), formerly used as an antipyretic-analgesic is now used to investigate hepatic drug metabolism since 95% of its metabolism is by microsomal enzymes in the liver. The plasma half-life of antipyrine in individuals of comparable age varies widely between 5 and 70 hours and is affected by liver, renal and malignant disease, by smoking and by alcohol consumption. While there is considerable variation between individuals, the mean plasma half-life of antipyrine is increased in the aged, reflecting a reduction in hepatic drug metabolizing capacity to one-half to two-thirds of that found in younger subjects.

Hepatic enzyme activity may be enhanced or inhibited by concurrently administered drugs. Stimulation of enzyme activities (enzyme induction) can occur as a result of ingestion or inhalation of a number of chemical agents administered therapeutically. The barbiturates, doxycycline, ethanol, phenylbutazone, phenytoin and rifampicin all induce enzymes thus bringing about their own metabolism as well as the metabolism of other drugs such as the antidepressants, sterorids and oral anticoagulants. Enzyme induction may afford some protective benefits to patients receiving several drugs metabolized by the liver by hastening drug metabolism. This protective effect of enzyme induction may be less in the elderly since the degree to which enzyme induction occurs with concurrent drug therapy is reduced in older patients (Salem *et al.* 1978).

Enzyme inhibition by a number of drugs delays hepatic metabolism. The H_2 blocker, cimetidine, is of particular importance in this regard because of its widespread use at present. Cimetidine delays the metabolism of concurrently administered chlordiazepoxide, diazepam, propranolol and warfarin not only by inhibiting enzyme activity but also perhaps by its effect on hepatic blood flow.

Hepatic blood flow

Hepatic uptake and metabolism of certain drugs is restricted to the unbound fraction and is not influenced by hepatic blood flow. Other drugs with a high hepatic extraction ratio, such as propranolol and lidocaine, are so rapidly removed from the plasma that hepatic blood flow is the rate-limited factor. Hepatic blood flow declines with age due to reduced cardiac output and redistribution of cardiac output which results in a disproportionate fall in splanchnic blood flow. Normally the reduction of hepatic blood flow which occurs in the elderly is of no clinical consequence, but when hepatic reserve capacity is further challenged by anoxia or by congestive heart failure, metabolism of drugs such as lidocaine is impaired and adverse effects such as cardiac and respiratory depression, confusion and convulsions may occur.

Hepatic drug metabolizing capacity declines with age but routine tests of liver function are often normal. Downward adjustment of dosage should be made for most drugs which undergo hepatic metabolism. Many drugs, such as H_2-blockers and β-blockers, impair metabolism of concurrently administered drugs by inhibiting enzymes or by reducing hepatic blood flow.

Renal excretion

The kidney shows an age-related decline in function in the absence of clinically or radiologically discernible disease, and even when serum creatinine or urea nitrogen levels are normal or only slightly raised. In contrast to the liver where the decline in drug-metabolizing capacity is variable and is not reflected in common tests of hepatic function, age changes in renal function are more constant and are reflected in changes in creatinine clearance.

Water-soluble drugs and their metabolites which undergo renal excretion may be handled by glomerular filtration or by tubular secretion.

Although both glomerular filtration and tubular secretion decline with advancing age, effects on glomerular filtration are more accessible to study.

Glomerular filtration

Glomerular filtration, measured by inulin clearance or more commonly by creatinine clearance, declines from values of around 140 ml/min/1.73 m^2 at age 30 to 97 ml/min/1.73 m^2 or less in the healthy 80-year-old (Rowe *et al.* 1976).

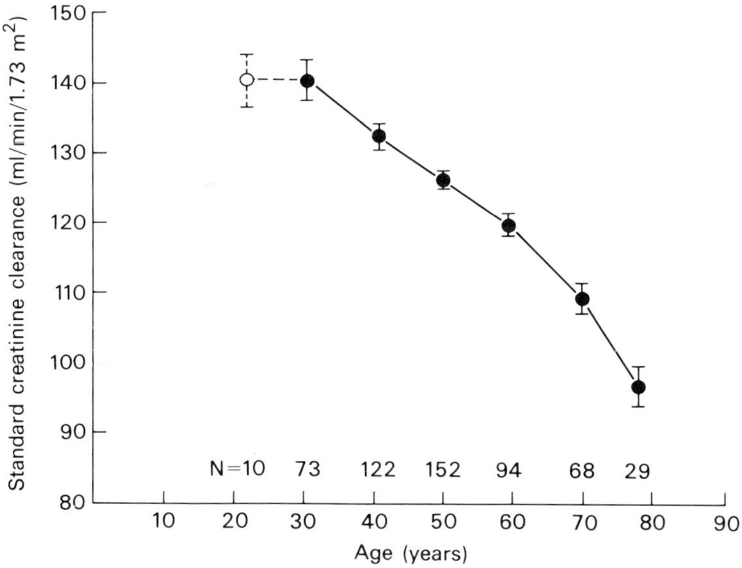

Fig. 4.6 Cross-sectional differences in standard creatinine clearance with age in men. (Redrawn from Rowe *et al.* (1976) by kind permission of the authors and the editor of the *Journal of Gerontology*.) (Values are for true creatinine clearance. To obtain values comparable to automated chromogen method ×0.8; Bennett *et al.* 1980b.)

The decline in creatinine clearance values results from a reduction in the number of intact functioning nephrons and from a reduced renal plasma flow. When dehydration or congestive heart failure is present or when drugs which reduce renal blood flow such as antihypertensives, β-blockers, and non-steroidal acute inflammatory drugs are given, the glomerular filtration rate may fall to 25–50 ml/min. Chronic renal disease, when present, is associated with even lower values. Fig. 4.7 is a nomogram from which the percentile rank for creatinine clearance may be calculated for different ages.

Drugs and their metabolites of low molecular weight existing unbound

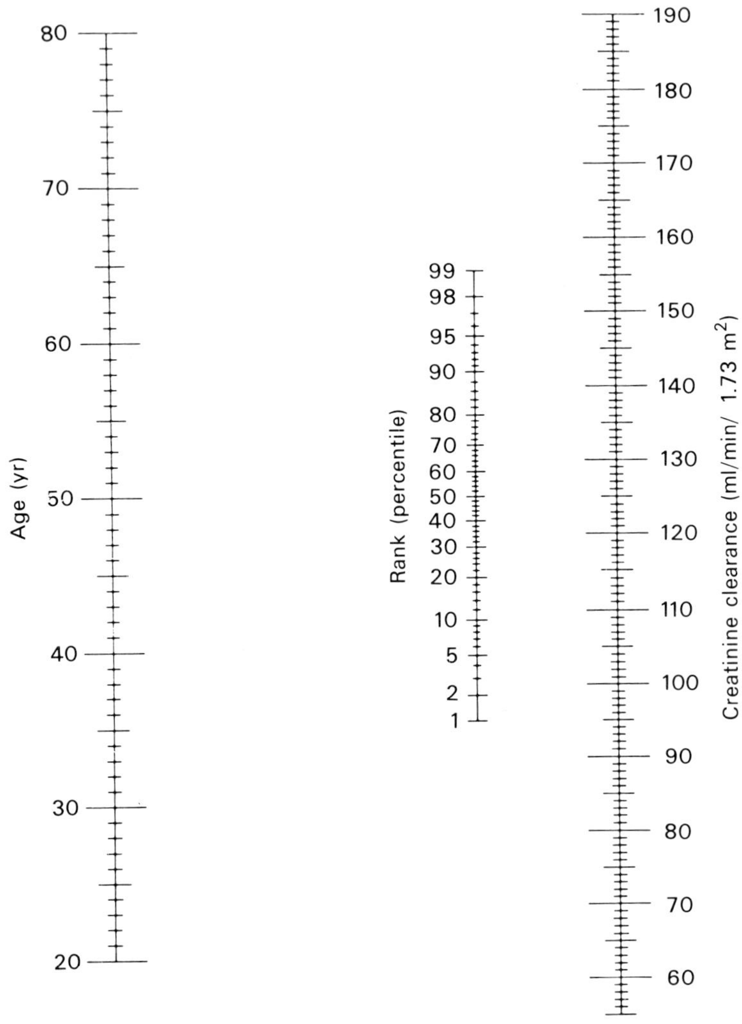

Fig. 4.7 Nomogram for determination of age-adjusted percentile rank in true creatinine clearance, values are based on total chromogen creatinine. Auto analyser values may be multiplied by 1.25 to obtain equivalent true creatinine clearance for use on the nomogram. (Reproduced from Rowe *et al.* (1976) by kind permission of the authors and the editor of the *Journal of Gerontology*.)

in the plasma are filtered at the glomerulus, pass through the tubules where some reabsorption may take place, and are excreted in the urine. Digoxin and the aminoglycoside antibiotics are examples of commonly used drugs which are excreted in this way. The rate of excretion of these drugs which are excreted primarily by glomerular filtration is proportional to the creatinine clearance. Clearance of digoxin has been extensively studied, and, while some digoxin is excreted by non-renal routes, Roberts and Caird (1976) have shown a close relationship between digoxin and creatinine clearance in elderly patients (see Fig 4.8)

Serum biochemistry results may give false reassurance to the prescriber since many elderly individuals with measured creatinine clearance of 50 or 60 ml/min or less have serum creatinine values within the normal range.

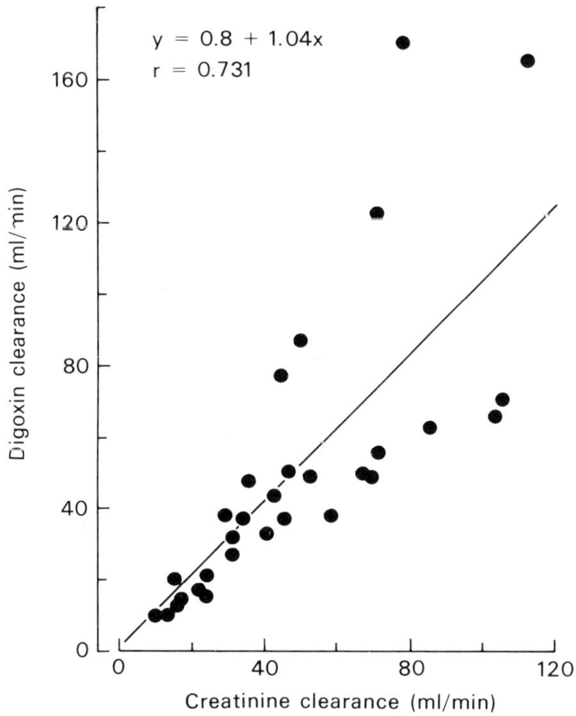

Fig. 4.8 Relationship between digoxin and creatinine clearance in elderly patients. (Redrawn from Roberts & Caird (1976) by kind permission of the authors and the editor of *Age and Ageing*.)

Endogenous creatinine production, which is related to body muscle mass, declines with age, thus the diminished excretory capacity of the kidney is compensated by decreased creatinine production resulting in normal or near normal values of serum creatinine. When age or disease-related reduction in renal function is observed or suspected then the frequency or dose of drugs should be modified in accordance with published guidelines. When available, the use of serial serum drug concentrations is helpful in determining appropriate dosage especially when using drugs such as the aminoglycosides, antibiotics and digoxin.

Tubular secretion

Renal tubular secretion is the major route of excretion of organic acids, particularly the penicillin and cephalosporin antibiotics. Although less extensively studied than creatinine clearance, it appears that tubular secretory capacity declines in parallel with the decline in glomerular filtration. Decreased renal tubular excretion in the elderly results in prolongation of the half-life of Penicillin G to values almost twice that of the young. Inhibition of tubular secretion may occur and this effect may be used therapeutically when probenecid is given with penicillin to maintain serum penicillin levels. Drug interactions at the renal tubular level occur with drugs which share common transport systems. Penicillin, oral antidiabetic agents, salicylates and thiazides share a common secretory system and when administered concurrently competition leads to blood levels higher than anticipated for each drug when administered separately.

Case Study 3

Mr H.M., an 81-year-old retired railroad worker, lived with his 75-year old wife. He had previous surgery for cataracts and benign prostrate hypertrophy, and had a large unoperated inguinal hernia and hydrocele. Drug treatment for chronic obstructure lung disease, atrial fibrillation and mild congestive heart failure included digoxin 0.25 mg daily, furosemide 40 mg daily and oral potassium supplement.

Over the course of a few weeks he became easily fatigued, 'grumpy', 'hard to manage', and wandered aimlessly. His wife was unable to manage his care at home and since nursing home admission was not immediately available, he was admitted to hospital where Haloperidol 2 mg t.i.d. and Largactil 25 mg t.i.d. were administered to control his behaviour. On admission digoxin dosage was reduced to 0.125 mg and several days later a serum digoxin level was drawn and reported at 2.5 ng/ml. Blood urea level and serum creatinine were slightly elevated. Endogenous creatinine clearance was 48 ml/min. Electrocardiogram showed atrial fibrillation at a rate of 55 per minute with digitalis effect.

Within one week of lowering the dosage of digoxin, Mr M's behaviour disorder resolved without the use of tranquillizers, he was oriented and functionally independent. Arrangements were made for surgical treatment of the hydrocele and hernia and he was discharged to his home on digoxin 0.125 mg daily and triamterene-hydrochlorothiazide (Dyazide) 1 tablet daily.

Mrs M. stated that she 'thought it was his heart pill all the time.'

Renal excretion of drugs is markedly impaired in the aged. Serum creatinine and urea nitrogen levels do not reflect accurately the reduction in glomerular filtration and tubular secretion.

Biliary excretion

Many drugs and their metabolites are excreted by this route and some are reabsorbed thus establishing an enterohepatic circulation. Ampicillin, certain tetracyclines and rifampicin are actively transported from the blood to bile by hepatocytes and the two former drugs are, therefore, of value in inflammatory disorders of the biliary tree. There are no data on age effects on biliary drug excretion.

Tissue responsiveness

The effect of a drug depends not only on the plasma level but also upon the responsiveness of the tissues. Physicians prescribing for the elderly have long suspected that the older patients exhibit altered responsiveness to certain drugs. Altered or increased sensitivity seems to affect the aged brain in particular, with the elderly person becoming confused and disoriented after the administration of doses of barbiturates, hypnotics, anticholinergics and dopaminergic drugs which would be well tolerated by younger adults. Nitrazepam (Mogadon), a benzodiazepepine which has similar pharmacokinetic characteristics in the young and the old, produced significantly greater impairment in psychomotor tests in the elderly compared with the young (Castleden *et al.* 1977a).

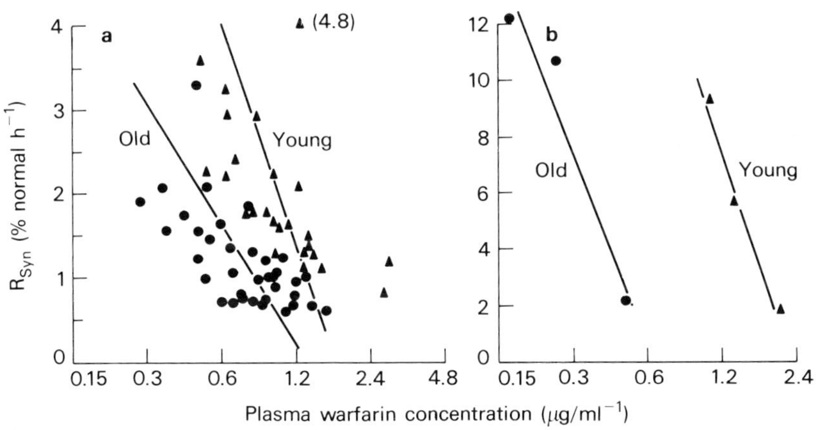

Fig. 4.9 Rate of synthesis of clotting factors (R_{Syn}) against log plasma warfarin concentration in young and old humans (a) and rats (b). (Redrawn from Shepherd *et al.* (1977) by kind permission of the authors and the editor of the *British Journal of Clinical Pharmacology*.)

In both humans and rats age changes in tissue responsiveness to oral anticoagulants have been found (Shepherd *et al.* 1977). No major difference in pharmacokinetics was found between the young and the old, however at the same plasma warfarin concentrations old subjects showed greater suppression of clotting factor synthesis (see Fig 4.9). When prescribing warfarin for the older patient, increased tissue sensitivity, as demonstrated by greater inhibition of synthesis of vitamin K-dependent clotting factors, must be considered as well as drug interactions between warfarin and concurrently administered drugs which may displace it from its protein binding sites.

SUMMARY

The effects of aging on drug handling are complex, and are further complicated by the effects of disease and multiple drug use. With the exception of drug absorption which is usually unaffected, age changes in pharmacokinetics lead to plasma level of free drug higher than anticipated and to prolonged drug action. For the healthy older person receiving short-term single drug therapy the clinical impact of these changes may be insignificant. For the very old, for those suffering from multiple illnesses and receiving several drugs concurrently, rational drug management demands knowledge of the pharmacokinetic and pharmacodynamic changes. When the reserve capacity of body systems is reduced by aging and by disease and when several drugs are used together, appropriate adjustment to dosage and frequency of administration must be made.

If the prescribing physician has access to a laboratory where serum levels of drugs such as acetylsalicylic acid, digoxin, dilantin, gentamicin and theophylline may be obtained, serial monitoring of the plasma drug level is useful in assessing the response to therapy.

This chapter opened with a challenge from the physician who coined the word 'geriatrics', Dr I.L. Nascher: '. . . ask yourself if you have any other rule for diminishing dose in old age than a rough guess.' Since Dr Nascher's paper was published in 1912 research in gerontology, pharmacology and medicine has expanded greatly our knowledge of drug handling in old age, thus enabling the prescriber to make informed decisions on drug use and drug dosage.

REFERENCES AND FURTHER READING

Bennet W.M., Muther R.S. & Parker R.A. (1980a) Drug therapy in renal failure: dosing guidelines for adults (Part 1). *Annals of internal Medicine* **93**, 62–89.

Bennet W.M., Muther R.S. & Parker R.A. (1980b) Drug therapy in renal failure: dosing guidelines for adults (Part 2). *Annals of internal Medicine* **93**, 286–325.

Castleden C.M., George C.F., Marcer D. & Hallett C. (1977a) Increased sensitivity to nitrazepam in old age. *British medical Journal* **1**, 10–12.

Castleden C.M., Volans C.N. & Raymond K. (1977b) The effect of ageing on drug absorption from the gut. *Age and Ageing* **6**, 138–43.

Divoll M., Ameer B., D.R. & Greenblatt D.J. (1982) Age does not alter acetaminophen absorption. *Journal of the American Geriatrics Society* **30**, 240–4.

Greenblatt D.J. (1979) Reduced serum albumin in the elderly: a report from the Boston Collaborative Drug Surveillance Program. *Journal of the American Geriatrics Society* **27**, 20–2.

Koch-Weser J. & Sellers E.M. (1971a) Drug interactions with courmarin anticoagulants (first of two parts). *New England Journal of Medicine* **285**, 487–98.

Koch-Weser J. & Sellers E.M. (1971b) Drug interactions with courmarin anticoagulants (second of two parts). *New England Journal of Medicine* **285**, 547–58.

Maninen V., Melin J., Apajalahti A. & Karesja M. (1973) Altered absorption of digoxin in patients given propantheline and metoclopramide. *Lancet i*, 398–400.

Nimmo J., Heading R.C., Tothill P. & Prescott L.F. (1973) Pharmacological modifications of gastric emptying: effects of propantheline and metoclopramide on paracetamol absorption. *British medical Journal* **1**, 587–9.

Parsons R.L. (1976) The absorption of drugs in malabsorption syndromes. *Hospital Update* 221–30.

Roberts M.A. & Caird F.I. (1976) Steady-state kinetics of digoxin in the elderly. *Age and Ageing* **5**, 214–23.

Robertson D. (1985) Pharmacology and ageing—pharmacokinetics and pharmacodynamics. In Brocklehurst J.C. (Ed.) *Textbook of Geriatric Medicine and Gerontology*, 3rd Edn. Churchill Livingstone, London. (In press.)

Rowe J.W., Andres R., Tobin J.D., Norris A.H. & Shock N.W. (1976) The effect of age on creatinine clearance in men: a cross-sectional and longitudinal study. *Journal of Gerontology* **31**, 155–63.

Rowland M. & Tozer T.N. (1980) *Clinical Pharmacokinetics: concepts and applications.* Lea & Febiger, Philadelphia.

Shepherd A.M.M., Hewick D.S., Moreland T.A. & Stevenson I.H. (1977) Age as determinant of sensitivity to warfarin. *British Journal of clinical Pharmacology* **4**, 315–20.

Salem S.A.M., Rajjayabun P., Shepherd A.M.M. & Stevenson I.H. (1978) Reduced induction of drug metabolism in the elderly. *Age and Ageing* **7**, 68–73.

Chapter Five
Adverse Drug Reactions in the Elderly

D. ROBERTSON

> I firmly believe that if the whole *Materia Medica* could be sunk to the bottom of the sea it would be all the better for mankind and all the worse for the fishes.
>
> *Oliver Wendell Holmes*
> Lecture at Harvard Medical School (1860)

OVERVIEW

Unwanted drug effects from prescribed and non-prescribed medications occur more commonly in the aged. They include idiosyncratic and allergic reactions and drug interactions. However, in the elderly impairment in cerebral or locomotor function, or impairment of self-care skills may be the presenting signs of an adverse drug reaction. Many such reactions could be anticipated and avoided if altered drug handling and increased sensitivity to drugs were recognized and appropriate adjustment to therapy made.

Adverse reactions to drugs are important problems and are commonly encountered in therapy of the elderly. Drug-induced illness may lead to hospital admission and while receiving treatment in hospital the elderly commonly experience adverse drug reactions. The World Health Organization has defined an adverse drug reaction (ADR) as 'any response to a drug which is noxious and unintended and which occurs at doses used in man for prophylaxis, diagnosis or therapy.' In this chapter the mechanisms by which adverse drug reactions occur and the reason why the elderly experience ADR more frequently than the young will be discussed. Common pathways of presentation of ADR in the elderly will be described, however, for detailed description of adverse effects of individual drugs the reader should consult standard reference texts.

With the exception of pure hormones given for replacement purposes, most drugs exhibit a spectrum of activity and a lack of specificity by affecting many organs and tissues other than the 'target tissue'. In this way, symptoms, disease and loss of function may be the unintended result of drug administration. Most adverse drug reactions encountered in the elderly are of this type, that is, non-allergic: they are predictable and potentially preventable since they are dose-related and represent an excess of the de-

Table 5.1 Types of adverse drug reaction (ADR).

Non-allergic	Excess of desired therapeutic effect	
	Pharmacologic spectrum of drug activity	
	Drug–drug interaction	
	Miscellaneous	
Allergic	Type I reaction	Immediate hypersensitivity
	Type II reaction	Cytotoxic
	Type III reaction	Immune complex disease
	Type IV reaction	Delayed hypersensitivity
Idiosyncratic		

sired therapeutic effect, actions which are part of the pharmacological spectrum of activity of the drug or interactions between drugs. Non-allergic adverse drug reactions include these examples: oversedation with hypnotics and sedatives, which is a manifestation of excess of the *desired therapeutic effect*; anticholinergic action of tricyclic antidepressants or sodium-retaining and potassium-depleting effects of corticosteroids, effects which are within the *spectrum of drug activity* but undesirable in a particular clinical situation; and displacement of anticoagulants from their binding sites by phenylbutazone and chloral hydrate which represent *drug–drug interactions*. Allergic and idiosyncratic reactions are generally non-dose-related and cannot be predicted unless the patient has previously experienced drug allergy (see Table 5.1). For a comprehensive review of allergic drug reaction, see References and Further Reading at the end of the chapter.

RISK FACTORS

Adverse drug reactions occur more commonly in the elderly due to age changes in pharmacokinetics and pharmacodynamics (see Chapter 4), and due to greater drug consumption than younger patients. The elderly in Western countries make up 10–15% of the population yet receive over one-third of all drugs prescribed. Risk factors associated with adverse drug reactions are listed in Table 5.2.

The older the patient, the more likely is an adverse drug effect to occur. This may reflect the compounded effects of reduced body size, and the effects of both aging and disease on drug metabolism. Elderly women are

Table 5.2 Risk factors for adverse drug reactions.

Age	Duration of therapy
Sex	Drug type(s)
Number of drugs	Non-compliance
Drug dosage	Underlying disease

said to be more prone to adverse drug reactions than elderly men. This may be a reflection of smaller body size and more frequent use of drugs, particularly those with central nervous system effects.

The greater the number of drugs prescribed the greater the risk of drug-induced illness. In a hospital population of elderly patients Hurwitz (1969) found that the frequency of ADR increased from 3.4% in patients receiving between 1 and 5 drugs to nearly 25% in those receiving 6 or more drugs.

The greater the amount of drug taken the more frequent the occurrence of ADR. Patients under 70 years of age receiving 15 mg of flurazepam daily experienced few adverse reactions, whereas 40% of those receiving 30 mg a day experienced adverse reactions such as drowsiness and ataxia.

The longer a drug is taken the greater the chance of developing ADR. This may result from accumulation of a drug such as a benzodiazepine in body tissues or from effects on organs or tissues which are particularly sensitive to a particular drug. An example of the latter is tardive dyskinesia which may follow phenothiazine use. The drugs most commonly implicated in ADR in the elderly are listed in Table 5.3.

Table 5.3 Drugs commonly associated with ADR.

Analgesics	Bronchodilators
Antibiotics	Digoxin
Anticoagulants	Diuretics
Antidepressants	Non-steroidal anti-inflammatory drugs
Antihypertensives	Oral hypoglycemic agents
Antiparkinsonian drugs	Sedative-hypnotic drugs
Antipsychotics	

Failure to comply exactly with a therapeutic regimen, or non-compliance, is probably the norm, since most patients fail to take medications exactly as directed. Non-compliance—that is failure to take a prescribed medication at all or potentially hazardous use of a prescribed medication—may occur in as many as one-quarter to one-half of elderly patients.

A number of conditions predispose to non-compliance: visual or hearing impairment may interfere with understanding of the directions for drug use; cognitive impairment or depression may interfere with understanding of instructions; arthritis may interfere with access to medications which are dispensed in child-proof containers which may also prove 'granny-proof'.

Non-compliance with therapeutic directions increases with the number of drugs prescribed. However, in such circumstances non-compliant behaviour may exert a protective influence against adverse effects. When victims of polypharmacy are admitted to hospital or to an institution they may receive for the first time full doses of medications which they were supposed to be receiving at home.

Many disease states, superimposed upon age changes in organ function, further compromise reserve capacity and affect drug handling or the response to drugs. The patient with dementia is more susceptible to the adverse effects of CNS drugs and the untreated hypothyroid patient is exquisitely sensitive to sedative drugs and narcotic analgesics. Mild heart failure may decompensate when a small dose of propranolol is used, and the patient in heart failure develops confusion and other signs of CNS toxicity when lidocaine or other antiarrhythmics are used even in modest doses.

The prescribing physician who is familiar with the action and adverse effects of drugs which he uses frequently will be alert to the possibility of non-compliance when treatment is inefficacious and of adverse reaction when new symptoms develop. The possibility that new symptoms represent adverse effects must always be considered.

Unfortunately, this is not always the case since adverse reactions may develop insidiously and in a non-specific fashion by affecting older persons' cognitive function, their locomotor skills or their capacity for self-care. When neither the physician nor the patient recognizes the role of prescribed and self-administered medications in causing these alterations in physical or mental function, and the functional decline is ascribed to 'aging' or 'dementia', a grave error is made. Since many drugs and combinations of drugs in common use lead to behavioral changes, locomotor impairment or decline in functional ability, and since patients, family members and professionals often ascribe any decremental change in an old person to aging, the prudent prescriber considers ADR in the differential diagnosis of any new symptoms.

The older person living in the community who suddenly develops disorientation, confusion, agitation, suspiciousness or aggressive behavior has not developed dementia overnight. He has developed an acute confusional state (delirium) which may occur in the cognitively intact older person as well as the individual with pre-existing dementia. Delirium is an acute or subacute change in central nervous system function in which disorientation, memory impairment, perceptual disturbance, disturbed sleep-wake cycle and altered psychomotor activity are associated with clouding of consciousness (American Psychiatric Association 1980). It may be precipitated by any physical illness, by pain or distress such as that caused by autonomic stimulation from a distended bladder or rectum, or it may result as an adverse effect of prescribed or non-prescribed drugs.

When the precipitating cause is identified and removed, former mental function and activity may be restored. If, however, the cause is not identified, the patient may be admitted inappropriately to hospital or to a long-term care facility. Psychoactive drugs administered to control the behavioral manifestations of an acute confusional state may simply mask symptoms, and an acute and potentially reversible ADR may, if unrecognized, lead to unnecessary permanent institutional care.

DRUG-INDUCED ACUTE BRAIN FAILURE

Sudden change in cognitive function or behavior in older patients may result from adverse reactions to a number of drugs. Most drug-induced delirium seen in geriatric practice is caused by cardiac glycosides, antiparkinsonian and antidepressant drugs, hypoglycemic agents, anti-inflammatory drugs, and analgesics.

Digitalis toxicity causes signs and symptoms in the elderly which may differ from those found in the young. The elderly brain appears to be more sensitive to serum levels of digoxin just above therapeutic levels and changes in mood and cognitive function may occur when the serum digoxin level is within the therapeutic range. Whereas the younger individual with digitalis toxicity more commonly develops gastrointestinal symptoms and cardiac dysrhythmias, the older person develops fatigue, anorexia and malaise, visual complaints such as blurring of vision and xanthopsia (yellow vision) and psychiatric symptoms such as confusion, depression and hallucinations.

Central nervous system drugs such as the barbiturates, antiparkinsonian drugs, antidepressants, and anticholinergics are commonly implicated in drug-induced confusion. Whereas most hypnotics in excess produce excessive sedation, a paradoxical reaction consisting of excitement, arousal and insomnia may result when barbiturates are given to old people. Because of the risk of addiction, the potential for abuse in suicide attempts and the occurrence of paradoxical excitation, barbiturates have no place in modern therapeutics in the elderly. A possible exception is their occasional use in the management of seizure disorders especially for patients who have received barbiturates for many years. In any case barbiturates should be withdrawn cautiously since withdrawal symptoms and seizures are likely following their abrupt discontinuation.

Acute confusion is more likely to occur in the older individual who is already suffering from dementia or who has previously experienced an acute confusional state. Drugs with anticholinergic activity, such as the antidepressants, anticholinergic and antiparkinsonian agents, antispasmodic drugs and, to a lesser extent, the phenothiazines may all lead to delirium by central anticholinergic action. It is unusual for central anticholinergic toxicity to develop when a modest dose of one drug with anticholinergic properties is administered. However, concurrent administration of two or more drugs with anticholinergic properties, such as an antidepressant, a phenothiazine and an antiparkinsonian agent, may lead to confusion, agitation and disturbed behavior. In mild cases all that may be required is to discontinue the offending drug(s); in more severe cases cautious parenteral administration of the physostigmine, a tertiary amine which is able to cross the blood–brain barrier, reverses the syndrome (Granacher & Baldessarini 1975).

Drugs used in the management of parkinsonism may cause confusional states. This applies not only to the anticholinergic agents such as benzotropine (Cogentin) and trihexyphenidyl (Artane) but also to amantadine, levodopa and bromocriptine. Since judicious use of these agents may make an enormous improvement in the function of the older patient with parkinsonism, therapy must be started cautiously. The initial dose should be low and careful observation should be made following each increment in dosage.

Acute confusion may result from hypoglycemia, occurring either spontaneously or induced by insulin or oral antidiabetic agents. Changes in neurologic or psychiatric state may range from headache and visual disturbance through paranoia and aggressive behavior to convulsions and coma. In order to avoid hypoglycemia, oral hypoglycemics should not be used concurrently with drugs which displace them from protein-binding sites (see Chapter 4) and long-acting oral agents such as chlorpropamide, which has a biological half life of around 36 hours, should be avoided.

Case Study 1

Mrs W.L., a 73-year-old married woman, took an annual winter vacation in Florida with her husband. She was in good health and was receiving no long-term drug therapy. While on vacation she visited a physician for a 'check-up' and was found to have slightly elevated blood glucose levels. Chlorpropamide was prescribed.

Within a week Mr L. noticed that his wife's behavior had changed. She withdrew from social contacts, became suspicious, hostile and verbally abusive. After a visit to an Emergency Department where haloperidol was prescribed, Mr L. was able to convince his wife to return to Canada, where she was admitted to a psychogeriatric unit.

Laboratory investigations showed hypoglycemia. Chlorpropamide was stopped and within a few days the tranquilizers were discontinued. Within a few weeks she had returned to her normal mental state and was discharged to her home.

DRUG-INDUCED CHRONIC BRAIN FAILURE (DEMENTIA)

Dementia is a syndrome characterized by loss of intellectual abilities of sufficient severity to interfere with social or occupational functioning. The syndrome comprises memory impairment and impairment in abstract thinking, higher cortical function and judgment without clouding of consciousness. This descriptive definition of the dementia syndrome does not imply progressiveness or irreversibility. However, some authors use the term dementia to imply a chronic and usually progressive condition when investigations have excluded reversible causes of impaired cerebral function. While it is true that the majority of elderly patients presenting with this syndrome will be found to have a primary cerebral degenerative disorder, usually senile dementia of the Alzheimer type, the adverse effects of drugs may simulate Alzheimer's disease.

Any drug with sedative properties may produce a 'hangover effect' on the day following administration. The increased sensitivity of the aging brain to drugs such as nitrazepam was discussed in Chapter 4. Hypnotics and tranquilizers which are slowly excreted tend to accumulate producing drowsiness, disorientation, confusion and inappropriate behavior. Over-the-counter hypnotic preparations containing antihistamines may cause confusion both as a result of sedation and anticholinergic effects.

Case Study 2 describes the development of benzodiazepine-induced confusion and locomotor impairment in an 86-year-old man.

Case Study 2

Mr N.G., an 86-year-old retired farmer, was in good health and lived with his wife in an apartment. He underwent prostatic surgery and developed an acute confusional state which resolved with mild residual memory impairment.

One year later, 30 mg of flurazepam was prescribed at bedtime for insomnia. A few days later he became unsteady on his feet and fell, lacerating his face. A week or so later he was incontinent of urine, incapable of caring for himself and became a management problem for his family. The degree of impairment of mental capacity was such that legal advice was sought regarding the management of his estate.

He continued to take flurazepam each night. However, he spent most nights awake, wandering aimlessly and unsteadily around his apartment, and occasionally insisting on leaving during the night. Since his wife was no longer able to cope with his care he was admitted to hospital.

Flurazepam was stopped and a small dose of thioridazine was prescribed to manage nocturnal agitation. Within one week his gait was stable, he was continent of urine and although the memory deficit persisted, his behavior was once again appropriate and manageable at home.

Adverse effects of central nervous system drugs are seen more commonly in the elderly who already exhibit mild cognitive impairment. In Case Study

2 a patient with mild, but manageable, dementia experienced more profound intellectual change and behavior disturbance as a result of adverse effects of flurazepam. Despite their unsuitability as hypnotics or tranquilizers in the elderly, long-acting benzodiazepines such as diazepam and flurazepam are widely prescribed. When a decline in mental function occurs in an older individual with or without underlying memory impairment the possibility of adverse effects of prescribed or over-the-counter CNS depressants must be considered.

DRUG-INDUCED LOCOMOTOR IMPAIRMENT

Postural instability and falls commonly result in morbidity and mortality in the aged. Even when they do not result in physical injury, falls, or the fear of falling, may lead to restriction of activity at home and may induce an old person or his family to seek admission to long-term care. Age-related changes in afferent sensory input, in central processing of proprioceptive information and in the musculoskeletal system render the aged more susceptible to falls although the adverse effects of drugs or disease usually precipitate the fall. Drugs may have their effect through direct toxic effect on peripheral nerves as is the case with hydralazine, phenytoin and isoniazid. More commonly falls are caused by drugs which alter consciousness or which lead to dizziness and orthostatic (postural) hypotension.

All hypnotic and sedative drugs may impair locomotor function by impairing consciousness, while benzodiazepine drugs appear to have an effect on balance and gait independent of their sedative effect. Ataxia, unsteadiness and falls as a result of flurazepam were described in Case Study 2. Aminoglycoside antibiotics and phenytoin impair balance by their effect on the labyrinth; acetylsalicylic acid, indomethacin and many of the nonsteroidal anti-inflammatory drugs may produce lightheadedness. Drugs may lead to syncope or to symptomatic orthostatic hypotension, they include drugs predisposing to cardiac dysrhythmias, such as β-agonists and theophylline, and drugs predisposing to orthostatic hypertension. The tricyclic antidepressants, L-dopa and other drugs may predispose to syncope by either of these mechanisms.

In practice, diuretics and antihypertensives are commonly implicated in iatrogenic locomotor impairment and falls. Diuretics are commonly prescribed for the elderly; appropriately for congestive heart failure and hypertension, and inappropriately for isolated dependent edema. Dependent edema often has a local cause and administration of a diuretic to a normovolemic patient results in dehydration, reduced intravascular volume and orthostatic hypotension. Metabolic effects of diuretics include hyperuricemia glucose intolerance and hypokalemia. Hypokalemia, if severe, may cause muscle weakness which increases further the risk of falling.

Rapidly acting 'loop diuretics' may result in orthostatic hypotension since cardiovascular reflexes are unable to compensate for the brisk diuresis. Urinary continence may be compromised by rapid diuresis and both incontinence and a fall may occur when an older patient with an unstable bladder hurries to the bathroom in an effort to maintain continence. Despite these important considerations which make rapidly acting diuretics unsuitable for long-term therapy, they are widely prescribed. Skoll *et al.* (1979) showed that persons aged 65 and over were 8 times as likely, and persons aged 85 and over, 20 times as likely to receive a prescription for frusemide as the middle-aged.

The indications for treatment of hypertension in the older patient are controversial and will not be discussed in detail. Injudicious prescription of antihypertensive agents, particularly to the very elderly produce symptomatic orthostatic hypotension which may result in falls, fractures and even death. Since hypertension is generally an asymptomatic condition and treatment is intended to prevent mortality and morbidity from cardiac, renal and cerebrovascular complications, the physician must weigh these expected benefits of treatment against the risks which have been described. The physician has limited experimental data to assist him in making a risk-benefit decision regarding treatment of hypertension in an elderly individual. While awaiting the results of prospective controlled trials of the treatment of hypertension in the elderly it is probably reasonable to treat diastolic hypertension similarly in the young and old. The prescriber must be familiar with the adverse effects commonly encountered in the elderly and should monitor patients carefully. When adverse effects occur it may be necessary to revise therapeutic goals as well as changing treatment.

DRUG-INDUCED DEPENDENCE FOR ACTIVITIES OF DAILY LIVING (ADL)

Modern geriatric care seeks to maintain and improve older persons' capacity for self-care. Many of the drugs which affect behavior and locomotion also affect self-care skills. Sedatives, by producing drowsiness and muscle weakness, may impair concentration and performance of ADL; phenothiazine-induced parkinsonism, akathesia and tardive dyskinesia may impair the motor skills required for self-care, and diuretics may render an individual incontinent. A number of drugs have adverse effects on the special senses: salicylates and ethacrynic acid produce hearing impairment; indomethacin and antitubercular drugs impair color vision and phenothiazines impair vision in dim lighting.

When an older person can no longer perform unaided the activities required for everyday living he becomes dependent upon another person or agency. The loss of self-care skills may result from disease or from adverse effects of drugs. Case Study 3 illustrates how a disabled older patient became unnecessarily dependent as a result of inappropriate drug therapy and how withdrawal of the offending drugs permitted return of self-care skills.

Case Study 3

Dr E.S., an 84-year-old retired physician, lived in an apartment with his 79-year-old wife who was a registered nurse. He had severe visual impairment due to macular degeneration and his left leg had been amputated above the knee as a result of an arterial embolus which followed a myocardial infarction. In order to relieve postoperative pain in the stump his wife administered merperidine (Demerol) 75 mg intramuscularly and Tuinal 100–200 mg orally each evening. He was totally dependent upon his wife and upon his former office nurse for 24-hour care, so when his wife was admitted to hospital for investigation of dysphagia and weight loss, Dr S. was also admitted to hospital.

During a six week hospital stay both merperidine (Demerol) and Tuinal were withdrawn. He became less dependent upon nursing staff, was soon able to participate in his self-care by washing and grooming himself and was able to transfer without assistance but with supervision. He was discharged home functionally improved but six months later when his wife was admitted to hospital for palliative care of carcinoma of the esophagus, Dr S. was admitted to a long-term care facility where he died two months later.

SUMMARY

This chapter opened with Oliver Wendell Holmes' view of the value of pharmacological treatments in ameliorating man's disease and distress. Since then many efficacious treatments for infection, central nervous system and cardiovascular system disorders have been developed and may be used with benefit in young and old alike. Since the elderly have so much to gain from appropriate drug therapy and so much to lose from inappropriate therapy or the adverse effects of drugs, the prescribing physician, armed with knowledge of altered drug handling and altered drug response in the aged, must weigh the anticipated benefits against the potential risks before prescribing any drug. In making a decision regarding drug therapy, the physician must consider the possible interactions between the drug to be prescribed and drugs already used by the patient (including non-prescribed drugs) as well as the interaction between the drug and active disease processes which are present in the patient. When drug therapy is indicated, the guidelines suggested in Table 5.4 may be helpful in reducing the possibility of adverse drug reaction.

Table 5.4 Guidelines for therapeutics in old age.

In general, use smaller doses of drugs than for younger adults
Set therapeutic goal and discontinue drug (if possible) when goal achieved
Simplify dosage schedule
Minimize concurrent therapy
Provide simple written instructions
Dispense in accessible containers
Monitor drug compliance
When appropriate, supervise drug taking

REFERENCES AND FURTHER READING

American Psychiatric Association, Task Force on Nomenclature and Statistics (1980) *Diagnostic and statistical manual of mental disorders.* (DSM III) 3rd edition, p. 107. American Psychiatric Association, Washington DC.

Criep L.H. (1982) Adverse reactions to drugs. In Conn H.F. (Ed.) *Current Therapy.* W.B. Saunders & Co., Philadelphia.

Friesen A.J.D. (1983) Adverse drug reactions in the geriatric client. In Pagliaro L.A. & Pagliaro A.M. (Eds.) *Pharmacologic Aspects of Aging.* C.V. Mosby Co., St Louis, Missouri.

Granacher R.P. & Baldessarini R.J. (1975) Physiostigmine. *Archives of general Psychiatry* **32**, 375–80.

Greenblatt D.J., Allen M.D. & Shader R.I. (1977) Toxicity of high dose flurazepam in the elderly. *Clinical Pharmacology and Therapeutics* **21**, 355.

Hurwitz N. (1969) Predisposing factors in adverse reactions to drugs. *British medical Journal* **1**, 536–9.

Medical Letter (1981) Adverse interactions of drugs. *Medical Letter on Drugs and Therapeutics* **23**, 17–28.

Skoll S.L., August R.J. & Johnson G.E. (1979) Drug prescribing in the elderly in Saskatchewan during 1976. *Canadian medical Association Journal* **121**, 1074–81.

Chapter Six
Cardiovascular System—
Digitalis Glycosides

M. D. W. LYE

OVERVIEW

The importance of treatable heart disease especially chronic cardiac failure in the elderly is emphasized. Physiological age changes in the cardiovascular system are contrasted with age-related cardiac pathology and the clinical importance of this differentiation of cardiac failure discussed. The difficulties of diagnosis of cardiac failure are discussed in detail. Due emphasis is given to the problem of misdiagnosis in cardiac disease.

The general management of chronic heart failure is detailed in relation to the underlying physiological compensatory factors and how these factors differ in elderly patients. The use and abuse of digoxin therapy is discussed with a description of its clinical value and limitations in the elderly patient.

EPIDEMIOLOGY

The demographic changes occurring in the UK and in other developed nations lead to increasing numbers of old people (see Chapter 1). It is worth stressing in the context of cardiovascular problems that the majority of cardiovascular diseases are age-related. Thus, the more elderly people in the population the more cardiovascular disease will be seen.

Every year nearly three-quarters of a million Americans over the age of 65 years will die of some form of cardiovascular disease and of these 75% will die of disease primarily affecting the heart. Altogether heart disease will cause 50% of all deaths in this age group.

As well as causing death in old age, heart disease leads to much morbidity which may not present to doctors until a late stage after many months or even years of disability.

AGING IN THE CARDIOVASCULAR SYSTEM

Because of the ubiquitous nature of arteriosclerosis in old age it may be difficult to differentiate the cardiovascular manifestations of universal aging from the highly age-related disease state. However, in spite of these interactions some general trends in physiological function must be recalled before instituting any cardio-active therapy in elderly patients.

In the resting state there is a significant decrease in the cardiac output with increasing age even in subjects with little or no evidence of arteriosclerosis. This reduction is in the main brought about by a smaller stroke volume. The overall reduction in output follows the reduced metabolic needs of the smaller lean body mass of the old person. Coronary arteriosclerosis, degenerative changes in the sinus node and increases in vascular rigidity leading to higher cardiac afterload, all contribute to age-related decline in cardiac performance. The reduced resting cardiac output has disproportionate effects upon the distribution of regional blood flow. Thus, that fraction of cardiac output distributed to muscles and kidneys falls to a greater extent than the fraction reserved for the heart and brain.

Histological myocardial changes include 'brown atrophy', lipofuscin and amyloid accumulation and an increase in fibrotic scarring. Some of these changes may not be true manifestations of biological aging; for example, scarring may be a consequence of previous virus infection (diphtheria) and amyloid deposition may have an immunological basis.

Increasing rigidity and decreasing elasticity of the major blood vessels, especially the aorta, with increasing age, are well documented. A more rigid vascular tree leads to an increase in systolic pressure, a widening of the pulse pressure and an increase in myocardial work required to eject the stroke volume. Increasing fibrosis, often leading to calcification of the cardiac valves, commonly occurs in the left side of the heart. The aortic valve is more readily affected than the mitral valve. Valvular changes lead to the common aortic and mitral murmurs found in otherwise healthy elderly subjects.

While at rest the healthy elderly person's cardiovascular system is not stressed. Unfortunately, physiological aging causes a reduction in cardiac reserve capacity. Thus, during exercise, pneumonia, surgery, etc., cardiac output cannot be sufficiently increased to match the increasing demand. Hence, the old person's overall cardiovascular equilibrium is more profoundly disturbed than in a young subject, equally stressed.

CARDIAC DISEASE IN OLD AGE

In old age, coronary arteriosclerosis leading to ischaemic heart disease is by far the most common cardiovascular problem. Community surveys have shown that approximately 20% of men and 12% of women over the age of 75 living at home have significant symptomatic ischaemic heart disease. In the majority of these people the problem will be of mild or moderate cardiac failure. Ischaemic heart disease manifests more commonly as myocardial infarction in people below the age of 65 years and as cardiac failure in those above 65 years—a phenomenon that warrants further study. Much ischaemic heart disease in the elderly is not reported to family physicians and these prevalence figures may well be underestimates.

Modern medical treatment and developments in cardiothoracic surgery mean that more people with valvular heart disease are surviving into old age. It is at this time that the decrease in cardiac output and decline in reserve capacity may bring about quite sudden cardiac decompensation leading to symptomatic expression of the condition. However, the sole occurrence of valvular calcification in old people may be a 'non-disease state' and over reliance should not be placed upon the finding of a single murmur in an otherwise healthy, elderly individual.

Diagnosis

Elderly people have, on the whole, low expectations and often attribute symptoms and significant disability to an inevitable aging process. This problem is compounded in the field of cardiovascular disease by the atypical manifestations of many cardiac states; for example, cardiac failure may present as confusion or extreme lethargy with no complaint of dyspnoea. Myocardial infarction is rarely manifest as crushing chest pain with its typical radiation. Indeed, it is often silent in the elderly. Oedema is often a sign of immobility.

The differential diagnosis of dyspnoea in the elderly often presents particular difficulty. Accurate differentiation of a cardiac from a respiratory aetiology demands a full clinical assessment—no easy task in a confused old man. A good history, possibly obtained from a relative or friend of the patient, is invaluable. Cardiac and pulmonary causes of breathlessness may coexist. Detailed and perhaps invasive methods of investigation of the patient at rest and during exercise are warranted if the possibility of a positive therapeutic intervention exists.

The diagnosis of acute left ventricular failure usually presents little difficulty in the elderly. Thus, dyspnoea, orthopnoea and paroxysmal nocturnal dyspnoea associated with tachycardia, pulmonary râles and a gallop rhythm point to the correct diagnosis. Biventricular (congestive) cardiac failure and chronic left ventricular failure may have many of these features but often in the elderly they tend to be much less dramatic and may indeed be on occasions entirely absent. Commonly the complaint is of weakness, lethargy or the patient 'just takes to his bed'.

The presence of peripheral pitting oedema in an old person is not an unfailing sign of fluid retention. The most common cause of dependent oedema in the elderly is immobility secondary to arthritis or central nervous system disease. Equally, the monitoring of oedema in an individual with cardiac failure whilst relatively immobilized in a hospital chair is of little practical benefit. Far better to weigh the patient.

In the elderly because of their lower cardiac output, overt failure may be produced by stress brought about by a non-cardiac cause. Respiratory infections in old people are a common cause of cardiac decompensation and resolution of the underlying infection leads to prompt resolution of the cardiac failure. Cardiac failure resistant to conventional treatment may be due to anaemia, thyrotoxicosis, bacterial endocarditis or, on rare occasions, Paget's disease.

Fluid retention from a renal lesion should also be considered but it must be remembered that the blood urea rises relatively rapidly in cardiac failure due to a decrease in renal perfusion; this combined with the nephron loss brought about by aging, may lead to excessive nitrogen retention. Adequate treatment of the cardiac failure invariably induces a prompt fall in blood urea to normal or near normal levels.

Management

Osler suggested 'once in heart failure, always in heart failure'. Hence the logical conclusion has been that treatment of heart failure should be lifelong. This concept is being increasingly questioned and therefore anti-heart-failure drugs, like all other drugs used in the treatment of the elderly, should be subject to regular review with the aim of eventual withdrawal or at least dosage reduction.

Equally important, it is necessary to be gentle with powerful drugs. No physician who has taken frusemide would give the drug without prior thought to an old man with prostatism or an old woman immobilized by arthritis.

Drugs may not be the most important therapeutic tools in the treatment of heart disease in old age. Consideration must be given to the choice of home or hospital, ordinary ward or coronary care unit, etc. Many senior physicians are themselves somewhat tremulous on approaching a modern intensive therapy unit, so spare a thought for the poor frightened patient. Often old people do remarkably well in familiar and, to some physicians, perhaps less desirable environments. This social factor should not be overlooked.

Provision of neighbourhood support to help with shopping may be more expeditious than squeezing the last drop of fluid or the last millimol of sodium out of a patient with high dose diuretics. Salt restriction or limitation is easily instituted in nursing homes as well as in the patient's own home. Allowing patients to sleep in chairs at night may be all that is needed to prevent paroxysmal dyspnoea in an otherwise well-controlled elderly patient with chronic cardiac failure.

The use of bed rest in the treatment of elderly patients with cardiac failure represents the utilization of a powerful but potentially toxic drug. Pressure sores, constipation and orthostatic pneumonia are some of its hazards. Its use should be limited, monitored and surrounded by much circumspection. Bed rest is so dangerous that it should be reserved only for very severely disabled cardiac patients with resistant failure. The judicious employment of modern diuretics makes this situation much rarer than it was in the past.

CARDIAC GLYCOSIDES

In one form or another the various cardiac glycosides have been known and used for therapy over the past 2000 years. In spite of this long and honourable history the place of the cardiac glycosides in the treatment of heart failure still arouses intense controversy. William Withering published the first clinical report of the efficacy of the Foxglove in dropsy though he maintained that its main action was on the kidney as a diuretic. He cautioned that the drug should be used properly and herein lies the problem. The cardiac glycosides are potent but dangerous drugs because the ideal therapeutic level is approximately 60% of the toxic level—a very precarious margin for safety. In the elderly this slim margin is probably further reduced.

Most pharmacopoeias list more than 20 digitalis preparations of cardiac glycosides derived from many natural sources. The differences between these compounds relate only to pharmacokinetic properties and their actions or presumed mechanisms of action are all essentially identical. For the purpose of this review the generic term digitalis will be used to encompass all types of cardiac glycosides and will not specifically relate to digitalis folia or prepared digitalis leaf.

Mechanism of action

Digitalis has a direct effect on the membrane of cardiac cells. It now seems apparent that digitalis directly inhibits Na, K-ATPase which acts as a specific receptor site for the drug. Membrane Na, K-ATPase is the energy source for the 'sodium pump', inhibition of which will allow sodium to diffuse into the cell and potassium to diffuse out. This finding has now been confirmed by direct intracellular ionic measurements.

Interestingly, it seems that the toxic effects of digitalis occur in situations where this process is overdone, suggesting a narrow band of efficiency at cellular level which is reflected by the clinically observed small therapeutic: toxic ratio.

Recent evidence suggests that it is not the efflux of potassium nor the influx of sodium *per se* which affects myocardial contractility but that these changes facilitate the intracellular influx of calcium and it is these ions which directly influence the formation of actin-myosin complex, giving rise to myocardial contraction.

Further elucidation of the mechanism of action of digitalis at cellular level is required to afford a rational explanation of the effects of systemic hypo- and hyper-kalaemia and the potentiating effects of hypercalcaemia upon digitalis toxicity.

Pharmacological effects

The effect of digitalis upon the function of the heart is twofold; action upon individual myocardial muscle fibres and action upon the myocardial conducting system. These two effects may be designated inotropic and chronotropic actions, respectively. Obviously, these two actions may overlap but in a theoretical physiological or clinical discussion they can be considered as being separate entities.

Inotropic actions

By its action on cell membrane digitalis facilitates contraction and increases the force of contraction of individual myocardial muscle cells. This has been demonstrated many times using isolated animal heart tissue (especially papillary muscle), in intact animal and human specimens and also in failing human hearts. Such experiments finally buried the idea, prevalent from the turn of this century, that the benefits of digitalis were solely due to a slowing of heart rate.

Digitalis increases the contractility of the heart whatever the condition but the increase is greater, the less the initial contractility. As the heart fails, the Frank–Starling mechanism initially compensates for the primary myocardial weakness by increasing contractility with increasing 'stretching' of myocardial fibres brought about by failure to empty the ventricle at the end of cardiac systole. This mechanism is obviously limited. Digitalis, by increasing contractility, alters the relationship between output and the end-diastolic pressure in such a manner that the heart functions on a different and more effective Frank–Starling relationship.

Thus, the 'effective efficiency', as measured by cardiac output for example, increases with no further increase in end-diastolic pressure. Indeed, most experiments show that the end-diastolic pressure actually falls to more normal values with digitalis whilst maintaining overall an improved cardiac output.

Additionally the increase in output produced by digitalis in the failing heart is not at the cost of an increased utilization of energy. Thus, myocardial oxygen consumption does not increase and may even decrease with digitalis—an important factor in coronary artery disease where oxygen delivery may be precarious.

Chronotropic actions

The action of digitalis upon cardiac conduction and myocardial electrical activity is complex, involving both direct cardiac effects and indirect reflex responses via the autonomic nervous system. A further chronotropic action in heart failure (slowing of heart rate) may be purely secondary to the inotropic action of digitalis. The main 'electrical' actions of digitalis on the heart can be considered in three main areas (other effects occur but they are of little physiological moment).

Automaticity. Digitalis in low or moderate doses decreases the automaticity of individual atrial fibres. In high or toxic dose levels this effect is reversed and atrial automaticity may be increased leading to supraventricular ectopic activity. However, even in moderate dosage digitalis increases the automaticity of ventricular tissue (Purkinje fibres) so that ventricular ectopic activity is not uncommon. If this occurs where the rhythm is basically regular (sinus or controlled atrial fibrillation), pulsus bigeminus is especially likely.

Effective refractory period. Digitalis prolongs the refractory period of Purkinje fibres and fibres of the atrioventricular (A-V) node. This is, in part, a direct action of digitalis on the A-V node and in part mediated by the vagus nerve. Again, the effect on the ventricular refractory period is in the other direction. A shortened ventricular refractory period may be measured on the ECG as prolongation of the $Q\text{-}T_c$ interval.

Conduction velocity. The speed of impulse propagation through the A-V node and Purkinje fibres is significantly prolonged by digitalis. This action is manifest on the ECG as prolongation of the P-R interval. For this reason digitalis should not be administered without suitable precautions to patients with any degree of heart block.

Toxic effects

Allergic reactions to digitalis are extremely uncommon considering the extensive prescribing of the drug. Urticaria does occasionally occur and may be associated with fever and malaise. Eosinophilia, with or without asthma, has been reported in allergic individuals. There is, however, no evidence that asthmatic subjects are more likely to be allergic to digitalis than others. It seems that allergy to digitalis is purely idiosyncratic.

Toxic manifestations of digitalis therapy are variably related to overdosage. It has been shown in animal studies that the lethal dose is only twice the dose that produces the earliest toxic signs and may be only five times higher than the minimum therapeutic dose. Little wonder then that between 10 and 20% of patients taking digitalis on a long-term basis exhibit toxic signs and symptoms.

The most important factor leading to intoxication is impairment of renal clearance of the drug. This is a particular problem in the elderly because of the age-related nephron loss discussed previously. The pharmacokinetics of digitalis have been reviewed in Chapter 4. There is no evidence of varying toxicity with the different preparations of digitalis, so claims that one product is safer than another product are unsubstantiated. The individual patient and his physician are the final determinants of toxicity (see Table 6.1).

Table 6.1 Factors predisposing to digitalis toxicity.

Old age
Impaired renal function
Reduced lean body mass
Hypokalaemia (diuretics)
Hypercalcaemia
Hypomagnesaemia (diuretics)
Chronic pulmonary disease (anoxia/acidosis)
Myocardial infarction
Hypothyroidism

Clinical use of digitalis

Digitalis preparations are the fourth most commonly prescribed group of drugs in Europe and the United States of America. Approximately one in five persons taking regular digitalis will be suffering some toxic side-effects. It is, therefore, necessary to examine the clinical as opposed to the physiological effects of digitalis in a critical manner.

Numerous experiments involving both animal cardiac tissue and human physiological studies *in vivo* demonstrate that digitalis can improve the contractility of the failing heart. As far as one can determine, this inotropic action is not at the expense of an increased myocardial oxygen consumption. Obviously, if this were the whole truth digitalis should be an almost perfect drug for the failing heart. As we have seen, however, this is not the whole truth and we must consider the role of digitalis as it works in the clinical situation.

Inotropic action

Digitalis exerts a positive, beneficial inotropic action in the short-term treatment of a failing heart. Is this benefit maintained?

Recent studies have been conflicting. Withdrawal of long-term digitalis treatment from patients with chronic heart failure has shown that the majority of such patients do not deteriorate clinically. Unfortunately, patients with sinus rhythm and patients with atrial fibrillation have not always been differentiated. A strong impression remains that it is patients with atrial fibrillation and other tachyarrhythmias in addition to their heart failure who deteriorate when digitalis is withdrawn.

The situation is further complicated by the recent development of potent oral diuretic agents. With these agents, properly administered, it is possible to 'dry out' patients with cardiac failure and indeed this procedure itself will improve cardiac performance. This factor alone should reduce the necessity for digitalis.

Between 1970 and 1972 the method of manufacture of standard Lanoxin tablets was changed by the manufacturers, resulting in a halving of therapeutic potency. This led to the recognition of the digoxin bioavailability problem. Interesting, however, is the fact that in the clinical situation no great change was noted at the time by physicians.

It will therefore be concluded that digitalis, because of its lack of proven long-term benefit and its high level of toxicity, especially in the elderly, can no longer be recommended for the treatment of elderly patients with heart failure and sinus rhythm. The drug should be restricted to the acute situation and even here with the advent of powerful diuretics it is not often required. It is believed that digitalis should be reserved for the treatment of rhythm disorders in old people with or without heart failure.

Chronotropic action

Atrial fibrillation remains the classical indication for digitalis. Approximately 5% of elderly persons have atrial fibrillation with or without other evidence of cardiac disease. Not all these patients will in fact require digitalis as atrial fibrillation in the elderly is often associated with a slower ventricular response than in younger people and hence no further slowing is required.

Patients with fibrillation and pulse rates above 85 beats per minute at rest will benefit from slowing. The aim should be to reduce the ventricular rate to between 70 and 80 beats per minute. If the expected slowing is not obtained with adequate digitalization, the arrhythmia should be considered as being secondary (see Table 6.2). Increasingly, patients with moderate or mild mitral stenosis are reaching old age and these patients may develop decompensation with the onset of atrial fibrillation. They respond well to digitalis.

The treatment of choice for atrial flutter is DC cardioversion but unfortunately many elderly patients have contraindications to cardioversion. In this situation digitalis may slow the flutter or even convert it to the more

Table 6.2 Atrial fibrillation refractory to digitalis.

Thyrotoxicosis
Infection especially with fever
Uncontrolled heart failure
Hypocalcaemia
Amyloid disease
Anaemia
Paget's disease
Recurrent pulmonary emboli
Impaired absorption (laxative)
Endocarditis
Myocarditis

manageable atrial fibrillation. Often large doses of digitalis are required so the institution of such therapy should be carefully controlled and monitored and not embarked upon lightly. Expert advice should be sought.

Digitalis in other arrhythmias is less satisfactory and, indeed, may be potentially dangerous; for example, in the Wolff–Parkinson–White syndrome or sick sinus syndrome. In the latter situation, which is not uncommon in the elderly, pacemaker implantation may allow subsequent suppression of tachyarrhythmias by digitalis.

Digitalis dosage regimens

Bioavailability. In the early 1970s it became apparent that different brands and different batches of the same brand of digitalis preparations could lead to a sevenfold difference in plasma level with the same tablet size given to the same patient.

Since 1975 the drug authorities in the UK and the USA have brought in regulations to standardize digoxin bioavailability. Fortunately, it has been found that a simple dissolution test *in vitro* can be used but the United States Pharmacopoeia and British Pharmacopoeia standards differ slightly. Thus, at one hour the USP requires a minimum mean dissolution rate of 65% whilst the BP requires 75% or more in the same period. Difficulties could arise with transatlantic travel. In spite of these statutory precautions it still seems wise to confine individual patients to the same brand of digitalis preparation throughout a period of therapy (see Table 6.3).

Oral. It is imperative to keep in mind the extreme variability of responses between individuals. The dosage schedules to be outlined do not remove the physician's responsibility to consider his patient as an individual who, if elderly, is more likely than most to 'break the rules'.

Table 6.3 Examples of different digitalis preparations referred to in the text.

Digoxin
Digitalis
Lanoxin
Ouabain
Medigoxin (Lanitop)
Lanatoside-C

In the past much emphasis has been placed upon the need for an initial or digitalizing dose. In the majority of cases this is unnecessarily dangerous. Equally, parenteral administration has been overemployed. Intramuscular injections cause severe local trauma, the rate of absorption following intramuscular injection is extremely variable and probably no faster than via the oral route. Intravenous administration should be reserved for life-threatening conditions such as acute pulmonary oedema associated with rapid atrial fibrillation. Powerful, rapidly acting diuretics have considerably reduced the frequency of intravenous digitalis administration.

Table 6.4 details certain pharmacokinetic data relating to 3 commonly used oral digitalis preparations. Several aspects are worth noting. First, the time to achieve peak plasma level after a single oral dose of digitoxin and digoxin is relatively short. Intravenous administration, whilst achieving peak plasma levels much more quickly than oral administration, does not make very much practical difference. Second, the extremely long half-life of all agents, but especially digitoxin, means that elimination after cessation of therapy will be prolonged also. Third, the high value of plasma protein binding of digitoxin may lead to large amounts of potentially toxic unbound

Table 6.4 Characteristics and dosage recommendations of some commonly used oral digitalis preparations in elderly patients.

	Digitoxin	Digoxin	Lantoside-C
Peak effect (min)	45	45–75	60–120
Half-life plasma (h)	192	36	33
Plasma binding (%)	97	23	25
Maintenance dose (mg)	0.005–0.150	0.0625–0.5	0.25–0.5
Tablet sizes (mg)	0.005	0.0625	0.25
	0.010	0.125	
	0.015	0.25	
	0.200		

drug activity in the plasma when the serum proteins are reduced. This is especially likely to be the case in elderly patients with chronic heart failure (cardiac cachexia).

The individual dosage recommendations are guidelines only and the physician must titrate individual response and dosage in the light of objectives he hopes to achieve; for example, to reduce the ventricular rate in atrial fibrillation to below 80 beats per minute. If the physician has no objective criteria by which he can monitor response he should critically question whether to use digitalis at all. The practice of pushing digitalis until toxic effects are produced and then reducing the dosage a little should be condemned. Unfortunately, the first toxic effect may be fatal.

Approximately 30% of digitoxin, 95% of digoxin and 90% of lantoside-C are excreted by the kidney. Thus, the state of the kidneys is crucially important in determining the dosage requirement. A number of simple formulae have been used to predict maintenance requirements. Most studies have examined digoxin elimination but other factors may be important. A useful formula for elderly patients incorporates serum albumin as well as creatinine clearance as a predictive variable.

$$\text{Daily dose } (\mu g) = 3.45\ Cl_{cr} + 2.7 \text{ albumin (mg/100 ml)}$$

(Dobbs *et al.* 1976)

Experience suggests that this particular formula is readily applicable to the elderly patient with cardiac failure.

Examination of Table 6.4 demonstrates that digoxin is the oral digitalis preparation of choice for use in the elderly. Thus, digoxin is quickly effective, does not have an unduly prolonged half-life, is poorly protein bound and has a suitable range of tablet sizes. A dose of 0.1875 mg daily (one 0.0625 mg and one 0.125 mg tablet) is particularly useful in clinical geriatric practice.

Intravenous therapy. Decreasing use of intravenously administered digitalis preparations have been noticeable over the last decade. The development and increasing use of powerful, rapidly acting diuretics, vasodilators and alternative inotropic agents have contributed to less reliance being placed upon intravenously administered digitalis. Occasionally, however, a very rapid action is required in an emergency.

Some average pharmacokinetic data for digitalis parenteral preparations are given in Fig. 6.1. Note that the axis is logarithmic.

If an intravenous preparation is really required, ouabain is the drug of choice. Even so this preparation may continue to affect the heart for up to 3 days after administration. Medigoxin (Lanitrop), a semi-synthetic digoxin which is highly lipid-soluble and can be administered orally or parenterally may in future be a useful alternative by virtue of its rapid onset of action (within 15 minutes of administration) and its short half-life.

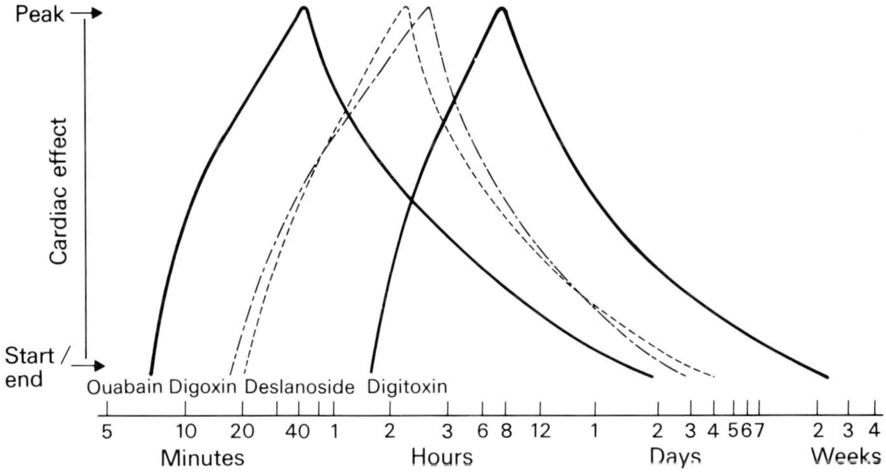

Fig. 6.1 Pharmacokinetics of intravenous digitalis preparations. Assumes normal renal function.

Clinical digitalis toxicity

Features of the patient particularly likely to develop digitalis toxicity have been listed previously (see Table 6.1). Table 6.5 describes clinical signs and symptoms of digitalis toxicity. In spite of the demonstration that digitalis is selectively concentrated in cardiac and renal tissues it should be recognized that many toxic effects relate to other organs.

Table 6.5 Clinical manifestations of digitalis intoxication.

Neurological	Lassitude/weakness Visual disturbances Headache/facial pain Depression—psychosis Dizziness Convulsions Confusion
Gastrointestinal	Anorexia Nausea } may be central Vomiting } Diarrhoea Abdominal pain Gastric stasis
Cardiac	Virtually any arrhythmia

Clinical features of intoxication

In the elderly the central nervous system is always particularly sensitive. The most common symptoms of toxicity, lassitude and general weakness are unfortunately so non-specific as to be often unrecognized by the patient or attributed to the cardiac failure by the physician. These symptoms are common in the intoxicated elderly and often progress to severe depression which may be of a psychotic or unipolar nature or indeed even progress to marked confusion. Such patients are at risk of being labelled as chronic dements.

Visual disturbances are not commonly recognized in the elderly. Perhaps this is because of inadequate clinical examination. Xanthopsia (yellow vision) is uncommon but detailed assessment of visual fields by perimetry reveals scotomata at quite early stages of intoxication.

Case Study 1

> An elderly woman was referred for psychogeriatric assessment because she had developed moderate confusion with an obsession that her lace window curtains were dirty and required frequent washing. Detailed questioning revealed that she thought they were yellowy-green and possibly mouldy. Observation showed that they were not. Stopping the excessive digoxin made the curtains appear whiter than white and the old lady became intelligent and self-caring again.

Many of the gastrointestinal effects, which tend to be more obvious in the younger patient, are due to central mechanisms involving poisoning of the mid-brain. Nausea and vomiting in elderly patients are not as common as anorexia and diarrhoea. By its vagal action digitalis may produce severe gastric stasis in patients of all ages with chronic peptic ulceration.

Digitalis intoxication may produce any type of cardiac arrhythmia. In short-term studies it has been shown that the inotropic and arrhythmogenic properties of digitalis are independent. Thus 'pushing' digitalis may continue to increment contractile force right up to the time the patient dies of ventricular fibrillation. Similarly, cardiac and non-cardiac toxic effects may be unassociated which means that the former and more dangerous manifestations may appear quite suddenly and without any previous warning. Thus, digitalis excess may produce atrial ectopic activity often associated with decreased atrio-ventricular conduction. Depression of sinoatrial node activity leads to an increasing P-R interval and the development of various degrees of heart block. Elderly patients with an underlying sick sinus syndrome are especially at risk of developing severe bradyarrhythmias in this situation.

Ventricular ectopic activity is enhanced by digitalis leading to the development of the classical manifestation of intoxication—pulsus bigeminus. Ventricular tachycardias are especially serious because they frequently herald the onset of ventricular fibrillation.

Management of intoxication

Correct diagnosis is of prime importance. Any patient taking digitalis, whether or not there has been recent dosage change, who subsequently develops any of the signs or symptoms listed in Table 6.5 should be assumed to be intoxicated with the drug until proved otherwise. In Table 6.1 (see p. 78) the features likely to be associated with the development of digitalis intoxication are listed but it must be emphasized that potentiating or precipitating factors may not be present in an individual.

The development of specific radioimmunoassay methods to measure plasma digoxin levels has unfortunately not been as useful as initially hoped. Plasma levels above 3.0 ng/ml are usually diagnostic of intoxication and in the elderly probably levels above 2.5 ng/ml represent intoxication. However, digitalis toxicity may be serious in some elderly individuals with much lower plasma levels. The significance of S-T depression in the ECG is less in elderly patients because of pre-existing ECG changes in most patients. No cardiac arrhythmia, including pulsus bigeminus, can be taken as conclusive proof of digitalis toxicity. The best diagnostic tool is the therapeutic trial—withdrawal of digitalis. Unfortunately, because of the long half-life of most preparations, the response takes time. Over this period the patient's ECG should be constantly monitored. Also the serum electrolytes should be measured and any degree of hypokalaemia promptly treated. Potassium administration may need to be continued for several days until lower digitalis levels have been produced.

Neither haemodialysis nor peritoneal dialysis is of any value in removing excess digitalis. Digitoxin which does undergo considerable enterohepatic recirculation may be bound in the gut with cholestyramine in an emergency.

The correction of any underlying aggravating factor (see Table 6.1) should be pursued vigorously. Elderly patients may well be hypokalaemic by virtue of diuretic usage and a poor dietary intake of the cation. In refractory cases intravenous supplementation may be needed. Care must be exercised because hyperkalaemia potentiates digitalis intoxication as well as hypokalaemia. Similarly, magnesium may be required but should only be used after correction of any hypokalaemia and the demonstration of a low serum magnesium level.

The treatment of digitalis-induced arrhythmias is difficult. Severe bradyarrhythmias may respond to frequent (2-hourly) injections of atropine but a transvenous pacemaker should be considered at an early stage. Phenytoin administered intravenously is probably the drug of choice for ventricular tachyarrhythmias induced by digitalis in the elderly. Quite large doses may be necessary. β-adrenergic blocking agents should be avoided in the elderly toxic patient because of their liability to reduce further the cardiac output and hence exacerbate cerebral perfusion. Lignocaine (lidocaine) may be a suitable alternative in cases refractory to phenytoin.

REFERENCES AND FURTHER READING

Demots H., Rahimtoola S.M., McAnultey J.H. & Porter, G.A. (1978) Effects of ouabain on coronary and systemic vascular resistance and myocardial oxygen consumption in patients without heart failure. *American Journal of Cardiology* **41,** 88–93.

Dobbs S.M., Mauwer G.E., Rogers E.M. & Woodcock B.G. (1976) Can digoxin dose requirement be predicted? *British Journal of Clinical Pharmacology* **3,** 231–7.

Flegg J.C., Gottlieb S.H. & Lahatta E.G. (1982) Is digoxin really important in the treatment of compensated heart failure? A placebo controlled crossover study in patients with sinus rhythm. *American Journal of Medicine* **73,** 244–50.

George C.F. (1983) Digitalis intoxication: A new approach to an old problem. *British medical Journal* **286,** 1533–4.

Haun W.B. (1983) Lanoxicaps—are they really worth it? *New England Journal of Medicine* **308,** 523–4.

Murray R.G., Tweddel A.C., Martin W., Pearson D., Hutton I. & Lawrie T.D.V. (1982) Evaluation of digitalis in cardiac failure. *British medical Journal* **284,** 1526–8.

Stults B.M. (1982) Digoxin use in the elderly. *Journal of the American Geriatrics Society* **30,** 158–64.

Chapter Seven
Cardiovascular System—
Diuretics

M. D. W. LYE

OVERVIEW

The intrinsic compensatory changes in fluid balance brought about by chronic cardiac failure are described in a simplified way to provide a basis for a discussion of the use of diuretic agents in this condition. The three major categories of diuretic agents (thiazides, loop and potassium sparing) are discussed and compared.

It is emphasized that the vast majority of old people with chronic cardiac failure will respond to simple low-dose therapy with a thiazide and it is unusual to have to use a more potent agent. The dangers and inconvenience of many diuretics given to old people are stressed. A special plea is made for the use of low dosage of parenterally administered loop diuretics even in acute cardiac failure.

A diuretic is any agent which increases urine production. The simplest is water itself. The osmotic agents, e.g. mannitol and glucose in moderate doses increase urine production simply by their physical presence in the glomerular filtrate. Unless used in very large doses they have no effect upon electrolyte excretion and are therefore of little use in the therapy of cardiac oedema.

The introduction of the thiazides and subsequently the high-ceiling (loop) diuretics heralded a revolution in the management of chronic fluid retention. They are effective orally, increase urine formation in a predictable manner and increase sodium excretion similarly. Naturally a price has to be paid for this potency and their other less desirable effects must be carefully monitored.

FLUID RETENTION IN CARDIAC FAILURE

Fluid retention in cardiac failure depends on a number of interacting feedback loops involving the kidney, the blood volume, the nervous system and various hormones. A much simplified schema is depicted in Fig. 7.1. We will assume that the prime lesion is myocardial failure due to ischaemic heart disease. Reduction in the pumping ability of the heart reduces cardiac output which is especially apparent on exercise and will cause lowering of the effective plasma volume. The volume reduction is sensed by arterial baroreceptors and the juxtaglomerular apparatus which respond by vasoconstriction and by a reduction in the renal excretion of salt and water. At the same time failure of cardiac pump action on the right heart increases blood volume (and pressure) on the venous side of the circulation. This reaction would also tend to decrease effective plasma volume. The accumulation of fluid in the venous circulation leads to extravasation of fluid which is recognized clinically as oedema.

The resultant decrease in sodium and water excretion by the kidney, potentiated by activation of the renin–angiotensin–aldosterone mechanism,

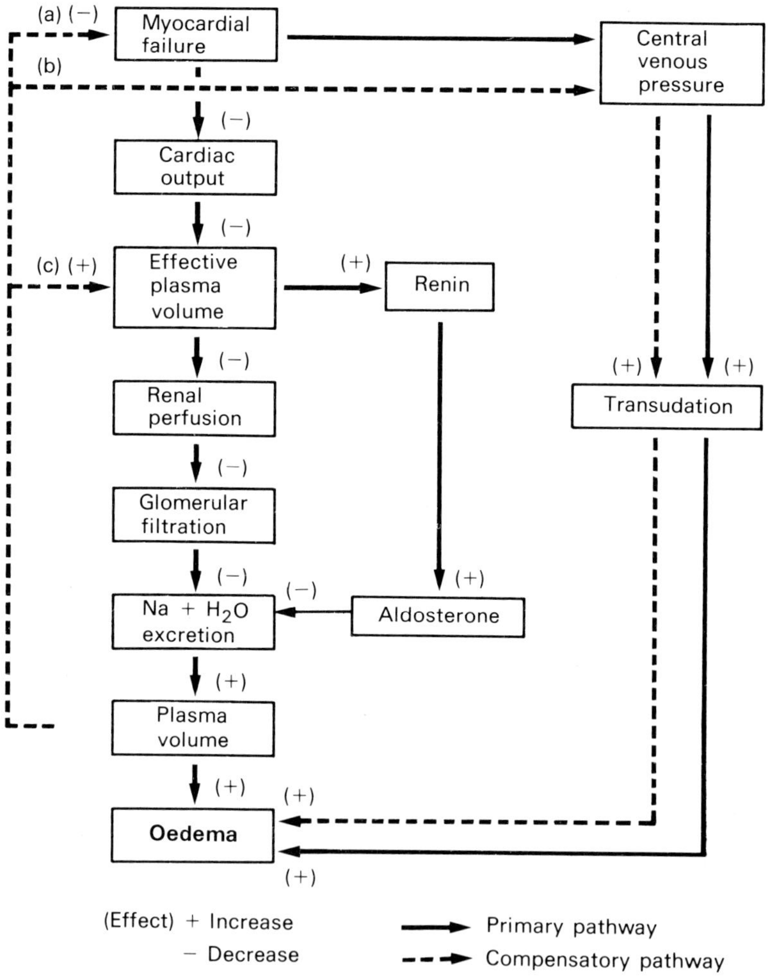

Fig. 7.1 Simplified sequence of events in congestive heart failure. See definitions of pathways (a), (b) and (c) in text.

will at least initially restore the effective plasma volume (pathway (c), Fig. 7.1). This pathway alone should reset the salt and water excretion threshold of the kidney at a new balance level. Unfortunately, the increase in plasma volume also increases the blood volume in the venous circulation (pathway (b), Fig. 7.1) leading to a further increase in oedema. The increase in venous volume does, however, have a beneficial effect (pathway (a), Fig. 7.1). By increasing venous tone and venous return to the heart the myocardial fibres are 'stretched' and the cardiac output will be increased via the Frank–Starling mechanism.

Obviously in the early stages of cardiac failure these feedback loops will lead to a form of compensation for the myocardial insufficiency. Often cardiac failure in the elderly is due to a transient decrease in myocardial function. This may be secondary to pneumonia and hence, all will be well when the precipitating cause has been resolved.

If, however, the prime myocardial insult is severe or chronic, the compensating pathways become out of phase or ineffective. Thus, there is a limit to the Frank–Starling effect (the Laplace phenomenon) and pathway (b), Fig. 7.1, predominates. The excessive fluid retention further potentiates the renin–aldosterone mechanism because hepatic congestion reduces the metabolic degradation of aldosterone. This simplified account of the pathophysiology of cardiac failure ignores natriuretic hormone (IIIrd factor) and anti-diuretic hormone. These obviously are important but it is difficult as yet to quantify their contribution to fluid balance in cardiac failure.

At this stage the salt and water retention mechanisms need to be turned off to prevent further deterioration. It is here that the diuretics can usefully be employed.

MECHANISMS OF DIURETIC ACTION

The glomerular filtrate is formed at a vast rate—about 125 ml/min in a healthy individual. Approximately 99% is then reabsorbed during passage down the renal tubular system. In an elderly person the amount of filtrate is much lower because of the age-mediated nephron loss but even in very old people most of the filtrate is reabsorbed, usually by energy-dependent mechanisms, though some transfer is passive. Equally a number of cations and anions are actively secreted by tubular cells into the filtrate. Water passively follows the osmotic gradients created by the more active movement of electrolytes, especially sodium. Thus, the composition of the ultimately voided urine can be actively varied by the kidney in response to the body's needs.

The majority of reabsorption takes place in the proximal tubule with progressively diminishing reabsorption down the tubule. Thus, approximately 70% of sodium is reabsorbed before the loop of Henle, 25% in the loop itself and only 5% by the distal tube. This latter reabsorption is controlled in the main by aldosterone.

The main groups of diuretic agents all work by inhibiting the active reabsorption of sodium or chloride at one or more segments along the renal tubule (see Table 7.1). The thiazides act principally on the proximal part of the distal tubule and to a lesser extent on the proximal tubule itself; loop diuretics have their main effect upon chloride reabsorption which leads to a secondary reduction in sodium reabsorption. They act primarily at the ascending limb of the loop of Henle—they also have a minor effect on proximal tubular function; the potassium-sparing diuretics are in the main only active in the distal tubule.

Table 7.1 Site of action of main diuretic groups.

	Main effect	Secondary effect
Thiazides	Proximal part of distal tubule	Proximal tubule
Loop diuretics	Ascending limb of loop of Henle	Proximal tubule
Potassium-sparing agents	Distal tubule	—

The vicious circle of ever-increasing fluid retention in chronic cardiac failure can be broken by the judicious use of diuretic agents. Diuretic agents by themselves can lead to significant and sustained improvement in cardiac function. There is no reason to believe and certainly no evidence to suggest that because renal function is reduced in old age due to nephron loss, the elderly are any less responsive to the renal action of diuretic agents.

As with all potent drugs a price has to be paid for the efficacy of diuretic agents. Complications and side-effects are not uncommon with diuretic agents and are especially frequent when prescribed for the elderly. These disadvantageous effects are related both to potency and dosage, though even mild diuretics used in moderate dose may lead to serious problems with long-term therapy in old people. Some complications are common to all diuretic agents and relate to their prime salt and water eliminating properties. Others relate to individual drugs and categories of drugs.

THIAZIDES

These were the first oral diuretics to replace the mercurials and they still remain the diuretics of choice in most circumstances. Table 7.2 lists some commonly available ones though this list is by no means exclusive. Their great advantage rests upon a smooth and prolonged duration of action. Pharmacologically they demonstrate predictable dose-response curves

Table 7.2 Some commonly used thiazide diuretics.

Drug	Duration of action (h) (onset–maximum)	Dosage range (mg/day)
Chlorothiazide	2–10	500–2000
Bendrofluazide	2–18	2.5–10
Hydrochlorothiazide	2–12	25–200
Polythiazide	2–36	4–8
Cyclopenthiazide	2–24	0.25–1
Metolazone	1–24	5–10
Chlorthalidone	2–48	50–100

which allow accurate individual titration of administered dose against renal response.

Except in cases of severe renal impairment or resistant heart failure, the thiazide diuretics are equal to the loop diuretics in potency, as measured by sodium and water elimination in 24 hours. Their average duration of action is about 10–12 hours and they show no catastrophic early peak effect which means that patient compliance is usally quite good. Patients often avoid taking more rapidly acting diuretics because of the social inconvenience produced by the initial and overwhelming urinary frequency. The choice of thiazide agent is a matter of personal preference. Become familiar with the effects of two or three agents rather than prescribing many different ones, as there are significant variations between them.

Chlorothiazide, the first-marketed diuretic of this group, has a relatively short maximum duration of action (approximately 10 hours) and is still quite useful. Of the newer thiazides, hydrochlorothiazide is similar in duration of action and is a much smaller tablet and is, therefore, probably more convenient for the elderly patient. In the author's opinion the best intermediate thiazide is bendrofluazide.

Chlorthalidone and polythiazide, two of the longer-acting thiazides, may be inconvenient because of sleep disturbance. They are, however, ideal for the treatment of hypertension where their prolonged action maintains a reduced blood pressure throughout the 24 hours with avoidance of swings. In this condition they do not seem to give rise to troublesome nocturia which is so often dangerous for an old person.

Side effects

Toxic side-effects of the thiazides are uncommon, taking into account their prolific use. Skin rashes, photosensitivity, gastrointestinal irritation, blood dyscrasias and jaundice have all been reported but their overall incidence is quite low. A form of necrotizing vasculitis affecting the skin and kidney is said to occur occasionally in elderly patients treated with thiazides.

The most important side-effects are related to the mode of action of the diuretic. Thus, by increasing the excretion of electrolytes and water, depletion of sodium, potassium, chloride and blood volume may be produced by prolonged or excessive dosage.

Hyponatraemia and hypovolaemia are much less common with the thiazides than with the potent loop diuretics. They may occur, however, presenting as weakness and postural hypotension. Stop the diuretic therapy for a short while, starting again at a lower dose. Occasionally water restriction may be required for persistent hyponatraemia but in this case the condition may be related to other diseases such as chronic respiratory infection or salt-losing nephritis. The angiotensin-converting enzyme inhibitor (Captopril) in low dose may restore diuretic responsiveness and correct the electrolyte imbalance. The blood pressure requires constant monitoring with this agent.

Thiazides increase the excretion of chloride and may produce a minor degree of alkalosis. The blood urea may rise owing to a reduction in glomerular filtration rate but this is usually a consequence of overdosage. By decreasing uric acid excretion hyperuricaemia and gout may occur in some predisposed patients but this does not seem to be a particular problem in the elderly. The development of hyperglycaemia, glycosuria and the uncovering of latent diabetes mellitus is a significant problem in the elderly. Diabetes may then continue after the diuretics are withdrawn. Thus, monitoring of blood and urine sugar is necessary at the commencement of therapy and should be repeated at 3–4-monthly intervals.

All thiazides increase the renal excretion of potassium and magnesium. In this respect they are *more potent* than the loop diuretics. They also tend to lower the plasma or serum potassium and may produce hypokalaemia. The relationship of plasma potassium to whole-body potassium is highly variable. The most up-to-date evidence suggests that diuretics have little part to play in depleting body potassium and further, potassium supplements have an even smaller role in increasing body potassium stores.

The interpretation of measurements of whole-body potassium in the elderly is confusing. Body potassium falls in cardiac failure due primarily to wasting of potassium-rich tissue (lean body mass). It is only in very severe or refractory cardiac failure that intracellular potassium falls and the evidence is that this condition cannot be reversed by potassium supplements or by any other means unless the cardiac function is itself improved. There is no doubt, however, that hypokalaemia potentiates digoxin toxicity and may in itself lead to cardiace arrhythymias.

Patients, even elderly ones, with untreated chronic heart failure have *elevated* plasma potassium levels. On average the thiazides will lower the plasma potassium by approximately 0.6 mmol/l (mEq/l) whereas a loop or high-ceiling diuretic will lower the plasma potassium by 0.3 mmol/l (mEq/l). There is some evidence that women are more sensitive to the kaliuretic effect of thiazides than men.

An important practical point is the observation that the change in plasma potassium with both thiazides and loop diuretics occurs early after the institution of treatment (usually within 1 month) and after this period a steady state is achieved, if the dose of diuretic is itself unchanged.

Bearing these points in mind, it is reasonable to measure the plasma potassium before starting diuretics because if it is low, there is a strong likelihood that it will fall further to a potentially significant level, i.e. <3.0 mmol/l (mEq/l). Thereafter, the plasma potassium should be measured twice, at approximately the same time of day to avoid diurnal variation, over the first month of diuretic therapy. If the level does not drop below 3.0 mmol/l (mEq/l) it is unlikely to fall subsequently and hypokalaemia will thus not be a problem. Further monitoring should take place at 3–4-monthly intervals.

If hypokalaemia is found initially or subsequently and the patient is taking concomitant digoxin, the hypokalaemia should be treated promptly with potassium supplements. For patients not taking digoxin the situation can be reassessed a week or so later. If plasma potassium remains low, it should be investigated and treated; if not, normal monitoring should continue. It is important not to ascribe the hypokalaemia to heart failure and diuretics; in the elderly other causes, gastrointestinal losses, laxative abuse, renal disease and secondary hyperaldosteronism are likely to be present and require specific treatment. Extreme hypokalaemia, i.e. plasma potassium <2.4 mmol/l (mEq/l) should be treated whatever the situation.

The treatment of established hypokalaemia may involve a reduction in thiazide dosage, use of potassium supplements or a change to a potassium-sparing diuretic. The first strategy is not considered frequently enough. Patients' requirements for diuretics change, usually downwards. They should be regularly reviewed and reduced if possible—especially in the elderly.

There are numerous fixed combinations of thiazide diuretics and potassium supplements. Without exception these combinations are useless in treating hypokalaemia and may, by inducing a false sense of security in the physician, be actually dangerous. The dose of supplement in the fixed combination drug is so low as to be invariably less than $\frac{1}{10}$ of the daily potassium dose. It is a personal view that 20 mmol (mEq)/day is the minimum requirement of potassium supplement required in treating hypokalaemia and not uncommonly 60 mmol (mEq)/day may be necessary for some individuals. The plasma potassium must be monitored at weekly intervals until normokalaemia is achieved. Thereafter the supplement can be reduced or even stopped as indicated by changes in the plasma levels.

Potassium supplements need to contain chloride in order to correct the metabolic alkalosis which itself potentiates extracellular potassium depletion. Unfortunately, many suitable preparations of potassium chloride are distinctly unpalatable and thus patient compliance may be poor.

There are numerous proprietary preparations of potassium (see Table 7.3). The original slow-release enteric-coated tablets have been virtually abandoned because of the serious risk of small intestinal and oesophageal ulceration and stricture formation. Slow-release tablets based on a wax matrix are preferred but a small risk of ulceration still remains with these tablets, especially if there is gastrointestinal hold-up or dysphagia. Five to six tablets daily are required to provide 40–48 mmol (mEq) potassium and it is often difficult to persuade elderly patients to take so many.

Table 7.3 Oral potassium preparations.

	Doses/day =40 mmol
Slow release KCl	5
Kloref eff	6
Kloref-S eff	2
Sando-K	4

Liquid preparations of potassium chloride are available but are not usually suitable for old people because of the unpalatable taste and the sensation of nausea they produce. The strong preparations, 10 and 20%, are particularly nauseating. Effervescent preparations are much preferred even though a few individuals remain intolerant. These preparations can be dissolved in various drinks to disguise the potassium taste. Kloref-S is particularly useful and being fruit flavoured is reasonably well tolerated by old people. Only two sachets daily are required to provide 40 mmol (mEq) potassium and 40 mmol (mEq) of chloride.

The plasma potassium should be regularly monitored in all patients taking potassium supplements. This action is imperative if there is any evidence of renal impairment. Equally, the development of a concomitant respiratory infection during long-term diuretic plus potassium therapy may compromise renal function further with the rapid development of potentially dangerous hyperkalaemia. It is rightly said that hyperkalaemia has killed more patients than hypokalaemia.

LOOP (HIGH-CEILING) DIURETICS

For the treatment of acute or life-threatening left ventricular failure the potent loop diuretics have brought about a minor revolution in medical practice. Before the advent of these fast-acting agents, the first episode of severe left ventricular failure was often the last. How many young physicians have seen the classic frothy, pulmonary oedema? There is unfortunately a tendency to use excessively high intravenous doses of these agents.

The commonly available agents are listed in Table 7.4.

Table 7.4 Commonly available Loop (High-ceiling) diuretic agents.

Drug	Duration of action (h) (onset–maximum)	Dosage range (mg/day)
Frusemide	1–4	20–600
Ethacrynic acid	0.5–6	50–150
Bumetamide	0.5–6	1–2

The prompt and desirable diuresis may cause acute retention of urine in old men with borderline prostatic hypertrophy and also in some elderly women. In patients with neuropathic bladders (e.g. due to cerebrovascular disease), sudden filling of the bladder may cause urinary incontinence if they are unable to respond quickly enough to the micturition reflex. If the use of potent loop diuretics cannot be avoided because of the severity of the cardiac state the prescription of an adjacent commode is as important as the prescription of the diuretic itself.

These potent agents also are prone to cause hypovolaemia by depleting the extracellular fluid volume. This may lead to hypotension with postural fainting. In some elderly patients the extracellular depletion can be so severe as to render the unfortunate patient bedridden.

The reduction in plasma volume as a consequence of diminished extracellular fluid reduces further the renal blood flow and hence glomerular filtration rate leading to significant increases in blood urea. Because of the age-related nephron loss this is especially likely to occur in elderly patients. If tetracycline is added (as in the management of acute heart failure secondary to bronchopneumonia), the increased protein catabolic state produced by the pneumonia may precipitate renal failure.

In general, the effects of loop diuretics on the plasma electrolytes, potassium, chloride and uric acid are *less* than those induced by the thiazides. Nevertheless, potassium status should be monitored as outlined previously. Similarly, the effect of frusemide and ethacrynic acid on the blood sugar level and the unmasking or precipitating of frank diabetes mellitus is reduced in comparison with the thiazide diuretics.

Ethacrynic acid, and to a lesser extent frusemide, may produce gastrointestinal upsets including anorexia and nausea, with or without vomiting, dysphagia and transient diarrhoea. Often a reduction in dosage is all that is required but a change to thiazide agents is sometimes needed. Intravenous administration of ethacrynic acid is potentially dangerous and is therefore not recommended.

Severe abdominal pain following parenteral administration is supposedly due to calyceal distension in the kidney and may be a problem though it is not usually sustained with subsequent oral therapy. Ethacrynic acid and frusemide in high doses may produce transient or occasionally permanent hearing loss of the sensorineural variety. This can be avoided by adhering strictly to the manufacturer's instructions concerning dosage and rates of infusion.

Long-term use of potent loop diuretics, even in moderate dosages, may lead to potentially serious osteopenia in elderly patients. Many old people have inadequate intake of vitamin D, and lack of exposure to sunlight. Sub-clinical, or indeed, frank osteomalacia may occur. The loop diuretics cause a significant increase in urinary calcium excretion, which continues for as long as the therapy. Additional calcium supplements may not reverse the negative calcium balance whilst these diuretics are used. The significance of the increased magnesium excretion induced by both ethacrynic and frusemide therapy is not clear but could be deleterious in the elderly patient. Hypomagnesaemia may potentiate potassium deficiency or render it resistant to replacement therapy.

POTASSIUM-SPARING DIURETICS

The so-called potassium-sparing diuretics primarily act on the distal renal tubule. On their own they are weak diuretics because only approximately 6% of sodium filtered by the glomerulus is reabsorbed by the distal tubule. Thus, they are usually administered in conjunction with more proximally active drugs whose diuretic action they will tend to potentiate. The 3 main members of this group are spironolactone, triamterene and amiloride (see Table 7.5).

Table 7.5 Potassium-sparing diuretic agents.

Drug	Duration of action (h) (onset–maximum)	Dosage range (mg/day)
Spironolactone	8–72	100–400
Trimaterene	2–6	100–250
Amiloride	2–24	5–20

Spironolactone

Structually spironolactone and its metabolites are similar to the natural adrenal hormone, aldosterone. Spironolactone acts as a competitive antagonist to aldosterone, blocking the latter's sodium and chloride reabsorption effect in the distal tubule. Spironolactone competes for aldosterone receptor sites in the distal tubule and the very high levels of circulating aldosterone which may thus occur (e.g. in severe hypertension or hepatic cirrhosis) may require correspondingly high doses of spironolactone.

Figure 7.1 shows the central role of aldosterone in promoting sodium and water retention in chronic heart failure. In individual cases, however, it is often difficult to assess the contribution of excess aldosterone to fluid retention. It should be suspected in the long-term cardiac patient who demonstrates increasing cachexia in association with a falling plasma potassium concentration. In this situation spironolactone can be usefully used to potentiate a thiazide or loop diuretic which has ceased to be effective. On its own spironolactone is a weak diuretic and except in cases of Conn's syndrome (primary hyperaldosteronism) is virtually useless. Spironolactone cannot be recommended as a routine addition to other diuretics for the treatment of elderly patients with cardiace failure. Spironolactone is a potent and dangerous drug in old people and if it is used the blood electrolytes must be carefully and continuously monitored.

The main danger is hyperkalaemia which may arise in up to 15% of patients taking the drug. This complication often arises in association with the continued use of potassium supplements and spironolactone in the presence of diminishing renal function. Having emphasized to the patient that he must take his potassium supplements with the thiazide or loop diuretic, subsequent instructions, following the addition of spironolactone to therapy, to cease supplementation are often ignored. Even if further supplements are not prescribed, old patients often have a horde of potassium supplements in the bathroom cabinet and continue to take them religiously.

Even healthy old people have diminished renal reserve because of the age-related nephron loss. When this is combined with low renal perfusion due to cardiac failure, the excretion of potassium will be impaired. It should be recalled that on average the plasma potassium of *untreated* patients with cardiac failure is *higher* than normal. If spironolactone is added in this situation, it may worsen the potassium retention and potentially cause significant hyperkalaemia.

Spironolactone may induce significant hyponatraemia and dehydration in some elderly patients. It is a gastric irritant and indeed may prevent the healing of peptic ulcers. Painful gynaecomastia in males and swelling of the breasts in females is a well recognized complication of spironolactone therapy. Fortunately it only occurs in a small proportion of elderly patients.

The mechanism by which spironolactone induces central nervous system disturbances (headaches, muzziness, confusion) is entirely unknown. A particular problem in the elderly is confusion—more likely in the patient with previous poor cerebral function but is also seen *de novo*.

Because of potentially dangerous side-effects spironolactone should be reserved for the minority of patients with resistant cardiac failure presumed to be related to secondary hyperaldosteronism.

Triamterene

In many ways triamterene is similar in action to spironolactone though it is not a competitive antagonist of aldosterone. Its site of action is in the distal renal tubule where it promotes sodium excretion and produces potassium and hydrogen ion retention. On its own it is a weak diuretic and is therefore usually combined with a thiazide diuretic agent to potentiate the diuresis whilst limiting potassium excretion. Apart from gynaecomastia, triamterene produces all the same adverse effects as spironolactone. However, in one serious way it is more dangerous than spironolactone. Trimaterene directly reduces glomerular filtration and leads to significant elevation in the blood urea. For this reason triamterene should not be used in elderly patients with cardiac failure.

Amiloride

Amiloride hydrochloride is a new distally acting potassium-sparing diuretic widely used throughout Europe in combination with a thiazide. Its mode of action is essentially the same as triamterene. In healthy subjects amiloride has no effect on glomerular filtration rate. This is not the case with elderly patients in whom significant elevation of blood urea and significant decreases in creatinine clearance can be regularly demonstrated.

Hyperkalaemia due to amiloride may arise in patients without significant renal impairment and without taking potassium supplements. This adverse effect is primarily dose-related. Amiloride is also particularly likely to produce significant and symptomatic hyponatraemia in elderly patients. The symptoms of hyponatraemia such as weakness and lethargy may be attributed to the heart failure itself and be inadvisedly treated by increasing the dosage of amiloride. The only treatment for amiloride-induced hyponatraemia is withdrawal of the drug and substution of a thiazide diuretic if necessary. Until more studies on older patients have been reported amiloride cannot be recommended.

Conclusion

Theoretically the potassium-sparing diuretics should be useful in the long-term management of old people with chronic fluid retention. However, their adverse effects on body electrolytes and renal function are so common and potentially so dangerous that it is the author's view that they cannot be generally recommended.

In the rare circumstances of secondary hyperaldosteronism and persistent hypokalaemia then spironolactone should be considered. It can be given orally and because of its long half-life only requires daily administration. However, the blood urea and plasma electrolytes require constant monitoring. If, during the course of long-term spironolactone therapy, the older patient should develop a catabolic state, for example, pneumonia, the drug should be stopped before hyperkalaemia develops.

ACUTE PULMONARY OEDEMA

Acute left ventricular failure is a dramatic event but invariably responds to quite moderate doses of parenteral loop diuretics. For example, 40 mg or even 20 mg frusemide intravenously initiates sufficient diuresis and reduction of pulmonary venous pressure to relieve promptly cardiac dyspnoea. Where patients are extremely agitated a small dose of intravenous morphine (10 mg) is also indicated. This can be repeated and may be especially useful in treating recurrent paroxysmal nocturnal dyspnoea due to left ventricular failure. However, this should not become a routine. Strenuous efforts should be made by promoting adequate diuresis to prevent the recurrence of this frightening and dangerous manifestation of heart disease.

It is a personal view that intravenous digitalis is not required for the emergency treatment of acute left ventricular failure unless there is an uncontrolled atrial tachyarrhythmia (see Chapter 9).

Whilst bed rest is often recommended, many elderly patients will find it more comfortable to be nursed, initially at least, in a semi-recumbent position in a chair. Often patients sleep much better in this position. Patients with left ventricular failure may be profoundly anoxic—this contributes to agitation and confusion—necessitating oxygen administration. If there is no pre-existing chronic obstructive airways disease (COAD), high (60–80%) concentrations can be administered via an appropriate mask. If there is any COAD or it cannot be excluded, low (24–28%) concentrations must be used.

After stabilization of the initial dyspnoea a search for precipitating factors should be undertaken. Myocardial infarction may be painless and hence unrecognized. A more common cause of acute failure in elderly patients is respiratory infection or pulmonary infarction, in which case signs of right heart failure would also be apparent. The sudden onset of an arrhythmia lowering cardiac output would be apparent on the electrocardiogram.

REFERENCES AND FURTHER READING

Huston G. (1979) Diuretics. In Hamer J. (Ed.) *Drugs for Heart Disease*, pp. 513–47. Chapman and Hall, London.

Kleit S.A., Hamburger R.J. & Martz B.L. (1970) Diuretic therapy: Current status. *American Heart Journal* **79**, 700–12.

Lye M. (1980) Body potassium content and capacity of elderly individuals with or without cardiac failure. *Cardiovascular Research* **16**, 22–5.

Montgomery A.J., Shepherd A.N. & Emslie-Smith D. (1982) Severe hyponatraemia and cardiac failure successfully treated with Captopril. *British medical Journal* **284**, 1085–6.

Oliver M.F. (Ed.) (1975) Modern Trends in Cardiology. Butterworths, London.

Chapter Eight
Cardiovascular System—Treatment of Hypertension

M.D.W. LYE

OVERVIEW

The enigma of hypertension in the elderly is discussed in relation to cost benefit in a clinical setting. It is concluded that hypertension in the elderly is a disease which if untreated may lead to morbidity and increasing mortality.

The management of raised blood pressure in the asymptomatic patient and in the patient with end-organ effects or other disease conditions is discussed in relation to the many drugs available. Due emphasis is given to side-effects and adverse reactions. Pharmacokinetic and pharmacodynamic data are provided. Personal recommendations for drug choice are described.

The continuing controversy concerning raised blood pressure and its management has become a long-term saga. The whole subject is beset by problems of definition, management and cost benefit. The distribution of attitudes among physicians ranges from 'treat all' to 'treat none' and follows a bell-shaped (Gaussian) curve reminiscent of the distribution curve of blood pressure itself. Thus, there are no clear divisions between a normotensive, a hypertensive and a hypotensive person. The addition of another variable, age, into the equation is likely to raise further the blood pressure of discussants.

DEFINITION

As there is no clear dividing line between normal blood pressure and an abnormally raised pressure an arbitrary definition is required. The Framingham longitudinal study of cardiovascular risk factors has provided important epidemiological information but, unfortunately, does not help in defining 'hypertension'. For practical purposes, however, we can clearly differentiate a group of subjects who show end-organ effects from a raised blood pressure. Thus, persons demonstrating left ventricular hypertrophy or strain, progressive renal or visual impairment and/or cerebral haemorrhage in association with a persistently raised blood pressure may be considered as suffering from hypertensive disease. It is before the development of end-organ complications that difficulties of definition arise.

There is, however, one exception and this is secondary hypertension (chronic pyelonephritis, collagen vascular disease, renal artery stenosis, primary aldosteronism, etc.) where cause and effect can be related. In the elderly these secondary causes of raised blood pressure are exceedingly rare. This is surprising as bacteriuria is common in old people and pyelonephritis is frequently associated with raised blood pressure in young and middle-aged patients. This is not the case in the elderly.

The Framingham study defined hypertension as a systolic pressure above 160 mmHg and diastolic above 95 mmHg. The World Health Organization chose 90 mmHg for the diastolic level. The European Working Party on High Blood Pressure in the Elderly also use the same definition of hypertension as WHO. With the exception of the latter group these definitions of hypertension do not automatically imply that such patients should be treated.

It is the author's view that asymtomatic hypertension in subjects above the age of 65 should be diagnosed after 3 separate estimates of blood pressure have recorded systolic levels of more than 190 and/or diastolic levels of more than 100 mmHg.

PREVALENCE

Numerous epidemiological studies have demonstrated that blood pressure increases with aging in both sexes. Estimates of the prevalence of hypertension naturally depend upon the arbitrary level of blood pressure chosen and thus vary from 10 to 70% of the population of elderly persons studied. Is the rise in average systolic and diastolic pressure 'normal' when more than half the population possess a particular characteristic, in this case the diagnostic label hypertension? Can this attribute then be called normal?

Certainly in many so-called underdeveloped societies increases in blood pressure with increasing age are not apparent. Equally, many individuals, though not the majority in the developed nations, fail to demonstrate an age-related change of blood pressure. It can, therefore, be concluded that the age-related rise in blood pressure seen in all developed nations though common is not inevitable and should be considered an atypical (? pathological) process. The financial implications, if it is decided that treatment is warranted, are outside the competence of the author to consider but may well influence, quite rightly, recommendations concerning treatment.

EFFECTS OF RAISED BLOOD PRESSURE

Numerous surveys have demonstrated that an increase of blood pressure in middle-aged persons is associated with increasing morbidity (mainly cardiovascular) and decreasing life expectancy. Insurance companies with their vested financial interests have known this for many years. Recent surveys have also demonstrated that this association applies to the elderly population. There is no denying that within the population with raised blood pressures there is a subgroup who seemingly suffer no ill-effects. The problem, however, is to identify these fortunate individuals at an early stage. The Framingham study demonstrates, unfortunately, that the proportion of 'protected' individuals with raised blood pressure actually decreases with increasing age. Thus, it can be concluded that raised blood pressure in the elderly is probably as dangerous as that in middle-aged individuals.

As in younger subjects, the organs at risk from high blood pressure are the heart, brain and kidneys. The kidneys in the elderly are much less affected by hypertension than in the young and it is rare to see the phenomenon of accelerated hypertension with renal failure in old people. Whilst the heart is affected by hypertension in all age groups, in broad terms young people sustain myocardial infarcts whereas old people gradually develop left ventricular failure.

TO TREAT OR NOT TO TREAT?

To date there have been no adequate long-term trials of antihypertensive therapy and its effect on mortality or morbidity reported which specifically relate to the elderly hypertensive. There is no doubt that the pharmacological lowering of raised blood pressure in young and middle-aged hypertensives is singularly effective in reducing morbidity and in increasing life-expectancy. There are no data available that suggest this beneficial situation would *not* apply to elderly hypertensive patients. There are, however, a number of unsupported anecdotal and theoretical objections put forward to suggest that the elderly would not benefit (possibly excuses for a nihilistic attitude towards this difficult problem).

Malignant or accelerated hypertension in the elderly should invariably be treated. Patients with the combination of cardiac failure and systolic blood pressure above 190 mmHg or diastolic levels above 100 mmHg should also be treated.

The patient with associated cerebral impairment, stroke or generalized cerebral arteriosclerosis presents a particular problem. In young and middle-aged stroke victims with sustained hypertension the lowering of blood pressure benefits a significant proportion. It is important, however, to remember that immediately following the ictus, blood pressure may be high and gradually settle spontaneously over a period of a month or more. It is suggested that such patients with systolic levels above 200 mmHg or diastolic levels above 110 mmHg should be cautiously treated. Patients with global cerebral disease causing gross mental impairment should probably not be treated because the generalized cerebrovascular insufficiency in such patients induces further confusion if the blood pressure is reduced. Equally, confusion in these individuals makes compliance difficult.

The elderly asymptomatic patient with sustained systolic pressures above 190 mmHg or diastolic pressures above 100 mmHg should be treated in the absence of specific contraindications. This conclusion, however, may require modification (up or down) in the light of further study.

MANAGEMENT

The management of the elderly hypertensive patient requires much more than the administration of potent hypotensive agents. It is important to treat the patient as a whole and not just the sphygmomanometer readings. Whilst this approach is of course important in managing all patients, it is particularly apposite to the care of the elderly.

Diagnosis

A single recording of a raised blood pressure measured in the general practitioner's surgery or hospital clinic does not imply that the blood pressure is chronically elevated. Many elderly subjects are very worried and fear the worst whenever they consult their physician. A friendly, reassuring atmosphere and approach by the physician and his staff will reduce the blood pressure of many an anxious patient.

The blood pressure should be recorded in the sitting position on 3 occasions after at least 5 minutes rest. The average rather than the highest level should be recorded as the initial or starting blood pressure. The systolic levels should be confirmed by palpation as a number of elderly patients may have a silent period just below the actual systolic level. Diastolic levels are best recorded as Korotkoff Phase V.

The days of extensive investigation of the asymptomatic hypertensive are long gone. Secondary hypertension in the elderly is particularly rare. This is perhaps surprising considering the effects of age upon the kidney. The search for iatrogenic causes of raised blood pressure is usually more fruitful than detailed biochemical or radiological investigations. Thus, steroids and other agents which produce sodium retention, indomethacin, phenylbutazone, carbenoxalone, etc., should be excluded if possible before determining the basal blood presure.

Renal infection in the elderly can be difficult to evaluate in terms of hypertension. Chronic pyelonephritis is relatively uncommon—it is possible that such patients do not survive into old age. The patient with chronic pyelonephritis who develops an acute infection may show raised blood pressure levels during the acute phase which settle with appropriate antibacterial therapy. Asymptomatic bacteriuria in the elderly is not associated with the development of pyelonephritic renal failure, nor with the development of hypertension.

Endocrine causes of hypertension, including primary hyperaldosteronism (Conn's syndrome) are extremely rare in the elderly. Occasionally thyrotoxicosis, which is so often atypical in the older patient, may give rise to transient elevation of the blood pressure.

The serum electrolytes, urea, sugar and uric acid levels of patients should be measured before starting therapy, to establish base-lines. Urinalysis and urine culture may disclose a renal abnormality. A chest X-ray and electrocardiogram should be similarly obtained. In the elderly, often the first manifestation of hypertension is cardiac failure. Its presence may well influence subsequent therapeutic decisions and should be looked for.

Treatment

The fundamental aim of hypotensive therapy is to reduce blood pressures to an acceptable level without incurring unacceptable side-effects. It is the balancing of this equation which provides such a challenge to the physician and to the pharmaceutical industry. The level of blood pressure aimed at will depend upon the initial levels and any accompanying complications. In the elderly asymptomatic hypertensive patient with moderately elevated pressures it should be possible to reduce the levels to less than 160 mmHg systolic and between 90–95 mmHg diastolic without side-effects. It is essential to do this slowly and gently, possibly 4 months may even be required. High initial levels may require acceptance of less than ideal results but even in such patients diastolic levels should be reduced to below 105 mmHg.

Non-drug therapy

Whilst the role of dietary sodium intake in the aetiology of essential hypertension remains controversial there is no doubt that a high intake is associated with an additive or even potentiating effect on elevated blood pressure. A no-added-salt diet and removal of table salt are all that most elderly patients will accept. Not many old people are obese, but some elderly hypertensives are. Weight reduction is beneficial to the hypertensive of all ages. Unfortunately, it is often extremely difficult to ask old people to change long-established feeding habits. However, modest reductions in weight are well worth pursuing.

Weight reduction may have a beneficial effect upon hyperlipidaemia, especially Frederickson types III, IV and V. Beyond this simple dietary reduction in calories the author does not recommend specific lipid-reducing diets or drugs for elderly patients with hyperlipidaemia. In the future with the development of more specific or effective drugs this statement may need reconsideration.

Drug therapy

The multiplicity of hypertensive drugs bears witness to the fact that there is no single effective agent useful in all cases.

The choice of an individual agent(s) is to some extent the physician's personal preference but should be overridingly dictated by the patient's own condition, compliance, cardiovascular state, other drugs, etc.

The scheme of classification used in Table 8.1 is an oversimplification. The precise mode of action of many hypertensive agents, even those which have been in use for many years, is not always known. Equally, many drugs have multiple levels of action, so their precise allocation to one category or another is impossible.

Table 8.1 Classification of oral hypotensive agents.

Natriuretic drugs	Thiazides Indapamide* High-ceiling (loop) Potassium sparing
β-blocking agents	Propranolol Oxprenolol Pindolol Atenolol Labetalol*
Centrally acting agents	α-methyldopa Clonidine Reserpine
Peripherally acting agents	Bethanidine Guanethidine Debrisoquine
Peripheral vasodilators	Hydrallazine Prazosin Minoxidil

* Not available in North America.

Natriuretic agents

Any agent that increases sodium excretion will lower blood pressure. However, it must be borne in mind that the hypotensive effect of many drugs is not simply related to their natriuretic activity. Thus, the loop, or high-ceiling diuretics, though powerful natriuretics are not as potent in lowering blood pressure as the weaker thiazides.

Thiazides

Advantage should be taken of those two agents with long half-lives (see Table 7.2, p. 91), allowing once-daily dosage. Large doses should not be used for two reasons. First, elderly hypertensives seem to be unduly sensitive to the effects of thiazides, and second, the dose-responsive curve, in relation to blood pressure is attenuated. Thus, if the blood pressure cannot be lowered sufficiently with a moderate dose of diuretic, further increases would be no more effective. Better to add some other agent.

The choice, use, precaution, side-effects, etc., of these agents are fully discussed on p. 90. A list of commonly observed adverse effects is given in Table 8.2.

Table 8.2 Adverse effects of thiazides.

Electrolytes	—hypokalaemia —hyponatraemia —hypomagnesaemia —alkalosis
Volume depletion	
Urea retention	
Hyperuricaemia	
Hyperglycaemia	
Urinary frequency	
Incontinence	
Retention	

An interesting and potentially very useful development in this area is the synthesis of indapamide. In low doses (2.5 mg/day) this drug, though related to the thiazides, has little or no diuretic action, but does have useful hypotensive activity. This feature avoids many of the diuretic side-effects listed in Table 8.2. The result of further evaluation of this drug and reports from long-term trials are awaited with interest.

Loop (high-ceiling) diuretics

Generally these agents are not used to treat hypertension because of their lack of potency, short duration of action and brisk diuretic properties. Occasionally they may be substituted for a thiazide agent if the latter is ineffective (in renal impairment), or is actually contraindicated (in diabetes, gout).

Potassium-sparing diuretics

Because these agents further impair compromised renal function in elderly subjects, they cannot be recommended for the treatment of hypertension.

The only exception would be the use of spironolactone in primary hyperaldosteronism where surgery is contraindicated.

β-blocking agents

Many *β*-adrenergic blocking agents (*β*-blockers) are now available (see Table 8.3 for some examples).

Table 8.3 Some commonly used *β*-blocking agents.

	Activity		
Drug	Cardioselectivity (*β*-2)	Intrinsic sympathomimetic activity	Membrane stabilizing activity
Acebutolol	±	+	++
Alprenolol	+	+	+
Atenolol	−	−	−
Labetalol*†	+	−	+
Metoprolol	−	−	−
Nadolol*†	+	−	−
Oxprenolol	+	+	+
Penbutolol	+	+	+
Pindolol	+	+	+++
Propranolol	+	−	+
Sotalol	+	−	−
Timolol	+	−	+

* exhibits α-adrenergic blocking actions.
† Not available in North America.

The classic study of Ahlquist demonstrated that within the sympathetic nervous system two types of response (α and *β*) could be elicited by various agonists. In essence stimulation of α-receptors led to peripheral blood vessel vasoconstriction whilst stimulation of *β*-receptors had the opposite effect. Later it was shown that *β*-receptors were located in cardiac and bronchial smooth muscle as well as blood vessels.

All *β*-blockers act as competitive antagonists of noradrenaline and adrenaline at the *β*-adrenergic receptor site. The competitive nature of this antagonism leads to varying responses due to alterations in the agonist: antagonist ratio with varying doses and different formulations. All act by blocking (to some degree) the action of natural catecholamines on adenylate cyclase which normally produces cAMP. The reduction in cAMP inhibits the transmembrane calcium ion current.

Table 8.4 Primary effects of β-blockade.

β_1	Heart
	Contractility ↓
	Conduction velocity ↓
	Automaticity ↓
	Effective refractory period ↑
β_2	Blood vessels
	Vasoconstriction
	Bronchial smooth muscle
	Constriction
	Glycogenolysis
	Reduction

The principal effects of β-adrenergic blockade are given in Table 8.4. The magnitude of these effects is related to the overall level of sympathetic tone. In general β-blockers decrease the heart rate though there are differences between the various agents. Equally, all decrease myocardial muscle contractility leading to a decrease in stroke volume. These two effects combine to reduce cardiac output. At rest this may not be significant but during exercise, when sympathetic activity is high this reduction may cause symptoms. Similarly, by reducing the adrenergic cardiac drive, compensated cardiac failure may become overt. This adverse reaction is more likely with elderly subjects.

Cardioselectivity

Lands, on the basis of differential response to the agonists noradrenaline and adrenaline, introduced the concept of specific β_1 and β_2 receptors (see Table 8.4). Thus, the β_1 receptors are mainly 'involved' with cardiac and β_2 receptors concerned with peripheral vascular and bronchial dilatation. There is much overlap between β_1 and β_2 selectivity possibly because β_1 and β_2 receptors are not organ specific—only the relative proportions of the two receptors vary in different tissues. Alternatively it is suggested on the basis of varying drug polarity (lipid solubility) of different β-blockers that there is varying protection of the same receptors by a lipid barrier. This latter concept might explain differences in central nervous system adverse effects of β-blocking agents.

In clinical practice it is probably best to use a so-called cardioselective agent for persons with bronchial hypersensitivity, insulin-dependent diabetes and peripheral vascular insufficiency—remembering that cardioselectivity is only relative.

Intrinsic sympathomimetic activity (ISA)

Some β-blockers (see Table 8.3) possess ISA or partial agonist activity (PAA) and pharmaceutical companies in their advertising lay great stress on this feature. Agents with this property, whilst blocking the action of the neurotransmitter, may actually themselves stimulate the receptor. This activity is said to be apparent when used in subjects with low sympathetic tone. It is difficult to demonstrate any significant effect when sympathetic activity is high due to exercise, cardiac failure or possibly hypertension. The clinical relevance of ISA is uncertain though new agents with very high ISA are being developed and in the future may make a significant contribution to the treatment of hypertension.

Membrane stabilizing activity (MSA) or quinidine-like activity (QLA)

This is a secondary property of the β-blockers, (e.g. propranolol) with local anaesthetic action, which limits transcellular ionic movement. It is assumed that they also stabilize the cell membrane of cardiac cells. If this were the case, agents with high MSA should be good anti-arrhythmics and cause less reduction in cardiac contractility. Unfortunately, the doses required to produce membrane stabilization are often excessive. The anti-arrhythmic properties of β-blockers are probably more related to reduction in sympathetic tone than to a direct effect upon cardiac conducting tissue via MSA.

Pharmacokinetics

With the exception of pindolol all β-blockers and their active metabolites are excreted by the kidney. Thus, as a general rule, dosage and frequency

Table 8.5 Pharmacokinetics of β-blockers.

	Plasma half-life (h)	Protein binding	Lipid solubility
Acebutolol	3	++	+
Alprenolol	2	+++	+
Atenolol	8	+	−
Labetalol*	4	++	+
Metoprolol	3	+	+
Nadolol*	15	++	−
Oxprenolol	2	++	+
Pindolol	4	+++	?
Propranolol	3	+++	+
Sotalol	16	+++	−
Timolol	4	++	+

* Not available in North America.

of administration should both be reduced in the elderly. The plasma half-life of these agents varies considerably from compound to compound (see Table 8.5). However, all show the effect of cumulative administration. Once daily slow-release preparations of oxprenolol and propranolol are available which may aid patient compliance. It should be emphasized, however, that the biological half-lives of these compounds are much longer than the pharmacological half-lives.

Certain agents (see Table 8.5) are particularly strongly bound to plasma proteins and their dosages require reduction if there is any evidence of hypoproteinaemia, e.g. reduction in plasma albumin. The β-blockers differ in degree of lipid solubility. The highly lipid-soluble agents tend to penetrate nervous tissue easily and are, therefore, more likely to give rise to troublesome CNS side-effects.

Lipid solubility also effects hepatic metabolism of β-blockers via the 'first pass' effect. The lipid-soluble agents such as propranolol undergo active hepatic metabolism producing breakdown products which themselves may be highly active. This effect is reduced in the elderly and also in patients with a low cardiac output so that the plasma levels of these agents may be up to 4 times higher in old people than in younger people.

Adverse effects

β-blockers may give rise to numerous unwanted and adverse effects (see Table 8.6). Reference to individual pharmacokinetic data and the additional properties (cardioselectivity, ISA) may aid a physician to avoid these potentially dangerous consequences. Most adverse effects are, however, produced by overzealous dosage regimens. Because of the age-related altered metabolism and excretion of β-blockers adverse effects are much more likely in

Table 8.6 Adverse side-effects of β-blockade.

Cardiac	Reduced myocardial contractility Increase heart block Decrease SA node output Decrease peripheral perfusion Paradoxical hypertension Heart failure
Pulmonary	Increase bronchomotor tone Potentiate CO_2 retention
Cerebral	Drowsiness Depression Hallucinations Dreams
Metabolic	Mask insulin hypoglycaemia Increase hyperglycaemia Potassium retention

the elderly. Multiple pathology is also a contributing factor. Unfortunately, even judicious selection of agent does not guarantee safety; all β-blockers, in spite of their classification, may give rise to any adverse effect listed in Table 8.6.

Choice of β-blockers

Overlapping of drug actions and variability of patient response make specific recommendations difficult. Become familiar with a few preparations, remembering that the longer the drug has been used, the more is known about its potential side-effects.

In uncomplicated hypertension in the elderly a cardioselective agent with low lipid solubility and low plasma binding affinity which also possesses intrinsic sympathomimetic activity is usually indicated. In spite of all the permutations in formulae such a β-blocker does not exist as yet. Thus, the choice must reflect a compromise based upon the clinical condition of the individual patient.

Centrally acting agents

Vasomotor centres exist within the medulla which are concerned with the short- and long-term regulation of arterial blood pressure. These centres are served by the autonomic nervous system but are also to a variable extent influenced by input from higher brain stem and cortical levels. The main input to this system comes from baroreceptors located in the carotid sinus, aortic arch and other major vessels. There is some evidence that with increasing age the sensitivity of these receptors is significantly modulated. Output from the system is mainly by the sympathetic nerves to the heart and resistance arterioles.

Interrelating feedback loops exist within the system. The neurotransmitters include catecholamines (dopamine, noradrenaline, adrenaline) and serotonergic neurones. Neurotransmitters may be inhibitory or excitatory, depending upon which site within the system is involved. Much further work is needed to elucidate the various pathways, nuclei and neurotransmitters concerned. It seems obvious that this new knowledge will lead to pharmacological exploitation with the development of newer centrally acting hypotensive agents.

Methyldopa

In the past α-methyldopa has enjoyed great popularity as a hypotensive agent. Originally α-methyldopa was thought to act entirely peripherally by depleting adrenergic nerve endings of noradrenaline. It is now obvious that the agent acts centrally by depleting serotonin, dopamine and noradrenaline within the brain itself. Its precise locus of hypotensive action is not known though the brain stem is the most likely site.

α-methyldopa is well absorbed following oral administration. It is actively metabolized within the body and most metabolites are excreted by the kidney. Thus, impaired renal function prolongs the otherwise short half-like of the drug, a point always to be considered during therapy of the elderly. Therapy should be started at a low dose; for example, 125 mg twice daily and increased gradually as the blood pressure comes under control. The dose-response curve flattens out at 2.5–3.0 g/day and no further blood pressure reduction would be apparent at higher doses than these.

Side-effects. Because of the high frequency of side-effects, especially in the elderly, α-methyldopa can no longer be recommended as a suitable hypotensive agent in the elderly (see Table 8.7). Whilst α-methyldopa is said not to cause postural hypotension in young or middle-aged patients, it certainly can do so in the elderly.

Table 8.7 Side-effects attributable to α-methylodopa.

Weakness and lethargy*
Drowsiness
Depression*
Weight gain
Nasal congestion
Diarrhoea
Malabsorption
Nocturia*
Parkinsonism*
Jaundice→hepatitis→cirrhosis
Coomb's positive haemolytic anaemia
Impotence

* Special problems with the elderly.

Methyldopa's hypotensive action may be significantly potentiated by L-dopa therapy for Parkinsonism. The combination of L-dopa with a decarboxylase inhibitor accentuates this effect. Conversely, hypotensive activity may be reduced by tricyclic antidepressants, sympathomimetics, phenothiazines and the monoamine oxidase inhibitors.

Clonidine

A relatively recently introduced centrally acting hypotensive agent is clonidine. On a weight basis it is extremely potent. Whilst much discussion surrounds its exact mode of action, it seems to exert a significant stimulant effect upon central pre-synaptic receptors and adrenoreceptors with less action upon post-synaptic receptors. It is suggested that agonist activity within the brain stem increases inhibition of vasomotor sympathetic output.

Clonidine is well absorbed, has a relatively short half-life and its metabolites, which themselves may be active, are excreted by the renal route. Onset of action appears within 30 minutes following oral administration but in spite of this its use in hypertensive crises cannot be recommended because it may give rise to a transient increase in blood pressure. Initial dosage is usually 0.2 mg in divided doses and can be increased to 2.0 mg per day. Because of its short half-life the drug has to be administered on a 6-hourly basis, though a slow-release formulation may be given at night.

Side-effects. Dry mouth is almost invariable with clonidine though tolerance may occur with prolonged usage. Similarly, patients tend to develop tolerance to the sedative effects. Postural hypotension, though not exercise hypotension, may be a particular problem with some elderly subjects. As clonidine causes salt and water accumulation, cardiac failure may be precipitated in the compromised patient. In the presence of significant myocardial ischaemia arrhythmias may be a particular problem.

The most important problem related to clonidine therapy is rebound hypertension. This usually occurs following abrupt withdrawal though occasionally it may occur with gradual dosage reduction. The phenomenon seems to be related to excessive catecholamine activity and can be treated by a combination of α- and β-adrenergic blocking agents. The notoriously frequent non- or poor compliance of elderly patients limits the use of this drug.

Reserpine

There are many pharmacologically active derivatives of the **Rauwolfia** alkaloid of which reserpine is the best known. The hypotensive action of reserpine is twofold. First, by direct central action on the vasomotor centre it reduces sympathetic drive, and second, the drug depletes postganglionic adrenergic nerve endings of neurotransmitting catecholamines. It is poorly absorbed from the gastrointestinal tract, and has a long half-life. It lowers cardiac output and glomerular filtration rate, both very undesirable in the elderly patient.

The most serious problem with reserpine and the other Rauwolfia alkaloids is the production of severe depression which may lead to suicide. Reserpine has also been associated with the development of breast cancer. For all these reasons reserpine cannot be recommended.

Peripherally acting agents

Hypotensive agents acting on the peripheral autonomic nervous system comprise 2 pharmacologically distinct groups. The first or unselective group include agents such as hexamethonium, pentolinium and mecamylamine which block both parasympathetic and sympathetic components. The former action produces the severe postural, bladder, bowel and visual problems associated with the use of ganglion blockers. They are now no longer used and will not be discussed further. They have been replaced in clinical medicine by the second group—the so-called adrenergic neurone blocking agents.

Adrenergic neurone blocking agents

These agents all act by inhibiting the release of noradrenaline by the post-ganglionic adrenergic neurone, thus preventing transmission between the sympathetic nerve terminal and the effector cell. Thus the sympathetic tone maintaining some degree of vasoconstriction in the periphery is reduced. The higher the sympathetic tone, the greater the reduction produced by adrenergic blocking agents.

The main representatives of this group which are still in use include bethanidine, guanethedine and debrisoquine. There seem to be no differences in mode of action between these agents. They are all equally effective as hypotensive drugs though there are some pharmacokinetic differences which may influence the choice of agents in treating a long-term disease.

Bethanidine is well absorbed from the gastrointestinal tract, is effective quickly and rapidly excreted by the kidney (half-life 2 hours). Starting doses for elderly subjects should be 5 mg (half a tablet) three times daily. Maximum dose should be less than 200 mg daily. In renal impairment doses should be reduced considerably.

Guanethadine is poorly absorbed after oral administration, is extensively metabolized by the liver and is excreted in the urine and bile. Its approximate half-life is 40 hours which allows once-daily dosage. In the elderly, therapy should be started at 10 mg daily and adjustments made at no less than weekly intervals.

Debrisoquine is well absorbed, relatively quick in onset (4 hours) and has a half-life of approximately 12 hours. It is mainly eliminated by the kidneys. In the elderly with their reduced glomerular filtration a once-daily dose is usually adequate. A 1 mg starting dose is preferred and increments can be made at weekly intervals.

Side-effects. Adrenergic blockers produce similar side-effects to α-methyldopa, though the central nervous system complications are less frequent (see Table 8.8). In spite of claims to the contrary there are few significant differences between the individual agents—those said to produce most side-effects have been used longer.

The single most important problem is postural or exercise-induced hypotension. This limits their use in the elderly especially in individuals with cerebrovascular insufficiency. Equally, renal impairment is often exacerbated. Diarrhoea, particularly said to be associated with guanethidine, can be an intolerable condition for older patients who may have reduced mobility from other causes.

Table 8.8 Side-effects of adrenergic neurone blocking agents.

Postural and exercise hypotension
Reduce cardiac output
Lower renal blood flow
Diarrhoea
Nasal stuffiness
Dizziness
Depression
Weakness and lethargy

Vasodilating agents

Orally acting vasodilators have their main effect directly on the vascular smooth muscle of the peripheral resistance vessel. This action does not significantly involve any component of the autonomic nervous system, nor is central activity apparent. Because activity is so localized to vascular smooth muscle, side-effects related to the hypotensive activity are predictable whilst other effects are less frequent. The ideal vasodilator is not yet available but it is foreseen that in this area lies one of the main avenues for future research into hypertensive agents.

Hydrallazine

Hydrallazine is rapidly absorbed from the gastrointestinal tract into the plasma where it is bound (85%) to albumin. It undergoes metabolism in the gut wall and liver and metabolites are mainly excreted in the urine. Whilst its plasma half-life is short (<6 hours) its pharmacological effect is much longer. It has been suggested that arteriolar muscle binding may account for this phenomenon. Because of this it only requires twice daily administration.

The main problem with hydrallazine as a hypotensive agent is its capacity to produce a reflex tachycardia and to increase cardiac output, thus largely nullifying the vasodilator effects upon blood pressure. However, the prior use of a β-adrenergic blocking agent largely overcomes this problem. Thus, in general, hydrallazine should not be used as a sole hypotensive agent.

Doses initially should be small, especially in the presence of renal impairment, though hydrallazine often improves renal function. A usual starting dose in the elderly with prior β-blockade would be 25 mg twice daily, increasing by 25 mg a day at weekly intervals. Maximum doses would be in the range of 150–200 mg per day because side-effects are related to total dose.

Side-effects. Many adverse effects of hydrallazine can be minimized by β-blockade, by limiting maximum dosage and increasing dosage at weekly or longer intervals. Some of the effects are related to excess sympathetic stimulation. These would include reflex tachycardia and palpitations, sweating, nausea, headache, flushing and tremors. Angina can be potentiated and myocardial infarction simulted. It is contraindicated in the presence of any tachyarrhythmia.

In spite of increasing glomerular filtration rate hydrallazine sometimes causes sodium and water retention which usually respond to a simple diuretic. Of more moment is the production of a syndrome resembling rheumatoid disease or systemic lupus erythematosus. These side-effects are related to dose and duration of therapy. In the elderly the latter should not be too much of a problem, and the former can best be met by keeping total dose to below 200 mg per day.

Prazosin

This recently introduced drug has actions upon both vascular smooth muscle and α-adrenoceptors though this latter action is somewhat transient and ill-sustained. It is well absorbed though individuals may vary. Like most vasodilators it is selectively concentrated in the peripheral vasculature so that plasma half-life is short but hypotensive action is prolonged.

Initial dosage should be low, i.e. 0.5 mg preferably given with food prior to retiring. This precaution is to avoid or lessen the effects of sudden α-blockade (first dose effect) which may give rise to severe hypotension. It is wise to try the drug in an institutional setting so that this effect can be promptly treated. It does not usually recur after the first few initial doses as tolerance rapidly develops to the α-blocking effects.

Side-effects. Few side-effects have been recorded with this drug but this may be more related to lack of experience than intrinsic safety. The most severe problem, especially in elderly patients, is postural hypotension. Whilst it is gaining in popularity for treating young hypertensives this common side-effect precludes its use in the elderly.

Minoxidil

Less is known about the action of this agent compared with prazosin with which it has much in common. In keeping with its direct vasodilatation properties, it induces reflex increase in heart rate and cardiac output. It has been specifically recommended for use in hypertension associated with renal impairment where it usually increases glomerular filtration rate. Conversely, it does tend to cause sodium and water retention. At present it can only be recommended for treatment of severe hypertension with renal impairment when it should be combined with a diuretic and β-adrenergic blocking agent. It does not seem to cause significant postural hypotension, an important feature in the elderly.

Captopril

The recent introduction of an oral angiotensin-converting enzyme inhibitor, captopril, has added a new dimension to the management of hypertension. Initially introduced for the treatment of severe or refractory hypertension it is becoming more commonly used in mild to moderate disease. The primary action of captopril is inhibition of angiotensin-converting enzyme leading to a reduction in levels of the powerful vasocontrictor angiotensin II. However, captopril also lowers blood pressure in patients with low renin hypertension and recent work suggests that this is due to a direct peripheral vasodilating property.

Captopril causes a reduction in serum sodium (natriuretic effect) and an increase in serum potassium (possibly related to a reduction in aldosterone secretion or to reduction in renal function). In patients with hypertension and renal impairment who require high dose captopril further deterioration in renal function has been a limiting factor. As yet the effect of the age-related reduction in renal reserve in response to captopril and its adverse effects have not been evaluated. Until such studies are available captopril cannot be recommended as a firstline treatment for the elderly hypertensive.

Choice of anti-hypertensive agent

Once the decision to treat raised blood pressure has been made, the arrays of drugs available seems to be bewildering. However, as shown above the number of agents suitable for elderly patients forms a small group. Choice will depend critically upon the general condition of the patient, the presence of complications, other diseases and other medication. The concept of 'stepped' therapy has much to commend it. It is very important to start 'low' and to build up only after allowing sufficient time for full effects to become apparent; for example, the effects of a change in the dose of hydrallazine may not be fully manifest for 4 weeks.

For the uncomplicated essential hypertensive, it is best to commence with a single daily dose of a long-acting thiazide such as chlorthalidone. If, after a month, satisfactory control is not achieved, a cardioselective β-blocker should be added. Probably the best agent would be atenolol, which may be given as a slow-release formulation once daily. In the very rare event of inadequate control with this regimen a peripheral vasodilator, hydrallazine or minoxidil, can be added.

The uncomplicated elderly hypertensive is however the exception. A detailed investigation of the patient should be carried out before commencing treatment. Unfortunately, the first appearance of cardiac failure may follow the institution of a β-blocker and this situation does little to ensure the

Table 8.9. Choice of agent for the complicated elderly hypertensive. (Modified from James (1979) with the author's permission.)

Disease	Stage 1	Stage 2	Stage 3	Comments
Angina	β-blocker	Thiazide	Clonidine	Avoid peripheral vasodilators
Anxiety	β-blocker	Thiazide	Vasodilator	β-blockers help symptoms
Arthritis	Thiazide	Vasodilator	Spironolactone	Avoid hydrallazine
Cardiac failure	Thiazide	Vasodilator	β-blocker	Spironolactone alternative Stage 2
Cerebrovascular insufficiency	Thiazide	Vasodilator	Atenolol	Avoid α-methyldopa, clonidine and lipid-soluble β-blockers
COAD or asthma	Thiazide	Clonidine	Spironolactone	Avoid β-blockers and reserpine
Depression	Thiazide	Vasodilator	Atenolol	Avoid central agents and lipid-soluble β-blockers
Diabetes	Loop diuretic	Vasodilator	β-blocker	Avoid thiazide
Gout	β-blocker	Vasodilator	Loop diuretic	Avoid thiazide
Parkinson's disease	β-blocker	Thiazide	Vasodilator	Avoid α-methyldopa and reserpine
Peptic ulceration	β-blocker	Vasodilator	Thiazide	Avoid potassium and reserpine
Peripheral vascular disease	Thiazide	Minoxidil	Labetolol	Avoid β-blockers
Prostatism	Inadapamide	β-blocker	Vasodilator	Avoid all diuretics

patient's confidence or his satisfactory compliance. In the light of present experience, stepped schemes for the complicated eldely hypertensive are outlined in Table 8.9. The recommendations here deliberately err on the side of conservatism. Drugs that have been in use for a number of years are to be preferred because contraindications, side-effects, etc., are well known. The routine clinical situation is no place for avant garde experimentation.

REFERENCES AND FURTHER READING

Ahlquist R.P. (1949) A study of adrenotropic receptors. *American Journal of Physiology* **153**, 586–600.

Breckenbridge A. (1982) Captopril—worldwide clinical experience. *British Journal of Clinical Pharmacology* **14** (Suppl. 2), 65S.

James I.M. (1979) Hypertension: selecting the right drug. *Modern Geriatrics* **9**, 80–5.

Kannel W.B. & Gordon T. (1974) *The Framingham Study: an Epidemiological Investigation of Cardiovascular Disease.* US Government Printing Office, Washington, D.C.

Lands A.M., Arnold A., McAinliffe J.P., Ludana F.P. & Brown T.G. (1967) Differentiation of receptor systems activated by sympathetic amines. *Nature (London)* **214**, 597–8.

MacGregor G.A., Banks R.A., Markandu N.D., Bayliss J. & Roulston J. (1983) Lack of effect of betablocker on flat dose response to thiazide in hypertension. *British medical Journal* **286**, 1535–8.

National Institutes of Health (1978) *Report of the Joint National Committee on Detection, Evaluation and the Treatment of High Blood Pressure.* DHEW Publ. No. (NIH) 77–1088: Bethesda, Md.

Opie L.H. (1980) Drugs and the heart. *Lancet* **1**, 693–8.

Thomas J.P. & Thomson W.H. (1983) Comparison of thiazides and amiloride in the treatment of moderate hypertension. *British medical Journal* **286**, 2015–18.

Chapter Nine
Cardiovascular System—
Treatment of Arrhythmias

M.D.W. LYE

OVERVIEW

The high frequency of both transient and sustained cardiac arrhythmias in the elderly is discussed in terms of symptoms and potential dangers. The high incidence of arrhythmias in the otherwise healthy elderly is described.

Non-drug management of cardiac arrhythmias is discussed in relation to particular precipitating factors. A classification of the more commonly used anti-arrhythmic agents is given with pharmacokinetic and pharmacodynamic data allowing a rational choice of treatment.

Disturbances of cardiac rhythm are common and of clinical importance in geriatric patients. In the elderly, whilst most arrhythmias are associated with intrinsic heart disease, they are often uncovered or potentiated by non-cardiac factors. Their significance may lie more in revealing the precipitating cause than representing severe heart disease. The opposite holds true for young and middle-aged individuals where arrhythmias are closely associated with underlying heart disease. Thus, arrhythmias in the elderly often carry a better prognosis and better possibilities for therapeutic intervention than they do in the young.

INCIDENCE

The prevalence of arrhythmias in the elderly varies considerably depending on the populations observed and methods used. Thus, hospital patients invariably show more arrhythmias than patients in the community, even after taking into account the higher prevalence of heart disease in the former. Continuous monitoring of the electrocardiogram (ECG) in coronary care units or by portable ambulatory monitoring systems reveals a very high incidence of significant arrhythmias which in the main increase with increasing age. It is useful, therefore, to separate arrhythmias found by standard ECG (sustained arrhythmias) from those recorded only by continuous methods (transient arrhythmias).

Sustained arrhythmias

Ectopic beats of varying frequency and of atrial or ventricular origin are quite common, perhaps occurring in approximately 1 in 4 elderly persons. They are sometimes, though not always, associated with underlying heart disease. Sustained atrial fibrillation occurs in approximately 5% of old people living at home and 15% of elderly patients admitted to hospital. A much lower incidence of atrial flutter is reported.

Ventricular arrhythmias are much less frequent than supraventricular ones and are invariably associated, even in the very old, with intrinsic cardiac disease (ischaemia or amyloidosis). Not infrequently ventricular arrhythmias, especially tachycardia, are associated with digitalis intoxication (see p. 84).

Bradyarrhythmias, sometimes associated with tachyarrhythmias—the sick sinus syndrome—increase with advancing age. There is perhaps one exception and that is first degree atrio-ventricular (A-V) block—this is more common in young adults, especially those of an athletic nature. Up to 3% of old people demonstrate right bundle branch block whereas only approximately 1% show the left variety.

Transient arrhythmias

The relatively recent introduction of portable methods of recording ECGs (which allows individuals to continue their normal everyday activities) has revealed a much higher incidence of arrhythmia in populations of all ages. It seems that many activities undertaken by both young and old cause considerable stress and precipitate significant tachycardia or arrhythmias. Recordings from a healthy individual driving through city traffic or delivering lectures have given the author considerable cause for personal concern! Ambulatory monitoring has shown that approximately 50% of elderly healthy subjects show atrial ectopics at a rate of one or more per thousand QRS complexes. The comparable figure for ventricular ectopics is about 30%. Many ectopics occur in small runs. Approximately 10% of healthy old people manifest significant runs of supraventricular tachycardia and 1% show runs of ventricular tachycardia. Many ventricular ectopic beats in these individuals are multifocal in origin.

Transient bradyarrhythmias are much less common in healthy elderly subjects than the tachyarrhythmias. Mixed tachy- and brady-arrhythmias are intermediate in incidence.

Carotid sinus syndrome is said to be common in the elderly and is invariably associated with severe atherosclerosis. Recently both these conclusions have been questioned. Carotid sinus hypersensitivity may be demonstrated in up to 10% of healthy people and whilst it is twice as frequent in men it probably does not increase significantly with increasing age.

SIGNIFICANCE OF ARRHYTHMIAS

The relationship of signs and symptoms to cardiac arrythmias is not simple. The important variable to be considered is the cardiac output which maintains haemodynamic integrity. Thus, a healthy young individual can maintain a normal cardiac output when the heart rate varies between 40 and 170 beats per minute by increasing or decreasing respectively the stroke volume. There is an age-related reduction in this range so that healthy old people can only maintain normal cardiac output between 45 and 120 beats per minute. Of more importance however is the state of the myocardium and its ability to respond to different heart rates. Thus, the ischaemic heart may be unable to respond to heart rates above 90 beats per minute so cardiac output drops and cardiac failure may be precipitated.

Loss of atrio-ventricular synchrony with atrial tachycardias, fibrillation or block may lead to reduction in cardiac output. Again the function of ventricular myocardium is crucial. Loss of coordinated A-V valve closure may be more important than loss of A-V filling in the absence of coordinated atrial contraction.

Sustained arrhythmias

The isolated finding of a sustained supraventricular arrhythmia unassociated with any haemodynamic deficit, nor with symptoms in old people probably requires no specific therapy. If there is associated pathology, either cardiac, e.g. congestive failure, or non-cardiac, e.g. respiratory infection, treatment of the underlying condition frequently resolves the arrhythmia without recourse to potentially hazardous anti-arrhythmic therapy.

Ventricular arrhythmias, apart from isolated ectopic beats, invariably indicate significant cardiac disease and contribute to the haemodynamic disturbance. Thus, they require treatment. Bundle branch block does not in itself require therapy, but indicates the need for further investigation. Thus, left bundle branch block is usually an indication of ventricular ischaemia and right bundle branch block may be the only sign of recurrent minor pulmonary emboli. If, however, bundle branch block and fascicular block occur together, the patient may well develop complete heart block after a variable time lapse, so follow-up is recommended.

First degree heart block (prolonged P-R interval) does not produce symptoms. It may be associated with heart disease but more often is related to digitalis or anti-arrhythmic therapy or with hypoxia. It is also non-progressive as is second degree block of the Mobitz Type I variety (Wenckebach). Both types therefore carry a good prognosis. Mobitz Type II block is, however, an indication of severe organic heart disease and often progresses to complete heart block.

Third degree or complete heart block is a serious condition usually producing symptoms requiring treatment. Occasionally, some individuals are asymptomatic for a variable time but they are the exceptions. The incidence of sustained complete block increases with advancing age. In the elderly the aetiology is most likely to be bilateral bundle branch fibrosis without significant ischaemia. Invariably complete block leads to Stokes-Adams attacks and treatment (pacemaker insertion) is thus urgently required.

Transient arrhythmias

The finding by ambulatory monitoring that transient arrhythmias occur frequently in otherwise healthy asymptomatic old people makes therapeutic or prognostic decisions difficult in symptomatic patients.

The initial thought that transient arrhythmias could account for the vast majority of 'funny turns', 'queer dos', falls, etc., in patients whose symptoms could not be related to other pathologies can no longer be sustained. The cause and effect in this situation are difficult to relate although lack of correlation between symptoms and arrhythmias does not exclude cause and effect. If there is good temporal relationship, however, it is worth instituting appropriate anti-arrhythmic therapy.

Third degree transient block, runs of supraventricular tachycardia or multifocal ventricular ectopics are most likely to cause symptoms. Runs of atrial fibrillation in the absence of cardiac failure are usually innocuous.

MANAGEMENT OF ARRHYTHMIAS

The identification of an arrhythmia in an asymptomatic patient does not warrant the immediate administration of an anti-arrhythmic drug. The type of arrhythmia and its relation, if any, to symptoms, signs or potential dangers must be considered (see above). In the elderly many arrhythmias are due to non-cardiac events. Thus, atrial fibrillation or tachycardia may be due to infection, especially respiratory or to thyrotoxicosis. Treatment of a precipitating cause usually resolves the arrhythmia. Hypertension and cardiac failure are potent arrhythmogenic conditions in the elderly.

Drugs are particularly likely to precipitate arrhythmias especially in old people with minor degrees of ischaemia. The most common arrhythmogenic drug in clinical practice is digitalis (see p. 83). Some other agents associated with arrhythmias are listed in Table 9.1, but this list is by no means exhaustive. Excessive or heightened sympathetic tone may be associated with arrhythmias, especially those arising above the ventricle. Thus, coffee, cigarettes and cigars, alcohol and sexual activity have all been shown to produce various arrhythmias. In this situation the patient must get his priorities in some sort of order.

Table 9.1 Non-cardiac causes of atrial fibrillation.

Drugs	Metabolic Anaesthetic agents Quinidine Tricyclic antidepressants Exogenous catecholamines Fluorocarbon propellants (inhalers)
Metabolic	Thyrotoxicosis Anoxia Hypercapnia Hypo- and hyper-kalaemia Acidosis Hypercalcaemia
Pulmonary emboli	
Chronic obstructive airways disease	
Cerebrovascular disease (acute)	

Mechanical manoeuvres

Carotid sinus massage has been used to terminate certain paroxysmal supraventricular tachycardias. Whilst often successful, it cannot be wholeheartedly recommended in the elderly because of carotid sinus hypersensitivity, or the not uncommon complication ventricular standstill or fibrillation. Further, in some elderly patients cerebral perfusion may depend on only one carotid artery which obviously should not be compromised.

Electroconversion

Electric counter shock (cardioversion) synchronized for the ECG is an effective method for converting atrial fibrillation/flutter or ventricular tachycardia to normal sinus rhythm. In the elderly, however, complications, cardiac or otherwise, are common and its use should, therefore, be restricted to serious haemodynamically compromised individuals or those who have not responded to drugs. This should be carried out only in a specialized centre.

Cardiac pacemakers have improved markedly in the last few years and have completely supplanted drugs in the treatment of bradyarrhythmias. Indeed, they are now so sophisticated that they are increasingly being used for treatment of tachyarrhythmias by overdrive suppression. This, however, still remains a specialized technique. No patient is too old, too ill or too confused not to be given the benefit of a pacemaker if indicated. If there is doubt about the significance of transient bradyarrhythmias, especially sick sinus syndrome, a week or two's trial of a temporary transvenous pacemaker will resolve the issue. Pacemakers may need to be used in conjunction with anti-arrhythmic drugs in such conditions as the bradycardia—tachycardia syndrome.

ANTI-ARRHYTHMIC DRUGS

The plethora of anti-arrhythmic drugs has spawned several classification schemes. Unfortunately, none of these is entirely satisfactory. The most general scheme is that proposed by Vaughan Williams (Table 9.2) and modified by Hoffman.

Table 9.2 Electrophysiological classification of anti-arrhythmic agents (after Vaughan Williams 1971).

Class	Agents
I	Local anaesthetics with membrane-stabilizing effects
	(a) Quinidine, procainamide, disopyramide, carbamazine
	(b) Lignocaine (lidocaine), phenytoin, mexiletine
II	β-adrenergic blocking agents and bretylium (also α-blocker)
III	Amiodarone (bretylium)
IV	Calcium antagonist, verapamil

Class I drugs in high concentration are local anaesthetics and have membrane stabilizing properties. Class IA drugs mainly work by inhibiting fast sodium channels and class IB drugs, in addition, shorten rather than prolong the phase III action potential and the refractory period.

Class II drugs all act by blocking β-adrenergic receptors thus reducing cardiac sympathetic stimulation. Bretylium also has an α-blocking effect.

The sole representative of the class III group is amiodarone which prolongs the action potential and refractory period without altering the rate of rise of the action potential. Bretylium acts like a class III drug on the ventricles but not the atria. Verapamil is a calcium channel antagonist which blocks the slow inward calcium ion current and is the main class IV anti-arrhythmic drug.

Choice of anti-arrhymic agent

There is no safe anti-arrhythmic drug which can be used for all types of arrhythmia. The choice of drug must be based upon the type of arrhythmia and its presumed (or known) electrophysiological pathogenesis, the clinical state of the heart, previous response to other anti-arrhythmics and other concurrent drugs. There is a wide individual variation in the response between patients with similar arrhythmias.

It cannot be over-emphasized that if an arrhythmia fails to respond to standard therapy expert cardiological advice should be sought. More detailed investigations often reveal that the arrhythmia is not what it seems to be. The wise geriatrician will also question compliance, perhaps by measuring drug blood levels.

Supraventricular tachycardias

The main aim of the treatment is to slow the ventricular response, usually with digitalis (the treatment of choice for fast atrial fibrillation). In atrial flutter digitalis may convert the arrhythmia to atrial fibrillation. If digitalis does not work, the addition of verapamil or a β-blocker is often useful.

In paroxysmal atrial tachycardia, where carotid massage is contraindicated, as usual in the elderly, intravenous verapamil is useful. After restoring sinus rhythm oral disopyramide should maintain it. In chronic or sustained supraventricular tachycardia digitalis usually controls the ventricular rate. If unsuccessful, oral verapamil should be added. In young patients the addition of a β-blocker is indicated, but in the elderly this often produces cardiac failure.

In the Wolff-Parkinson White syndrome with episodes of paroxysmal tachycardia, digoxin must not be used as it is likely to precipitate ventricular fibrillation. Verapamil or amiodarone may be beneficial but it is wise to seek expert advice at an early stage.

Ventricular tachycardia

In the acute form especially in association with left ventricular failure (the usual situation), direct current counter-shock is indicated even in elderly patients. Oral disopyramide should be continued prophylactically. If there are contraindications to countershock or there is no overriding urgency, intravenous disopyramide should be administered.

Recurrent ventricular tachycardia, not responding to disopyramide is best managed with a β-blocker or procainamide. In the presence of heart failure the latter drug would be preferred, though if available amiodarone is more effective. Bretylium may be a useful alternative. In the phase of acute myocardial infarction lignocaine (lidocaine) infusion is used both in treatment and prophylactically against ventricular arrhythmia. Verapamil or disopyramide may be similarly used for suppressing supraventricular activity in this situation.

Bradyarrhythmias

In the acute form following myocardial infarction, subcutaneous atropine remains useful, though it may occasionally provoke ventricular ectopic activity. Isoprenaline in effective dose invariably does. If the bradyarrhythmia persists, it is best treated by transvenous pacing which is the treatment of choice for all heart blocks producing symptoms. If the condition becomes chronic, a permanent pacemaker should be inserted.

In the sick sinus or bradycardia—tachycardia syndromes it is important not to abolish the ectopic activity without first maintaining a good underlying heart rate by a pacemaker. Whilst man cannot live on ectopics alone, they are certainly useful if the basic ventricular rate is 20 per minute!

Dosage schedules for the various agents discussed are given in Table 9.3, with their non-cardiac side-effects. It is beyond the scope of this review to discuss cardiac side-effects. Details of doses are given as a guide only. The manufacturer's literature and the individual patient's condition should be considered. Regimens for digitalis and β-adrenergic blocking agents are considered on p. 80 and p. 110, respectively.

Table 9.3 Details of some commonly used anti-arrhythmic agents.

Drug	Route	Dose	Comments
Amiodarone	Oral	200–600 mg daily	CI in A-V block SE deposition in skin and cornea. Thyroid function
Atropine	i.v. or s.c.	0.25–2.0 mg 2-hourly	SE initial tachycardia occasionally ventricular fibrillation. Atropinism
Bretylium	i.v. or i.m.	5 mg/kg bolus and 12-hourly	SE hypotension, weakness, parotid pain
Disopyramide	i.v. Oral	2 mg/kg 100 mg 6-hourly	SE anticholinergic, gastric upsets
Isoprenaline	i.v.	2 mg infusion	SE ventricular arrhythmias
Lignocaine (lidocaine)	i.v.	50 mg load 1–5 mg/min infusion	CI liver dysfunction SE drowsiness, confusion (dose related)
Procainamide	i.v. Oral	100 mg load 2–20 mg/min infusion 1.0 g load 1.5 g daily	CI shock, heart failure, A-V block SE hypotension, drug fever, lupus
Verapamil	i.v. Oral	5–10 mg bolus 80–240 mg daily	CI A-V block SE gastric upset, postural hypotension

CI = contraindication
SE = side-effect

REFERENCES AND FURTHER READING

Harrison D.C., Fitzgerald J.W. & Winkle R.A. (1976) Ambulatory electrocardiography for diagnosis and treatment of cardiac arrhythmias. *New England Journal of Medicine* **294,** 373–80.

Jaffe A.S. (1980) Cardiac arrhythmias. In Freitag J.J. & Miller L.W. (Eds) *Manual of Medical Therapeutics*. 23rd Edition, p. 99. Little Brown & Co, Boston.

Kumana C. & Hamer J. (1979) Anti-arrhythmic drugs. In Hamer J. (ed.) *Drugs for Heart Disease*, pp. 44–147. Chapman & Hall, London.

Melman K.L. (Ed.) (1974) *Cardiovascular Drug Therapy*. F.A. Davis & Co., Philadelphia.

Opie L.H. (1980) Drugs and the heart: IV Antiarrhythmic agents. *Lancet* **1,** 861–8.

Sherman H., Sandberg S., Fineberg H.V. (1982) Exponential increase in age-specific prevalence of ventricular dysrhythmia among males. *Journal of Chronic Diseases* **35,** 743–50.

Vaughan Williams E.M. (1971) Electrophysiological basis for a rational approach to anti-dysrhythmia drug therapy. In Di Palma J.R. (Ed.) *Advances in Drug Research*, p. 824. McGraw-Hill Book Co. Inc., New York.

Chapter Ten
Central Nervous System—Anxiolytics and Hypnotics

D.E. HYAMS

OVERVIEW

This chapter discusses many drugs which may affect cerebral function and therefore the mental and psychomotor state of elderly patients.

A short account of the present usage of such drugs is followed by a systematic presentation of various groups of drugs, punctuated by paragraphs describing the management of relevant clinical problems in the elderly. The aim is to place the use of drug therapy in a proper clinical perspective, discouraging unnecessary administration of medications where other methods of management are more appropriate, and indicating the best ways to approach drug therapy where it clearly is appropriate.

PSYCHOTROPIC DRUGS

Patterns of usage in the elderly

Chapters 10–13 consider a wide variety of drugs which are capable of affecting cerebral function: they comprise the most common group of drugs prescribed in general medical practice. In the USA family physicians see clinically significant psychiatric features in 15% or more of their patients and prescribe 40% of all psychotherapeutic agents used in that country. In the UK 61% of psychotropic drugs are first prescribed by general practitioners; of all patients taking tablets in the UK, during a 2-week survey in 1972, 10% were taking tranquillizers, sedatives or hypnotics and 1% antidepressants. The rate of prescribing such drugs was said to be increasing faster than for any other drug group; in 1972, 27.2% of all NHS prescriptions written in the UK were for 'central nervous system' drugs; of these, two-thirds (17.7% of the total 256 million prescriptions for all drugs) were for psychoactive drugs. It is interesting to compare this figure with that for the USA for the same year: psychoactive drug prescriptions comprised 16% of the total 1400 million prescriptions for all drugs; it was estimated in 1972 that 22% of American adults used a psychotropic prescription drug, and 12% more used an over-the-counter drug for similar indications.

Focusing now on the elderly, in the USA people aged 65 and over comprise 11.4% of the population but receive 31% of all prescriptions written. It is likely that over one-third of these are for psychoactive drugs, particularly minor tranquillizers, sedatives and hypnotics, which are used by greater proportions of elderly persons than other age groups. American men aged 60–74 years are 4 times as likely to have used psychoactive drugs as are those aged 18–29 years; women show similar but less pronounced differences.

Only 5% of Americans aged 65 and older are in institutions, but 60–75% of the institutionalized elderly are said to be receiving psychotropic medications, and 60% of these are antipsychotic drugs. A recent Department of Health, Welfare and Education (DHEW) report on over a quarter of a million nursing home patients in the USA showed an average use of 6.1 drugs per patient per day; 40% of patients were receiving 7 or more drugs. 46.9% of the patients were receiving antipsychotic drugs. A one-year study of 5902 Medicaid patients in 173 Tennessee nursing homes revealed that 43% of them received antipsychotic drugs, 9% on a regular daily basis.

In Canada a survey of 1431 chronically ill elderly persons referred for long-term institutional care revealed that psychoactive drugs had been prescribed for about one-quarter of them, mainly to provide night-time sedation or sleep. Antidepressants were prescribed infrequently, even in severely depressed patients, and inappropriate use of tranquillizers was noted. In another Canadian survey of geriatric out-patient practice, 26% of 226 patients were found to be on psychotropic drugs; in 10% of these the drugs were regarded as the cause of the patients' symptoms. In a study of 731 persons in continuing care institutions in London, Ontario, nearly 20% were receiving 6 or more medications daily.

In the UK 15% of the population are aged 65 and over, but about 30% of prescriptions are written for them. Psychotropic drug prescribing increases sharply with age and features prominently in published surveys.

General principles

Diagnosis of mental disorders in old age

At any age, psychiatric diagnosis may be difficult; witness the effort put into the classification of psychiatric illness over many years. Clinical pictures are rarely 'pure', and the multiple pathology of old age may include overlapping mental disturbances as well as physical disorders; furthermore, the drugs used for physical disease may interact with those used for mental symptoms, and vice versa. The interaction may or may not be deleterious.

Accurate diagnosis is, therefore, of utmost importance in elderly patients; the aphorism 'diagnosis before treatment' is never more mandatory than in the practice of geriatric medicine. It must be appreciated that many different diseases (including drug-induced disease or symptoms) may present in non-specific ways in old age, quite differently from the 'standard' textbook descriptions; but the difficulties of making a diagnosis are no excuse for neglecting to arrive at one (or, more likely, at several). Only then can rational drug treatment be prescribed and only then is it possible to live up to one of the most fundamental principles of medicine at any age: 'the patient should never be the worse for seeing a physician'. One salutary example of what may otherwise happen was the finding that in four mid-Western state hospitals in the USA the major tranquillizers thioridazine and chlorpromazine were the most commonly used psychotropic agents, but with little regard for diagnosis.

Choosing the therapeutic regimen

Age-related changes in the pharmacokinetics (absorption, distribution, metabolism, excretion) and pharmacodynamics (target organ responsiveness) may influence the response of the elderly to drugs and the nature and incidence of side-effects.

Most physicians agree that the elderly brain appears to be more responsive ('sensitive' is an unsatisfactory term) to drugs acting on the central nervous system. Various explanations have been offered: progressive loss of cerebral cortical neurons, accumulation of lipofuscin pigment in brain cells, changes in neuronal metabolism, cerebral blood flow, neuro-endocrine changes, and changes in receptor number. It must always be remembered that alcohol interacts with many commonly prescribed psychoactive drugs and may enhance their toxicity, even to the point of death. The frequent use of over-the-counter medications, especially analgesics, must also be noted.

Dosage

It will be obvious from the foregoing that great care must be taken with regard to dosage in the elderly. Small doses are usually required, at least initially, and increments should be small and gradual. Exceptions might include phenytoin for epilepsy (see below).

In some circumstances, side-effects may be put to good use but in general they are unwanted and may limit the usefulness of the drug.

Wise choice of a drug will include consideration of how much of an unwanted side-effect can be accepted in order to achieve the main desired effect; for example, some antidepressants have less anticholinergic properties than others in the same chemical class or group. On the other hand, overall clinical experience with the former may be much greater than with the latter, and this will allow a balanced judgement to vary according to the individual patient.

It is a good general rule to know how to use a few of these drugs well and these chapters will concentrate on those drugs for which there is sufficient experience or promise in regard to use in elderly patients. They are best used individually and the usual principle of minimal drug regimen in the elderly should apply, i.e. use the least number of drugs, in the smallest effective doses, for the shortest possible time. Combinations of psychotropic drugs should be avoided: it is preferable to use a drug with beneficial secondary properties; for example, an antidepressant may also have a sedative effect and thus be useful in the management of agitated depression.

In one study from a psychogeriatric service, 16% of 236 patients admitted had adverse effects from psychotropic drugs and improved rapidly when the drugs were withdrawn. It is clear that frequent review of the prescription of psychotherapeutic agents in the elderly is mandatory, and routine repeat prescriptions should be avoided.

ANXIOLYTIC DRUGS, SEDATIVES AND HYPNOTICS

Anti-anxiety drugs (see Table 10.1) are primarily central nervous system depressants which may be sedative in low or moderate doses and act as hypnotics in higher doses.

The World Health Organization definition of 'anxiolytic sedatives' is: 'substances which reduce pathological anxiety, tension and agitation without therapeutic effects on cognitive or perceptual processes'.

Table 10.1 Anxiolytic drugs.

Benzodiazepines
Meprobamate
Miscellaneous (β-blockers, antihistamines, etc.)

Anxiety in the elderly usually presents in a different way from anxiety at younger ages: it is more likely to produce somatic complaints (restlessness, hypochondriasis, insomnia, and perhaps anorexia or compulsive eating). Severe acute anxiety is rare in old age. Agitation may accompany depression and these two disorders need treatment together and will be dealt with later in this chapter.

Benzodiazepines (see Table 10.2)

This group of drugs is the major class of anxiolytic agents used at all ages. The widespread popularity of these drugs in the 20 years since their introduction may be attributed to their relative safety at normal doses (and even in overdose); their versatility as anti-anxiety agents at sub-hypnotic doses, and their infrequent interference with hepatic drug-metabolizing enzyme systems (which means that problems due to interaction with other drugs are unlikely). All these properties are advantages over barbiturates, especially in the elderly (in whom barbiturates should be avoided), and account for the 'benzodiazepine bonanza' of recent years, with new introductions becoming ever more frequent.

Benzodiazepines may be divided into long- and short-acting drugs (see Table 10.2). The long-acting group have long plasma half-lives and/or form long-acting active metabolites with half-lives up to 200 hours; by contrast, the short-acting drugs are conjugated to form inactive substances which are excreted by the kidneys. It is obvious that the most appropriate benzodiazepines for the elderly are the short-acting ones; this is especially true in view of the evidence that the elderly brain is more responsive to certain of

Table 10.2 Benzodiazepines.

				Pharmacological changes in old age	
Class by duration of effect	Drug name	Plasma half-life ($T_{\frac{1}{2}}$ (h))	Active metabolite(s)	Increased receptor sensitivity	Pharmacokinetics
Short-acting	Oxazepam	5–10	No	Probably	No change
	Temazepam	6–8	Very little oxazepam	Probably	No change
	Lorazepam	8–20	No	Probably	Conflicting evidence
Long-acting	Diazepam	20–90	Yes*	Demonstrated	Decreases in protein binding, rate of metabolism and free plasma clearance
	Chlordiazepoxide	5–30	Yes*	Probably	Increased elimination $T_{\frac{1}{2}}$
	Nitrazepam	20–38	Probably	Demonstrated	No change
	Flurazepam	1–4	Yes**	Probably	Probably changed
	Medazepam	10–24	Yes*	Probably	Probably changed
	Prazepam	100	Yes*	Probably	Not known
	Chlorazepate§ (pro-drug)	—	Yes*		
	Clobazam	48	Yes†		

* Longest-acting metabolite is nordiazepam (desmethyldiazepam), plasma $T_{\frac{1}{2}} = 36–200$ h.

** Desalkylflurazepam, plasma $T_{\frac{1}{2}} = 47–100$ h.

§ Absorbed after conversion to nordiazepam at acid pH, absorption slowed in achlorhydric subjects.

† Desmethylclobazam; multiple doses lead to washout half-life 69 h in elderly women, 326 h in elderly men.

the long-acting agents (diazepam, nitrazepam and flurazepam). In the Boston Collaborative Drug Survey (1973), the incidence of drowsiness following diazepam and chlordiazepoxide increased with age, and was more than twice as common in patients over 70 years as in patients below 40 years. This effect is less apparent in smokers. Thus, the short-acting drugs oxazepam, lorazepam or temazepam are being increasingly recommended for elderly patients requiring benzodiazepine therapy.

Nevertheless, diazepam continues to be used extensively: in the UK it accounted for 4.3% of all prescriptions written in 1977, making it the most widely prescribed of all drugs in the UK. In the USA, where benzodiazepines are by far the most common anti-anxiety agents prescribed, it has been estimated that 1 in 10 adult Americans will receive a benzodiazepine (most often diazepam) during any given one-year period. Clorazepate potassium has effects akin to those of diazepam, and is too long-acting to be appropriate for the elderly. Clobazam does not impair psychomotor performance and coordination, but its long duration of effect is a disadvantage. Nitrazepam and flurazepam will be discussed later, as hypnotics.

Short-acting benzodiazepines

Oxazepam (Serax, *USA;* Serenid-D, *UK*). Synthesized in 1961, and available in the USA since 1965, this drug is of intermediate potency between chlordiazepoxide and diazepam, but is less toxic than either—repeated administration does not lead to significant drug accumulation. Its half-life is 5–10 hours and its metabolites are inactive. Its pharmacokinetics show no change in old age or in the presence of parenchymal liver disease.

There are few studies directly comparing oxazepam against another benzodiazepine or a placebo in geriatric patients.

Dose: 10 mg up to 4 times daily; if necessary, cautiously increase to 15 mg.

Lorazepam (Ativan, *USA*, *UK*). This drug is a 2-chloro-derivative of oxazepam; much of what has been said about oxazepam applies to lorazepam also, but it is much more potent on a mg-for-mg basis and has a plasma half-life of 8–20 hours. Unlike oxazepam, it may also be given intravenously for premedication purposes; but for routine oral use oxazepam is to be preferred, since its onset of action is faster and its duration of action less prolonged.

Oral dose: 0.5–2 mg daily in divided doses.

Temazepam (Euhypnos, *UK* Restoril, *USA*). This drug is N-methyloxazepam, and is also the 3-hydroxy derivative of diazepam. A little oxazepam is formed as an active metabolite of temazepam, but the overall effect is still that of a short-acting benzodiazepine, half-life 6–8 hours. Its use as a hypnotic will be considered further below.

New benzodiazepines which may prove to have use in particular anxiety situations include *halazepam*, *clobazam*, *ketazolam*, *camazepam* and the triazolobenzodiazepine *alprazolam*; but halazepam may impair motor co-ordination in the elderly and clobazam has a long half-life.

General principles in the use of benzodiazepines

Do not prescribe until it is clear that such medication is really needed. Look for underlying mental and physical problems (depression or dementia may be aggravated by benzodiazepines), and use reassurance and psychotherapy as far as possible before resorting to these drugs. Remember that one eminent psychiatrist sees only 'the rarest justification' for the use of benzodiazepines during daytime hours (Oswald 1979). Be aware of any other central nervous system-depressant drugs the patient is taking.

Use short courses; do not prescribe benzodiazepines for long periods continuously since dependence is well recognized, if uncommon.

Avoid:

(a) antacids, since absorption falls off when gastric pH exceeds 7.4;
(b) alcohol, which potentiates sedative side-effects;
(c) driving until dosage is stabilized.

Withdraw the drug gradually rather than suddenly.

Meprobamate (Equanil, Miltown)

This drug, derived from the muscle relaxant mephenesin, was the first modern anxiolytic agent, introduced a quarter of a century ago. It is weaker than benzodiazepam which has largely superseded it; but it still finds favour as a hypnotic (see below).

Miscellaneous

Antihistamines are best reserved for allergy. They often produce confusion in the elderly.

Barbiturates should be avoided in the elderly.

β-blockers modify peripheral physical aspects of anxiety but do not improve the anxiety itself.

Thioridazine (Mellaril, *USA*; Melleril, *UK*) may help but is best used for the agitation which may be associated with depression.

MANAGEMENT OF INSOMNIA AND USE OF HYPNOTICS

Before considering the use of hypnotic drugs it is essential to evaluate most carefully a complaint of 'insomnia' in an elderly patient. Sleep patterns alter in middle life: sleep lessens and is more interrupted, and insomnia becomes a more common symptom thereafter. One result is that 39% of all hypnotics prescribed in the USA in 1977 were for patients aged over 60 years. Yet the incidence of complaints of insomnia does not decrease proportionately with the increase in the prescription of hypnotic drugs; and morbidity increases as the side-effects of the hypnotics take their toll. It is worth noting that in one survey in the UK 70% of the prescriptions for hypnotics in general practice had been written by the receptionist on behalf of the practitioner, compared with 22% for other drugs.

Judicious management as indicated by an analysis of 'insomnia', as set out in Table 10.3, will often obviate the need for hypnotic drugs. In some

Table 10.3 Causes of insomnia in old age.

Bodily discomfort	Pain, pruritus, distended bladder or rectum, dyspnoea, nausea, uncomfortable bed/room, room temperature
Over-stimulation	Tea, coffee late in the day
Sedation or 'cat-napping' during the day	
Chronic obstructive lung disease	
Sleep-apnoea syndrome	
Affective disorder	Anxiety, depression
Acute confusion	Underlying disease or inappropriate medication
Dementia (chronic brain syndrome)	Any or all of the above may coexist
	Restlessness

instances the need will be more for a tranquillizer than for a true hypnotic; for example, in anxiety a sub-hypnotic dose of a benzodiazepine may be adequate; and for motor restlessness meprobamate may be useful (see below). If chronic obstructive lung disease or sleep-apnoea is present, sedative-hypnotics may be dangerous, even lethal; protriptyline may be of benefit for sleep-apnoea.

Before resorting to hypnotics, it should be appreciated that they do not necessarily produce a 'physiological' sleep, i.e. sleep of normal quality. This is particularly important in regard to rapid-eye-movement (REM) sleep, during which dreaming occurs, and slow-wave (deep or Stage IV) sleep. Both REM and slow-wave sleep are reduced in the elderly; most hypnotics will decrease these stages even further. Does it matter? Consider the following points.

(a) Decreased REM sleep is highly correlated with impairment of memory and intelligence.
(b) Nightmares may be shifted to become 'day terrors'.
(c) Withdrawal of the hypnotic leads to rebound increase in REM sleep, which may lead to nightmares or delirium.
(d) In sleep laboratories, chronic insomniacs sleep as poorly on drugs as off drugs.

On the other hand, nocturnal incontinence, sleep-walking and nightmares occur mainly during slow-wave sleep, and carefully chosen hypnotics may help some patients with such problems.

Nevertheless, the physician may wish to prescribe a hypnotic for a particular patient, in which case he should always try to use only occasional doses, or short courses.

Hypnotics

Benzodiazepines

Nitrazepam (Mogadon) was introduced in 1965 as a safe and effective non-barbiturate hypnotic and quickly found favour for the elderly. However, it became apparent that the recommended dose of 10 mg produced considerable hangover effects, which could last for several days in the elderly even after a single dose. Even 5 mg has been shown to cause undesirable effects in the elderly and if this drug is to be used in old age it should be given in a dose of only 2.5 mg. As indicated previously, the reasons for this prolonged effect are the long half-life (20–38 hours) together with increased responsiveness of the elderly brain to the drug.

Flurazepam (Dalmane) was introduced in 1970 and has become the most widely prescribed hypnotic in the USA: in 1977, 53% of all prescriptions

Table 10.4 Hypnotics for the elderly.

Benzodiazepines	Nitrazepam Flurazepam Clorazepate potassium Temazepam Triazolam Fosazepam Flunitrazepam
Meprobamate	
Chlormethiazole	
Chloral	Chloral hydrate Triclofos (Tricloryl) Dichloralphenazone
Miscellaneous	

for hypnotics were for flurazepam, i.e. 13.6 million prescriptions for this one benzodiazepine alone. It is metabolized very rapidly but the metabolite is active and has a half-life of 47–100 hours (see Table 10.2). As a result, flurazepam causes prolonged effects, with undesirable hangover.

The blood level of active agent after a week of daily treatment with flurazepam is likely to be 5 or 6 times that found after the first day's treatment. The usual dose recommended is 15–30 mg, but the 30 mg dose should never be used in the elderly, and even the 15 mg dose may have adverse effects with continued use in old age.

Withdrawal may be easier than after nitrazepam.

Clorazepate potassium (Azene, *USA*; Tranxene, *UK*) is long-acting and resembles diazepam in its effects.

Temazepam (Restoril, *USA*; Euhypnos and Euhypnos forte, *UK*). Restoril capsules 15 mg and 30 mg; Euhypnos 10 mg soft gelatin capsule; forte 20 mg capsule. Hypnotic doses have ranged from 10 mg to 60 mg and hangover is not commonly a problem. In a study in geriatric patients 10 mg was usually sufficient; a few patients required 20 mg, and the drug appeared superior to chlormethiazole syrup (500 mg in 10 ml) in terms of quality and duration of sleep, ease of awakening and carry-over effects. Rebound insomnia, however, has been reported as a problem after withdrawal of short-acting hypnotics.

Triazolam (Halcion, *USA*, *UK*). A more complex structure characterizes this newer benzodiazepine which has been claimed as superior to flurazepam in adult out-patients and in geriatric patients. However, evidence of cognitive and intellectual impairment has followed its use, and rebound insomnia may be a problem on withdrawal. Some patients on triazolam have developed a complex psychiatric disturbance which has cleared after withdrawal of the drug, but this appears to be largely confined to the Netherlands and there is no clear evidence of causality.

Dose: 0.125 mg, increasing to 0.25 mg, if necessary.

Other benzodiazepines

Fosazepam is similar in efficacy and tolerability to flurazepam in psychogeriatric patients.

Flunitrazepam is an effective hypnotic in elderly patients. 0.5 mg being as effective as meprobamate 200 mg.

Meprobamate

This drug is used as a hypnotic in the elderly by some geriatricians because it reduces motor restlessness moderately and consistently during the satisfactory period of sleep it induces; by contrast, promazine and amylobarbital sodium may produce alternating immobility and restlessness. To avoid pressure sores it is important not to sedate the patient to a degree that produces long periods of immobility.

Dose: 200–800 mg.

Clormethiazole (UK, Europe)

This drug is derived from vitamin B_1, and is a central nervous system depressant, having sedative/hypnotic and anticonvulsant properties. It has been used in elderly patients for over 15 years and is generally well-tolerated as a hypnotic, having a short half-life (4 hours), no active metabolites, and producing little or no hangover. However, there may be reduced hepatic first-pass metabolism in the elderly, leading to raised peak plasma levels and associated with reduced plasma and red-cell binding of the drug. The usual care must therefore be taken with regard to dosage in the elderly; chlormethiazole then compares well with other sedative agents such as dichloralphenazone, meprobamate and thioridazine; it is preferred to nitrazepam.

Chloral

This was the first synthetic hypnotic, introduced in 1869, and has long been regarded as useful in the elderly. In solution, as chloral hydrate, it has an unpleasant taste; it is rapidly absorbed and metabolized (by alcohol dehydrogenase) into the active hypnotic trichlorethanol, and the overall effect lasts for 6–8 hours, with little hangover. Hepatic conjugation precedes urinary excretion of the inert glucuronide; the latter gives a positive result in urine tests for sugar but not in the glucose oxidase enzyme test.

Chloral should be avoided in the presence of hepatic or renal impairment, or peptic ulcer. It may interact with alcohol, which potentiates the hypnotic effect, and displaces some protein-bound drugs in the plasma, causing increased free levels of them and increasing their effect (e.g. warfarin). Hypersensitivity occasionally develops, with a skin rash.

Tolerance may develop after 1 to 2 weeks of regular use, with decreasing effect. Increasing the dose may be dangerous: the fatal dose is only 4–10 times the hypnotic dose.

Dose of chloral hydrate: 0.5–2 g.

Other formulations are available:

Triclofos (Tricloryl) is a stable ester of trichlorethanol. Dose: 0.5–1 g.

Dicloralphenazone (Welldorm) is a combination of chloral and the analgesic phenazone. It has proved to be a popular hypnotic in the elderly.

Dose: 650 mg–1.3 g.

Miscellaneous hypnotics

Barbiturates should be avoided in the elderly. They have many disadvantages as hypnotics, may cause paradoxical excitement or confusion in the elderly; prolonged use may cause or aggrevate dementia and ataxia.

Undesirable non-barbiturate hypnotics. Carbromal can cause bromism, and, like bromides themselves, is obsolete.

Ethchlorvynol (Arvynol), glutethimide (Doriden), methaqualone (Melsed) and methyprylone (Noludar) all share the addicting, REM-sleep suppressing and withdrawal problems of the barbiturates. They cannot be recommended.

Paraldehyde has many disadvantages and can be replaced by other medications.

Antihistamines such as promethazine (Phenergan) and trimeprazine (Vallergan) have hypnotic effects. Trimeprazine may have an advantage over benzodiazepines in that it increases both REM and slow-wave sleep, and is free of REM-rebound on withdrawal.

REFERENCES AND FURTHER READING

Drug usage

The Aging Process and Psychoactive Drug Use (1979) Menlo Park, California: Stanford Research Institute. Nat Inst. on Drug Abuse Services Research Monograph Series Publication, G.P.O. 79-813.

Hyams D.E. (1984) Drug usage in the elderly. In Roe D.A. (Ed.) *Drugs and Nutrition in the Geriatric Patient*, pp. 1–26. Churchill Livingstone, New York.

Clinical pharmacology in the elderly

Crooks J. & Steveson I.H. (Eds) 1979 *Drugs and the Elderly: Perspectives in Geriatric Clinical Pharmacology*. Proc. Sympos, Dundee. Sept., 1977, pp. 13–14. University Park Press, Baltimore.

Benzodiazepines

Bellantuone C., Reggi V., Togoni G. & Garrattini S. (1980) Benzodiazepines: Clinical pharmacology and therapeutic use. *Drugs* **19,** 195–219.

Committee on the Review of Medicines (1980) Systematic review of the benzodiazepines. *British medical Journal* **280,** 910–12.

Dement W.C. (1983) Rational basis for the use of sleeping pills. *Pharmacology* **27** (Suppl. 2) 3–38.
Oswald I. (1979) The why and how of hypnotic drugs. *British medical Journal* **1,** 1167–8.
Tyler P.J. (1984) Benzodiazepines on trial. *British medical Journal* **288,** 1101–2.

General reviews

Ban T.A. (1980) *Psychopharmacology for the Aged.* S. Karger, Basel.
Salzman C. (1982) A primer on geriatric psychopharmacology. *American Journal of Psychiatry* **139,** 67–74.
Thompson T.L., Moran M.G. & Nies A.S. (1983) Psychotropic drug use in the elderly. *New England Journal of Medicine* **308,** 134–8; 194–9.

Chapter Eleven
Central Nervous System—Antidepressants

D.E. HYAMS

OVERVIEW

Depression is a common and often occult condition in old age. It is very amenable to treatment. The range of anti-depressants now available is considerable and knowledge of their side-effects and interactions is essential for the prescriber. Nowhere is the importance of 'knowing a few drugs well' applied with more force.

Depression is one of the most common problems met with in old age; there are 3 major reasons for this:
(1) the physiological depletion of biogenic amines in old age, together with an increase in monoamine oxidase;
(2) environmental deprivation factors such as loss of loved ones, narrowing of contacts and of interests, loss of role and possibly financial problems;
(3) drug-induced depression is more likely in old age.

This is not the place to enter into questions of classification of depression, but it is essential to appreciate how important the problem of depression is in old age.

The significance of depression in old age is not attributable merely to its frequent incidence, but to three other factors:
(a) depression is frequently undiagnosed;
(b) depression may lead to suicide, the incidence of which is well-known to increase in old age;
(c) depression is usually treatable and to miss its presence is truly a disservice to the elderly patient.

THE DIAGNOSIS OF DEPRESSION IN OLD AGE

Although the clinical picture may resemble that seen at younger ages, there may be more apathy, gloom, inertia, withdrawal, loss of initiative, and more physical symptoms in elderly depressed patients than in younger ones. Severe motor retardation may mimic aspects of parkinsonism and 'pseudo-dementia' is a well-recognized presentation of depression in old age—often rewarding because of the dramatic disappearance of the 'dementia' on anti-depressant treatment. 'Masked depression' is a confusing term, sometimes used to refer to masking by somatic symptoms, but surely better applied to a broader canvas; depression in the elderly is often 'masked' by mimicking other diseases (physical or mental) or by being attributed simply to 'old age' by the patient or, worse, by the physician.

Antidepressant drugs for the elderly (see Table 11.1)

Table 11.1 Antidepressant drugs in geriatric practice.

Class and generic names	Some trade names	
	USA	UK, Europe
(a) In common use		
Tricyclics		
Dihydrodibenzazepines		
Imipramine	Tofranil	Tofranil
Clomipramine	—	—
Desimipramine	Pertofrane	Pertofran
Trimipramine	—	Surmontil
Dibenzocycloheptenes		
Amitriptyline	Elavil	Tryptizol
Nortriptyline	Aventyl	Aventyl
Protriptyline	Vivactil	Concordin
Dibenzoxepins		
Doxepin	Sinequan	Sinequan
Monoamine oxidase inhibitors(MAOI) (not for routine use—see text)		
Psychomotor stimulants		
Amphetamine	Dexedrine	Dexedrine
Methylphenidate	Ritalin	Ritalin
Pemoline	Cylert	Ronyl
Pentylenetetrazol	Metrazol	Cardiazol
Others		
L-tryptophan	Trofan	Optimax
Lithium	Eskalith	Camcolit
Flupenthixol	Flaxol	Flaxol
(b) Newer agents		
Tetracyclics		
Maprotiline	Ludiomil	Ludiomil
Mianserin	—	Bolvidon
Bicyclics		
Viloxazine	—	Vivalan
Tricyclic		
Amoxapine	Asendin	Moxadil
Tetrahydroisoquinoline		
Nomifensin	—	Merital
Triazolopyridine		
Trazodone	Desyrel	Molipaxin

ANTIDEPRESSANTS IN COMMON USE

Tricyclics (see Table 11.2)

The tricyclic antidepressants are closely related chemically to the phenothiazines; imipramine was discovered during a search for a drug to replace chlorpromazine. Replacement of the central nitrogen atom of imipramine by a carbon atom gives amitriptyline.

Table 11.2 Some characteristics of tricyclic antidepressants.

	Rapidity of onset of response	Sedative or alerting effect	Anticholinergic effects
Imipramine	2–3 weeks	Alerting	++
Desimipramine	2–3 weeks	Alerting	+
Amitriptyline	2–3 weeks	Sedative	+++
Nortriptyline	2–3 weeks	Sedative	++
Protriptyline	Within 1 week	Alerting	++
Doxepin	Within 1 week	Sedative	+++

Tricyclics are among the most effective anti-depressants available, and may benefit more than two-thirds of patients treated, although the aetiology of the depression appears to influence the outcome. In old age, 'endogenous' or 'unipolar' depression responds as well as at younger ages. Response decreases as 'reactive' or 'neurotic' factors increase in importance in causation of the depression.

Tricyclics are readily absorbed from the gastrointestinal tract but first-pass metabolism is extensive; binding to plasma protein is high.

Plasma half-life may be much increased in the elderly; therefore steady-state plasma levels, which are reached in 5–10 days in the general population, may take 2–3 weeks to be achieved in elderly depressives. These steady-state levels show very wide (but consistent) variation between different patients given a similar dose, regardless of age; but elderly patients show significantly higher levels, and this helps to explain the increased susceptibility of the elderly to adverse effects of these drugs. It also emphasizes the need to use lower dosages of tricyclics in elderly depressed patients, especially in the early stages of therapy.

These pharmacokinetic age-differences do not seem to apply to nortriptyline itself; but in any case it is difficult to relate plasma levels of tricyclics to therapeutic response. There appears to be a 'therapeutic window', above *and* below which response is suboptimal, at least for endogenous depression; this applies to amitriptyline (which is slowly demethylated in the liver to nortriptyline) and may apply to protriptyline as well as to nortriptyline itself. By contrast, there appears to be a linear plasma level response for imipramine, which is rapidly demethylated to desimipramine; however, it is probable that response will plateau at higher dose-levels. This type of relationship may also apply to doxepin; but data are lacking. The situation is complicated by the fact that the demethylated metabolites are themselves active anti-depressants, with longer half-lives than the parent substances.

Thus, monitoring of plasma levels of tricyclics is not generally recommended as a routine, but may be of use in occasional elderly patients to help avoid failures of treatment or to avoid toxicity.

Choice of tricyclics

In general, all tricyclics have similar antidepressant efficacy; however, individual patients may well respond to or tolerate one better than another. Table 11.2 shows several properties of the various drugs which may be of particular use in individual patients. Thus, depressed patients with agitation or insomnia would be suitable for a trial of amitriptyline or doxepin rather than imipramine; conversely, retarded patients may well do better on protriptyline or imipramine. Protriptyline offers the advantage over imipramine of a more rapid onset of effect, but no diminution in anticholinergic or cardiovascular side-effects. Parenteral administration has no greater speed of onset of effect.

Dosage and regimen (see Table 11.3)

In elderly patients it is wise to begin treatment very circumspectly, when the clinical situation allows this. Initial doses should be as small as possible and given about 2 hours before bedtime; increments, if needed, should be made gradually and at longer intervals than in younger patients. The maximum daily doses are shown for 'adults' but are rarely indicated or tolerated in the elderly. The maximum dosage used must be decided on an individual basis; it will rarely be more than one-third to one-half those shown. Once

Table 11.3 Dosage of tricyclic antidepressants.

Drug	Starting dose (mg)	Initial dosage interval (days)	Maximum 'adult' daily dose (divided)
Imipramine	10–25	1–7	300
Desimipramine	25	1–7	300
Amitriptyline	10–25	1–7	250
Nortriptyline	10	1–7	100
Protriptyline	5	1–7	60
Doxepin	10	1–7	300–400

a satisfactory response is obtained, the dose may be reduced by about one-third. Full remission may be slow. Medication should continue for several months after remission has been obtained, and then the dose should be gradually reduced and the drug withdrawn. If there is no adequate response to full or maximum doses after 3–4 weeks, the drug should be withdrawn gradually. Too rapid a response should alert the physician to the possibility that the patient may have decided to commit suicide.

Adverse effects and drug interactions

Anticholinergic effects are the most common side-effects, and may be particularly troublesome in the elderly, especially when initial dosage is high or increased rapidly.

The effects may be central or peripheral.

Central effects show as clinical deterioration with the development of lability of mood and mild confusion. Cognitive loss follows, and later there may be severe confusion with delusions and hallucinations. Clearly, the patient may be thought to be developing dementia. This situation is particularly likely to occur in patients who are concurrently taking other drugs with anticholinergic properties (e.g. antipsychotics of antiparkinsonism drugs). The susceptibility to this syndrome increases with age after 40 years.

Peripheral effects consist of a progressive series of organ disturbances: early features are decreased salivary and bronchial secretions, decreased sweating, constipation, postural hypotension and a tendency to hypothermia; later, blurred vision and cardiac arrhythmias may occur (see below), and then urinary retention and ileus may develop. The risk of glaucoma is present.

These anticholinergic effects may remain mild and may be tolerated for the sake of the antidepressant efficacy of the drug; and they may improve to some degree spontaneously. They may be avoided to some extent by giving the drug in unequal divided doses, the larger dose being near bedtime; but side-effects are correlated with plasma drug levels and reduction in dosage may be needed. For more acute toxicity, physostigmine 1–2 mg may be injected intramuscularly or intravenously.

Cardiovascular side-effects

These are considered separately because of their clinical significance. Postural hypotension and cardiac arrhythmias have been mentioned. Tachycardia and palpitation have long been recognized as side-effects of these drugs, but arrhythmias and electrocardiographic (ECG) abnormalities were described more recently.

In therapeutic doses, ECG abnormalities such as prolonged P-R, QRS and Q-T_c have been recorded, as well as reduced amplitude of T waves. With larger doses, and in overdose, conduction defects and ventricular tachyarrhythmias may develop, but at more modest therapeutic doses the quinidine-like effects may prevail, and the tricyclics may actually exert anti-arrhythmic effects such as reduction or disappearance of pre-existing ventricular premature contractions. However, in the elderly there is some evidence that undesirable cardiac side-effects may occur during long-term tricyclic therapy whether or not there is a previous history of cardiac abnormality. Obviously, if there is such a history, particularly careful evaluation and observation of the patient is mandatory during tricyclic therapy.

Interactions with other cardiovascular drugs

Antihypertensive drugs such as guanethidine, bethanidine and debrisoquine are taken up into presynaptic neurons by the same 'amine pump' which is responsible for norepinephrine uptake. Tricyclics act in part by interfering with this 'pump' and so, in addition to blocking norepinephrine uptake, they will prevent the uptake of those antihypertensive drugs; the antihypertensive effect is lost and blood pressure will rise. This interference can persist for 2–3 weeks after a longer-acting tricyclic such as amitriptyline has been stopped. Doxepin causes less interference than the other tricyclics. Other antihypertensive agents may also be antagonized, e.g. clonidine by desimipramine.

Hypertensive episodes may occur if methylphenidate is given to patients on tricyclics, or if other sympathomimetic substances are given.

Diuretics may predispose to postural hypotension in tricyclic-treated patients.

Anti-arrhythmia drugs and anticoagulants may also be involved in drug interactions with tricyclics, causing (respectively) undue depression of cardiac conduction or increased anticoagulant effect. Note that thioridazine has the same type of effect on the heart as the tricyclics, and should not be given with the latter drugs.

Other side-effects include precipitation of hypomania in patients with bipolar depression; weight gain; and, rarely, fits. A tremor may occur with therapeutic doses.

Tricyclics may impair the bioavailability of concurrently administered drugs with a large first-pass metabolism, e.g. chloropromazine and levodopa. Conversely neuroleptics may inhibit the metabolism of tricyclics.

MAOIs*

These drugs are, in general, less effective than tricyclics, and their use carries the risk of hypertensive crises if an interaction with tyramine is allowed to occur. Tyramine occurs in certain foods and drinks (e.g. cheese, beans, yeast products, chicken livers, chocolate, beer and red wine). It may be very difficult to ensure compliance with the strict exclusion of such food and drink in the elderly. Certain other drugs may interact with MAOIs and produce a similar crisis (e.g. sympathomimetic amines in cough and cold remedies or nasal drops, levodopa) and potentiation of tricyclics, antihypertensive agents and narcotics may also occur.

MAOIs should not be used in geriatric patients if an alternative treatment is likely to succeed. If they are to be used they should be given only to patients who can understand and remember the hazards and who can be relied upon to follow the stringent rules.

Psychomotor stimulants in depression

These drugs have limited efficacy in depression (see Table 11.2). **Amphetamine** is best avoided altogether; some elderly patients become worse on amphetamines, with dysphoria rather than euphoria, other adverse effects and rapid development of tolerance. A related, safer compound is **methylphenidate,** which has a mild mood-elevating effect. Overstimulation may occur and may produce or aggravate confusion. As an antidepressant for elderly patients, this drug is usually reserved for those who fail on other therapy or who refuse (or are unfit for) electroconvulsive therapy.

Pemoline may lessen apathy, but in the elderly it is more often used in attempts to improve psychological performance. Methylphenidate, pemoline and pentylenetetrazol are discussed in more detail in Chapter 12.

Lithium

Lithium carbonate was reported to be effective in manic patients in 1949 and this was quickly confirmed. About 75% of manic patients respond within 6–10 days of the start of lithium treatment without sedation.

The use of lithium in depression has become established more recently, following earlier conflicting reports. Its main value here is in the prevention of recurrent endogenous depression, whether unipolar or bipolar. Its indication for an existing depression is less clear, but it may be used to poten-

* *Note on MAOIs.* It is usual to contraindicate the use of tricyclics within 14 days of taking a MAOI. Psychiatrists have in fact used both drugs concurrently with success in selected patients, but the family practitioner and the general physician are warned against this practice for out-patients or in non-psychiatric hospital environments.

tiate tricyclics in cases refractory to the latter drugs. Improvement may be rapid or very gradual, but the preventive effect is eventually marked; prolonged maintenance therapy is likely to be needed.

Lithium does not impair mental or emotional function, even after years of treatment. However, lithium does have somatic effects: it can substitute for sodium, potassium, magnesium or calcium ions at various cellular sites and alter physiological processes: it blunts responsiveness of the distal renal tubules to antidiuretic hormone, i.e. it causes a nephrogenic diabetes insipidus. The compensatory increase in vasopressin may play a part in the mechanism of lithium's effect on the brain. An effect of lithium on brain choline turnover has also been described; this is of interest because choline can induce depression and because the cholinergic agonist physostigmine is effective in the treatment of mania. Lithium influences cardiac repolarization and may cause S-T prolongation and T-wave depression. There is no increase in mortality in patients on long-term lithium therapy, but to avoid the toxicity (confusion and coma may develop rapidly above a serum lithium level of 1.5 mEq/l; at lower levels gastrointestinal irritability may occur) it is necessary to monitor serum levels regularly, which makes this therapy troublesome in general practice.

Dosage: In elderly patients, low doses are recommended—150–600 mg/day, in divided doses after meals, rather than the 600–1800 mg used at younger ages. Serum levels of 0.5–0.6 mEq/l should be high enough in old age (as against 0.6–1.2 mEq/l for younger subjects), as symptoms of toxicity may occur in the elderly even at 'normal' therapeutic levels: the half-life of lithium in the elderly may increase to 36 hours, as against the 18–30 hours in younger patients.

Precautions: Lithium should not be used with diuretics, and renal function should be kept under review. Periodic ECGs are advisable. An interaction with chlorpromazine causes reduced plasma levels of the latter. Lithium may potentiate MAOIs. Thyroid function tests should be performed once or twice a year to detect possible hypothyroidism.

L-*tryptophan*

This amino acid is a precursor of serotonin and has been used with variable results in mixed groups of depressive patients, on the hypothesis that some forms of depression may be due to serotonin deficiency. Patients with bipolar depression are more likely to respond to L-tryptophan than are unipolar patients; mania may also be improved on such therapy. However, the evidence is not yet firm enough to allow a clear picture to be seen of the value of L-tryptophan in the management of depression or mania.

Thioxanthenes

Flupenthixol has been discussed earlier as an anxiolytic drug; it has also had some success in the management of depression. It has the advantage of good tolerance, rapid onset of effect (within one week) and a high therapeutic index. No interactions with tricyclics or benzodiazepines have been reported, but the drug has been shown to induce hepatic enzyme activity.

NEWER ANTIDEPRESSANT DRUGS

Tetracyclics

In general the tetracyclics resemble the tricyclics, but certain advantages are claimed and they are useful in particular situations.

Maprotilene resembles desimipramine in selectively blocking norepinephrine reuptake into neurons, without affecting serotonin uptake; these two drugs also share a lesser tendency to cause anticholinergic side-effects. However, maprotilene had the advantage of a more rapid onset of effect. It has also been shown to have an anti-arrhythmic effect in therapeutic doses. Dosage is as for imipramine.

Mianserin resembles amitriptyline in having a sedative effect in addition to its antidepressant effect; the two drugs have similar efficacy, but it has been claimed that mianserin is less likely to produce anticholinergic or cardiotoxic side-effects than amitriptyline or imipramine. It appears to be well-tolerated by the elderly in doses of 30–60 mg daily. No clinically significant interactions with antihypertensive or anticoagulant drugs have been reported. There have been a few instances of depressed bone marrow with mianserin.

Bicyclics

Viloxazine is a bicyclic drug which, in doses of 150–300 mg daily, has shown antidepressant efficacy within 7 days in geriatric patients, without anticholinergic side-effects. Headaches, nausea, vomiting, loss of weight and a transient early rise in blood pressure have been reported as side-effects. A rebound of depression may follow its withdrawal. If given to patients on phenytoin, the dose of the latter may need to be reduced.

Tetrahydroisoquinolines

Nomifensine is chemically distinct from all other antidepressants. It inhibits neuronal reuptake of dopamine as well as of norepinephrine, and is a relatively weak inhibitor of serotonin uptake. Its antidepressant efficacy is comparable to that of amitriptyline or imipramine, but it causes little or no sedation, fewer and milder anticholinergic side-effects, and is less likely to be cardiotoxic on overdose. It is well-tolerated by elderly patients. It may aggravate schizoid tendencies.

Triazolopyridine

Trazodone has virtually no anticholinergic side-effects but has serotoninergic properties. It has proved useful in depression associated with anxiety, and has a relatively rapid onset of action (3–7 days in some cases). Side-effects are fewer than with tricyclics. This drug may prove to be of particular value in some geriatric patients with depression. It may, however, be cardiotoxic in patients with pre-existing heart disease.

The introduction of predominantly serotoninergic drugs as antidepressants (zimelidine, trazodone) is of interest; amitriptyline has some serotoninergic properties, but these are much less than the effects on noradrenergic transmission.

A NOTE ON ELECTROCONVULSIVE THERAPY (ECT) IN THE ELDERLY

For those patients refractory to drugs, or in whom drugs are contraindicated, or when there is not time to wait for the drugs to begin to have an effect, ECT still has a place. In recent years this form of treatment has lost popularity: in New York State there was a 49% reduction in its use between 1972 and 1977. For 40 years ECT has been used without understanding of its mechanism of action, and little research has been directed towards making good that deficit. This situation is now changing, although slowly.

An important advance in the use of ECT in old age came when it was shown that unilateral ECT to the non-dominant hemisphere offered advantages over bilateral treatment: shorter recovery time and less anterograde and retrograde amnesia, but equal efficacy. Further, one method of electrode placement for unilateral treatment has been shown to require less electrical energy, and to allow even shorter recovery times and even less amnesia than another method.

PSYCHOSTIMULANTS

These drugs were considered briefly above. A few more details follow.

Amphetamine. Amphetamine has been used for various conditions since its introduction as a stimulant half a century ago but the possibility of addiction and of the development of psychoses has led to its virtual abandonment. It has not been shown to improve cognitive processes in geriatric patients, but may have a limited use in the rehabilitable elderly with apathy and poor motivation, although methylphenidate is preferable.

Methylphenidate (Ritalin, *USA* and *UK;* Methidate, *Canada*). This is an amphetamine derivative which has been shown to improve psychomotor performance in some elderly patients. Its effect on cognition has been variable but it is preferable to amphetamine.

Dosage: 5 mg, gradually increased if necessary to 15 mg, morning and midday.

Sympathomimetic side-effects may occur; a β-blocker has helped to suppress these, and allowed patients to continue to benefit from methylphenidate treatment.

Hepatotoxicity is rare. Long-term use has led to cardiomyopathy.

Pemoline (Cylert, Volital, *USA* and *UK;* Ronyl, Kethamed, *UK*). The stimulant effects of pemoline resemble those of amphetamine, but it is a safer drug to use. It enhances cerebral ribonucleic acid (RNA) synthesis, and has been used in patients with memory impairment (since RNA synthesis is associated with learning and memory); the results have, however, been disappointing.

Dose: 5–20 mg daily in two divided doses, given morning and midday. Larger doses may cause agitation, confusion and insomnia.

Meclofenoxate (*centrophenoxine*) (Lucidril, *UK*) is popular in Europe and has undoubted effects on the brain, but has given mixed results in clinical practice. However, a pilot study in geriatric patients, using a teaching machine, suggested that cognitive function could be improved by the drug; and normal old people showed a highly significant improvement in delayed free recall after taking the drug. It is not available in North America.

Fencamfamin (Reactivan, *UK* and *Europe*) is related to camphor and its stimulant effect resembles that of amphetamine, but without the peripheral effects. It has been used mainly in fatigue states, but has been claimed to improve mental function in mild to moderate cases of dementia. It is not available in North America.

Pentylenetetrazol (Metrazol, *USA*) is still popular in the USA as a stimulant for elderly patients; it may be combined with nicotinic acid (as in Menic, *USA*), possibly with vitamins added (as in Cerebro-Nicin, *USA*). Its use lacks validation by clinical studies.

REFERENCES AND FURTHER READING

Hicks R., Funkenstein H.H., Davis J.M. & Dysken M.W. (1980) Geriatric psychopharmacology. In Birren J.E. & Sloane R.B. (Eds) *Handbook of Mental Health & Aging*, pp. 753–9. Prentice Hall, New Jersey.

Post F. (1984) The Emotional Disorders. In Brocklehurst J.C. (Ed.) *Textbook of Geriatric Medicine and Gerontology*, 3rd ed, Ch. 16. Churchill Livingstone, London; Longman, New York.

Chapter Twelve
Central Nervous System—Dementia

D. E. HYAMS

OVERVIEW

While drugs seem, on present evidence, to have a very limited role in the prevention of dementia, the condition is so prevalent and produces so much dependency among the aged, that the place of drugs needs careful review. The principal use of neuroleptic drugs is in the management of the behavioural disturbances associated with dementia. Many neuroleptic drugs have serious side-effects.

THE MANAGEMENT OF DEMENTIA

Perhaps one in ten persons aged 65 and over have some degree of dementia, and its prevalence increases steeply with age, exceeding 20% in those aged 80 and over. While the numbers and proportions of the elderly are increasing in developed countries generally, by far the largest 'population explosion' throughout the rest of this century will be in the age group 80 and above. In this context the management of dementia (including preventive aspects) takes on a significance which has enormous sociomedical implications.

DRUGS AND PREVENTION OF DEMENTIA

Drugs used in attempts to improve mental function in elderly demented patients have been reviewed several times in recent years. It is important not to expect too much of pharmacological intervention, but to set up an overall management plan for each patient and his or her particular environmental situation; the patient needs mental and physical activity during each day, and a role, without which there can be no hope of success. Drugs may be involved in the aetiology of dementia (e.g. bromides, barbiturates, tranquillizers).

Drugs play a very limited therapeutic role in dementia and should be used only in carefully selected patients who are not so severely demented that small improvements cannot possibly be recognized. Problems of memory and compliance need to be tackled; optimism must be tempered with realism, but the physician should keep an open mind and organize careful surveillance of the therapy and its possible effects. Even a small improvement in a patient's mental performance and/or mood and behaviour can sometimes make a disproportionately great difference to the pattern of care and its success: increased manageability and arrest of deterioration may be very reasonable rewards for these therapeutic endeavours.

The idea that what is needed for these patients are cerebral vasodilator drugs is now recognized as obsolete. Most dementia is *not* due to cerebral atherosclerosis, and increasing cerebral blood flow can only rarely be correlated with improved cerebral function. The emphasis has shifted now to metabolic effects which may be produced by drugs, acting either on cerebral cells or on the physical properties of the blood, both effects alleged to improve cerebral microcirculation as a secondary phenomenon. Thus in many instances any increase in cerebral blood flow (CBF) will be secondary to increased demand due to enhanced metabolic activity in cerebral cells.

Table 12.1 A classification of drugs used in the treatment of impaired cerebral function in old age.

DRUGS MAINLY VASODILATOR

Acting via autonomic nervous system

(1) α-adrenergic blockers, e.g. ergot derivatives, raubasine
(2) β-adrenergic stimulants, e.g. isoxsuprine, nylidrin

Acting directly on vascular smooth muscle

e.g. papaverine, cyclandelate, betahistine, nicotinic acid and its derivatives (nicotinyl alcohol tartrate, inositol hexanicotinate, xanthinol nicotinate)

Acting indirectly on vascular smooth muscle

e.g. calcium-flux blockers (cinnarizine, flunarizine, nimodipine)

DRUGS INFLUENCING CEREBRAL CELL METABOLISM

Drugs with mixed vasodilator and metabolic effects

(1) Ergot alkaloids, e.g. codergocrine mesylate
(2) Ergolines, e.g. nicergoline (metergoline)
(3) *Vinca minor* alkaloids, e.g. vincamine, eburnamonine
(4) Synthetic derivatives of vincamine, e.g. ethyl apovincaminate
(5) Methyl xanthines, e.g. pentoxifylline
(6) Miscellaneous synthetic drugs—suloctidil; naftidrofuryl; hexobendine

Drugs with mainly metabolic effects

(1) Pyritinol (pyrithioxin)
(2) Agents enhancing cerebral acetylcholine levels, e.g. physostigmine, lecithin, choline, deanol, dopaminergic drugs
(3) Piracetam
(4) Neuropeptides, e.g. ACTH4-10, vasopressin
(5) Agents enhancing cerebral RNA concentrations, e.g. pemoline
(6) Psychomotor stimulants
(7) Procaine (H_3)
(8) Oxygen—normobaric or hyperbaric

AGENTS WITH MAINLY HAEMORHEOLOGICAL EFFECTS

e.g. Dextran 40

The discussion that follows will concentrate on the relatively few drugs which are available in North America as well as in Europe (Table 12.2) and will touch upon the many others, which are widely used in Europe, but usually on the basis of conflicting data, often derived from unsatisfactorily designed studies.

Table 12.2 Some cerebroactive drugs used in Europe and North America.

	Trade names		
Generic name	USA, Canada	UK	Europe
Isoxusprine	Vasodilan	Duvadilan Defencin-CP Vasotran	Vasoplex (Germany)
Papaverine	Parabid Pavakey Therapav Vasospan, etc.	—	Panergon (Germany)
Ethaverine	Ethatab Circubid etc.	—	Cardiostron (Germany)
Cyclandelate	Cyclospasmol	Cyclospasmol	Spasmocyclon (Germany)
Nicotinic acid	Nico-400 Nicobid Nicolar, etc.	Pernivit	Niconacid (Germany) Nicyl (France)
Nicotinyl alcohol (β-pyridylcarbinol)	Roniacol	Ronicol	Ronicol
Codergocrine mesylate	Hydergine Deapril-ST Circanol	Hydergine	Hydergin
Pentylenetetrazol	Metrazol	—	Cardiazol (Germany)

Isoxsuprine

This drug is a derivative of adrenaline. It is said to increase CBF, to improve EEG patterns during cerebral vasoconstriction, and to improve flow properties of blood (lowers viscosity and inhibits red-cell clumping). Its use has been accompanied by a decreased incidence of transient ischaemic attacks (TIAs). Two small double-blind studies in elderly patients showed significant improvement in psychometric test results (including the use of a teaching machine).

Dosage: Isoxsuprine hydrochloride, 20 mg q.i.d. **or:** Isoxsuprine resinate, 40 mg b.d.

Papaverine

Papaverine is an opium alkaloid, but can be synthesized. It relaxes smooth muscle generally and has some metabolic effects, e.g. improved glucose and oxygen uptake in the brain, as well as an ability to increase CBF. Clinical improvement may or may not follow these effects; double-blind studies in the elderly have produced very mixed results: in 9 good studies, 6 included some improvements but only 1 study claimed to show practical benefit from the therapy. Papaverine was judged inferior to Hydergine in 5 studies in which these 2 drugs were compared. Despite its popularity in North America, its value appears to be questionable; however, there is so much individual variability, not only in old age but also in the clinical manifestations of dementia within each patient, that a therapeutic trial of papaverine may be justified in certain cases.

Dosage: In USA sustained release formulations of papaverine (150 mg) may be less bioavailable than the regular soft gelatin capsules (75 mg). The latter need to be given up to 4-hourly to maintain therapeutic blood levels, since the half-life of papaverine is no more than 2 hours due to rapid hepatic metabolism. In the UK and Europe, a sustained-release tablet has proved far superior to a capsule presentation, therapeutic blood levels being reached within 1 hour and sustained for 10–12 hours: 12-hourly dosage produced no accumulation.

Side-effects are those of vasodilators in general, but abnormal liver function tests probably occur more commonly than hitherto realized, and intravenous papaverine has produced cardiac arrhythmias. Ethaverine (*USA*) is a related compound with similar properties.

Cyclandelate

Structurally related to papaverine, cyclandelate is 3 times as potent in its effect on vascular smooth muscle, while being a less toxic drug. As for papaverine, improved cerebral metabolism has been reported. In the elderly, CSF may increase but few clinical correlations are available. Well-designed studies have shown inconsistent results; improvement is most likely below the age of 75. A significant improvement in intellectual function was reported in healthy elderly women given cyclandelate for 2 months; elderly men deteriorated despite the drug. A prophylactic effect in TIAs has been reported. Patients who were started on large doses at least 2 months after a stroke showed improved sensorimotor recovery.

Dosage: 400 mg t.i.d. or q.i.d., increasing to 800 mg t.i.d.

Nicotinic acid

This alone has not been of significant benefit in the elderly with cerebral impairment; but some of its derivatives have been claimed to be of use in this indication.

Codergocrine mesylate, UK; Ergoloid mesylates, USA

This long-established agent is a mixture of three hydrogenated alkaloids of ergotoxine dihydroergocornine, dihydroergocristine and dihydroergokryptine as their mesylates. It is widely known as dihydroergotoxine mesylate, or DHE; in the UK it has recently been given the generic name of codergocrine mesylate.

Dihydrogenation eliminates the vasoconstrictor effects of ergotoxine and enhances its α-blocking properties. However, its principal actions are now considered to be a wide range of improvements in cerebral metabolism, including enzyme activities and energy balance; these effects are thought to lead to improved cerebral aerobic metabolism, enhanced cerebral protein synthesis and improved EEG patterns. Cerebral microcirculation may be influenced secondarily.

Clinical experience with this drug has been reported for over a quarter of a century and over 20 well-planned studies show significant improvement in 1 or more psychological or behavioural feature of benefit to the patient. Memory appears to be least likely to show improvement, but the patient may feel better and this may make a large difference to the quality of life for the patient and/or his relatives. Useful effects may take up to 3 months to appear, and this should be the minimum duration of any therapeutic endeavour with this drug.

Dosage: 1.5 mg tablet (*UK*), 1 mg tablet (*USA*). The drug is irregularly absorbed, and doses should be increased up to 4.5–6 mg daily (in 3 divided doses) if clinically indicated.

Side-effects are rare: in 1593 elderly patients in 25 studies the incidence of dizziness or hypotension was less than 2%.

Other drugs

Betahistine (Serc), a histamine analogue, dilates the labyrinthine microcirculation and has been used successfully in Ménière's disease. It has been claimed to improve CBF particularly in the vertebrobasilar arterial system, but the incidence of TIAs was not reduced.

Inositol hexanicotinate (Hexopal) is popular in the UK and Europe, but the evidence for any benefit in cerebral function is scanty.

Xanthinol nicotinate (Complamex, Complamin) has metabolic effects and improves microcirculatory flow.

Nicergoline (Sermion) resembles DHE: it is made by combining a modified ergoline nucleus with nicotinic acid.

Cinnarizine (Stugeron, Stutgeron, Midronal) is a piperazine derivative related to cyclizine. It has antihistamine properties and is effective in motion sickness. It antagonizes the contraction of vascular smooth muscle by blocking calcium entry into the depolarized muscle cells; it also reduces blood viscosity. Clinical studies in dementia have given mixed results.

Flunarizine (Sibelium) is a fluorinated derivative of cinnarizine and is more potent than the parent compound.

Nimodipine is a new calcium-entry blocker selective for cardiac and cerebral arteries which looks promising pharmacologically.

Vincamine was introduced as a mild antihypertensive agent; it may increase CBF and has been marketed mainly as a cerebral vasodilator. More recently it has been claimed to improve cerebral metabolism as well.

Ethyl apovincaminate is a more potent, synthetic derivative of vincamine.

Eburnamonine is another vinca minor alkaloid, structurally similar to vincamine but claimed to have more beneficial effects on cerebral metabolism.

Pentoxifylline (Trental) is a methylxanthine derivative and *suloctidil* (Sulocton) is a synthetic agent; both have direct vasodilator effects and several biochemical effects which are said to improve the flow properties of the blood and to improve cerebral metabolism. Suloctidil is also claimed to have antiplatelet-aggregating and antithrombotic properties.

Naftidrofuryl (Praxilene) is a synthetic drug which is popular in Europe. It too has direct vasodilator properties and various biochemical actions involving neurotransmitters and enzymes, and, it is claimed, the energy balance of cerebral cells. Clinical evaluation of this drug in chronic brain syndrome has been more satisfactory than that of many other drugs mentioned in this review but the usual variability as regards details of the studies makes it difficult to state its potential value with any certainty; nevertheless it seems one of the more promising agents.

Pyritinol (Encephabol) is derived from pyridoxine: it may improve cerebral metabolism and may secondarily increase CBF, though in chronic brain syndrome the former effect has been found without the latter. It has been claimed to improve short-term memory and other aspects of mental function.

Agents enhancing cerebral acetylcholine (ACh) levels

These are being intensively studied in view of the current interest in selective failure of cholinergic function as the possible basis for senile (and presenile) dementia of the Alzheimer type. *Physostigmine* may improve mental function in such patients but has to be given by injection, is short-acting and has troublesome side-effects. Oral *choline* and *lecithin* have given some promising results. Deanol (Deaner) is a choline precursor which, however, has not been very helpful in demented patients. *Dopaminergic drugs* increase ACh levels in the brain and may increase CBF; L-dopa has resulted in cognitive improvement in some patients with and some without parkinsonism.

Piracetam (Nootropyl, Normabrain) is a derivative of the major inhibitory neurotransmitter, γ-aminobutyric acid (GABA). It is claimed to have several beneficial effects on cerebral energy and metabolism, and to help protect the brain from chemical insults (including hypoxia) as well as facilitating cerebral function. It has been used successfully to shorten recovery time after neurosurgery, concussion and alcoholic pre-delirium. In mild dementia, it has improved some aspects of mental function, but not memory.

Neuropeptides present another field of intense current research. ACTH 4-10 and vasopressin have been shown to improve memory, but are cumbersome to administer (injection and nasal spray respectively). The endorphins are potent psychotropic agents and provide a vast potential source of fruitful research.

Procaine (Gerovital—H_3, GH_3, KH_3) has not lived up to the early claims made for it as an 'anti-aging' drug. It has weak monoamine oxidase activity and may act mainly as a mild antidepressant, improving the well-being of some of its elderly recipients. It has had a great vogue but lacks scientific support for its efficacy and safety.

Oxygen has been used to improve psychomotor performance in stroke patients and elderly subjects with memory impairment. Normobaric and hyperbaric administration have produced mixed results. Hyperbaric oxygen is dangerous, expensive and impracticable; normobaric oxygen does help in frank dementia, but healthy old men who had noted some memory impairment showed improved psychometric and memory test results after a period of continuous portable oxygen therapy.

Dextran 40 (Rheomacrodex) lowers blood viscosity and increases CBF. It is of no practical value, however, in the management of organic brain syndrome in the elderly, since it must be administered by intravenous infusion; it may have some value in acute cerebral ischaemia and embolism.

NEUROLEPTIC DRUGS

This group of drugs is used mainly as antipsychotic therapy, in the management of agitation, behaviour disturbances, delusions and hallucinations. They also reduce tension and anxiety.

There are 3 major classes of neuroleptics of particular value in elderly patients: phenothiazines; thioxanthenes, and butyrophenones. Their main features are shown in Table 12.3.

Table 12.3 Some neuroleptic antipsychotic drugs.

		Examples of some trade names	
Chemical class	Generic name	USA	UK, Europe
Phenothiazines			
Aliphatic	Chlorpromazine	Thorazine	Largactil
	Promazine	Prazine	Sparine
Piperidine	Thioridazine	Mellaril	Melleril
Piperazine	Fluphenazine	Prolixin	Moditen
	Perphenazine	Trilafon	Fentazin
	Prochlorperazine	Compazine	Stemetil
	Trifluoperazine	Stelazine	Stelazine
Thioxanthenes			
Aliphatic	Chlorprothixene	Taractan	Taractan
Piperazine	Flupenthixol	—	Depixol, Fluanxol
	Thiothixene	Navane	—
Dibenzazepines	Loxapine	Loxitane	—
Butyrophenones	Haloperidol	Haldol	Serenace
Diphenylbutylpiperidines (long-acting)	Fluspirilene (i.m.)	—	Redeptin, Imap
	Penfluridol (oral)	—	Semap
	Pimozide (oral)	Orap	Orap
Indolones	Molindone	Moban	—
Orthopramides	Sulpiride	Dogmatil	Dogmatil

The neuroleptics are the most frequently prescribed drugs in elderly institutionalized patients; in the USA thioridazine is the most popular of these agents and this may well be true in the UK as well. The reason is the relatively low incidence of extrapyramidal side-effects, although sedation, hypotension and anticholinergic side-effects may occur, as with chlorpromazine. It may be noted here that the adverse effects of neuroleptics are dose-related; the halogenated compounds are often more potent but tend to be more toxic than the others, although there is much overlap. Phenothiazines potentiate all cerebral depressant drugs.

The main side-effects of particular importance in old age are as follows:

CNS—Extrapyramidal side-effects
- acute dystonia
- akathisia
- parkinsonism
- perioral tremor ('rabbit syndrome')
- tardive dyskinesia
- oversedation

Gastrointestinal
- constipation
- jaundice

Genitourinary
- retention of urine

Ocular
- glaucoma
- corneal opacity
- retinal damage

CVS
- hypotension
- arrhythmia
- conduction defects

Dermatological
- photosensitivity
- melanomatosis

Metabolic
- hypothermia

Haematological
- agranulocytosis

Phenothiazines

The phenothiazines are by far the most common neuroleptic drugs used; the introduction of chlorpromazine in France in 1952 revolutionized the practice of psychiatry, and heralded the explosive development of psychopharmacology over the next 5 years. It is of interest that promazine, which has its proponents in geriatric medicine, was introduced as a new drug in 1956, yet was known in 1950 and its value not appreciated until its chlorinated derivative was made and tested; incidentally, promazine is an analogue of imipramine.

Chlorpromazine causes side-effects sufficiently often to warrant careful supervision if it is used in the elderly. Casual use is unwarranted. Initial dosage should be low (10 mg orally) and built up gradually if required.

Plasma levels are higher in the old than the young. Parenteral administration should be avoided.

Promazine is more suited to mildly agitated ambulant patients; it is less likely to cause jaundice or hypotension. The dose is 25 mg upwards.

Thioridazine is usually considered the phenothiazine of choice for the elderly. From an efficacy standpoint, there is little evidence for any superiority, but it has been claimed that extrapyramidal side-effects and jaundice occur relatively rarely with this drug.

Prochlorperazine has been used with some success in the elderly with paraphrenia and other paranoid states; it can cause severe dystonia and is better replaced by flupenthixol (where available).

Fluphenazine decanoate (Modecate) is a long-acting depot preparation given by intramuscular injection which has been used successfully in elderly patients with paranoid psychoses; moderate or severe dementia is a contraindication, predisposing to severe extrapyramidal reactions. Fluphenazine enanthate is another depot form given successfully in doses of 5 mg 2-weekly to elderly patients with late paraphrenia. Few adverse effects occurred in these cases.

Thioxanthenes

Flupenthixol (Fluanxol, 0.5 and 1 mg tablets; Depixol, 3 mg tablets; depot injection—flupenthixol decanoate, 20 mg and 40 mg ampoules—all *UK*, *Europe*; not in the USA).

This drug is useful in the management of psychoses, including paranoid states in the elderly, in whom depot injections of 20–90 mg every 3–4 weeks have been well tolerated, even in the presence of moderate dementia. Rather than sedating the patients, flupenthixol has activating and alerting effects. This is an advantage over fluphenazine or prochlorperazine. The drug is also useful in depression in lower oral doses.

Butyrophenones

Haloperidol has a number of advantages over the phenothiazines: it shares much of their efficacy but is more likely to improve alertness, interest, sociability and sometimes memory. It is particularly useful in elderly patients who are agitated, restless, hallucinated and paranoid, and in withdrawn uncooperative patients. By injection, it is valuable for calming wildly hyperactive patients, and may be preferable to (if not more effective than) phenothiazines in this respect. It does not cause cardiac arrhythmia or autonomic disturbance. However, its major adverse effects are neurological, and extrapyramidal disturbances are relatively common. When injected, an antiparkinsonism drug should be injected at the same time. Very low dosage may be obtained by using haloperidol drops, and this may prove effective therapy for certain elderly patients without producing significant parkinsonism. The onset of effect may be slow after low oral doses.

Dosage: Oral: Manufacturer's recommended doses are 0.5–2.0 mg two or three times a day for geriatric patients (0.5 mg tablets and capsules and 1.5 mg and 5 mg tablets are also available). Liquid preparations contain 2 mg/ml and a dropper is available so that single drops (0.1 mg each) can be given.

Parenteral: A 5 mg/ml solution is supplied; the initial dose ranges from 2–10 mg intramuscularly or intravenously (but up to 30 mg if needed); 6-hourly injections may be given but oral therapy should be instituted as soon as possible.

Prevention and treatment of side-effects of neuroleptic drugs

Since the likelihood of adverse effects in general increases with dose, duration of therapy, and age, the mainstays of prevention are: wise choice of therapy; low dosage; short courses—'drug holidays' (withdrawal for periods short of relapse of the psychosis); careful surveillance.

There are certain important exceptions. Chlorpromazine may cause cholestatic jaundice with no warning; it usually appears after 2–4 weeks of treatment, but on re-exposure to the drug at a later time it may appear very quickly. It is not dose-related, and usually clears; however, it may be slow to clear and occasionally causes severe liver damage which may be fatal. Age is a more important factor with phenothiazines than with flupenthixol.

Constipation may lead to distention, discomfort, restlessness and insomnia; intestinal slowing may affect the absorption of concomitantly administered drugs.

Of all the possible adverse effects, some of the most distressing and intractable are the extrapyramidal syndromes, which are 5 to 6 times more common in the elderly than at younger ages.

Drug-induced parkinsonism may appear from 1 to 4 weeks after the start of neuroleptic drug therapy. It may then gradually diminish, but some antiparkinsonian therapy is frequently required. Care is needed, however, since the latter therapy usually consists of an anticholinergic drug, which may rapidly lead to signs of toxicity, with restlessness, agitation, confusion and peripheral features such as flushed dry skin, tachycardia and acute retention of urine. If this syndrome occurs, the antiparkinsonian drug must be stopped and physostigmine may be given by injection.

Routine administration of antiparkinsonian drugs to prevent extrapyramidal side-effects of neuroleptic therapy may produce similar problems; it is often unnecessary, and may increase the risk of the development of tardive dyskinesia.

Tardive dyskinesia is difficult to treat pharmacologically and is most likely to occur with prolonged neuroleptic therapy but may appear sooner if high doses are used. It is seen in about one-third of patients on long-term neuroleptic treatment. Withdrawal of the causative drug usually aggravates the dyskinesia, but ultimately may be the best policy and the dyskinesia may recede, particularly if the withdrawal is very gradual—over years if need be. Of course, the original disorder may then relapse. Attempts at drug therapy have been based on attempts to understand the underlying mechanism: all have given variable and conflicting results. In intractable cases, the following may be used in short trials: choline, benzodiazepines, tetrabenazine and baclofen.

By contrast, acute dystonia may occur within the first few days of treatment, and usually responds rapidly to injection of an antiparkinsonian drug.

THE MANAGEMENT OF CONFUSIONAL STATES

Confusion and dementia may coexist but they are not the same thing. Dementia is loss of cognitive function and judgement; confusion implies loss of reality orientation and may exist without dementia. Indeed, acute confusional states are delirium and should be managed accordingly—good nursing, familiar surroundings and people, avoidance of the dark; and absolutely minimal use of drugs, which may aggravate the confusion. Many confusional states in the elderly are actually due to drugs, and this cause must always be excluded first in assessing the patient. Physicians in geriatric medicine probably stop drugs more frequently than they start them in their patients.

However, for severe agitation and restlessness it may be necessary to use drugs judiciously: haloperidol and chlormethiazole are useful; oxazepam may help in less disturbed cases. Phenothiazines are best avoided, but if considered necessary, thioridazine should be the first choice in this group.

Chronic confusion is more likely to be part of an organic chronic brain syndrome, and should be treated very circumspectly; in most instances a drug will be neither necessary nor wise, but if one is to be used oxazepam should be tried first. However, attention to dementia should be of prime importance. Some cases will be part of a psychiatric illness and will need more specialized management.

REFERENCES AND FURTHER READING

Baldessarini R.J. (1979a) The 'neuroleptic' antipsychotic drugs: Mechanisms of action. *Postgraduate Medicine* **65,** 108–19.

Baldessarini R.J. (1979b) The 'neuroleptic' antipsychotic drugs: Neuroleptic side effects. *Postgraduate Medicine* **65,** 123–8.

Cook P. & James I. (1981) Cerebral vasodilators. *New England Journal of Medicine* **305,** 1508–13; 1560–4.

Corkin S., Davis K.L., Growdon J.H., Usdin E. & Wurtman R.J. (Eds) (1982) *Alzheimer's Disease: A Report of Progress in Research* (Aging vol. 19). Raven Press, New York.

Hyams D.E. (1984) Cerebral function and drug therapy. In Brocklehurst J.C. (Ed.) *Textbook of Geriatric Medicine & Gerontology* 3rd edition, Ch. 17. Churchill Livingstone, London. Longman, New York.

Thompson T.L., Moran M.G. & Nies A.S. (1983) Psychotropic drug use in the elderly. *New England Journal of Medicine* **308,** 134–8; 194–8.

Yesavage J.A., Tinklenberg J.R., Hollister L.E. & Berger P.A. (1979) Vasodilators in senile dementias. *Archives of General Psychiatry* **36,** 220–3.

Chapter Thirteen
Central Nervous System—Antiparkinsonian and Antiepileptic Drugs, Use of Drugs in Stroke

D. E. HYAMS

OVERVIEW

Sinemet is the treatment of choice for parkinsonism. Amantadine may be added in difficult cases—anticholinergic drugs being used as a last resort. Many drugs are now available in the treatment of epilepsy—for grand mal phenytoin still retains primacry, although side-effects are not infrequent and may require alternative medication. In acute stroke glycerol may be useful (and is harmless). In transient ischaemic attacks opinion is still divided as to whether anticoagulants or aspirin should be used first.

ANTIPARKINSONIAN DRUGS

Parkinsonism is due to deficiency of dopamine in the brain. Administration of dopamine does not help because it does not cross the blood-brain barrier.

L-*dopa*

L-dopa is a dopamine precursor which crosses the blood-brain barrier and is rapidly converted (in brain and in peripheral tissues) to dopamine by an enzyme called dopa decarboxylase. However, large doses of L-dopa are needed in order to achieve adequate concentrations in the brain, since peripheral (especially hepatic) decarboxylation occurs rapidly. These large doses (several grams daily) led to major side-effects (postural hypotension, vomiting, involuntary movements and adverse mental changes) which effectively prevented this revolutionary new treatment from benefiting large numbers of elderly patients with parkinsonism.

The breakthrough for the elderly came with the introduction of drugs which inhibited the decarboxylase: carbidopa and benzserazide (the latter

Table 13.1 Drugs in the treatment of parkinsonism.

Dopamine precursors
L-Dopa
Sinemet
Ergot derivatives
Bromocriptine
Lysuride
Pergolide
Amantadine
Anticholinergic drugs
Benzhexol
Orphenadrine hydrochloride
Deprenyl

is not available in the USA). These enzyme-inhibitors prevent the peripheral loss of L-dopa, thus allowing much smaller doses of L-dopa to be given in order to produce as much brain penetration and clinical efficacy as the fourfold doses previously required. Many of the toxic effects of L-dopa are thus avoided, and this combination therapy has transformed the management of parkinsonism in old age.

Sinemet

Sinemet is a combination of L-dopa and carbidopa, originally in a 10:1 ratio, but currently also being made available in a 4:1 ratio since it has become appreciated that carbidopa is most valuable if given in a dose of not less than 70 mg/day. Sinemet is the most effective drug available in the USA for the treatment of parkinsonism. (In Europe, Madpar is an alternative, consisting of L-dopa and benzserazide.)

In the elderly the initial dose of L-dopa (in combination with the inhibitor) should not exceed 50 mg; this may be given once or twice a day and increased by a similar amount every 4 or 5 days until therapeutic efficacy or intolerance appears.

L-dopa used in this way has been associated with improved cognitive function in elderly patients with dementia, whether or not this was associated with parkinsonism; earlier reports of mental deterioration in elderly patients on L-dopa were generally associated with large doses of L-dopa. The situation requires further study before firm conclusions can be drawn.

Long-term L-dopa therapy may gradually lose its effect; and an 'on-off' syndrome is well described, in which sudden fluctuations in performance may be seen. This syndrome occurs with increasing frequency in patients who have been on the drug for 5 years or more; the clinical features vary and may include end-of-dose akinesia or stiffness, or hypotonic 'freezing' as well as rapid swings in functional level ('yo-yoing'). Small dose regimens minimize the likelihood of this syndrome, which is not common in the elderly. Adjustment of dose, regimen and drug preparation used may help; the addition of small doses of bromocriptine (see below) had also been of benefit in a few patients with end-of-dose deterioration. Deprenyl, a monoamine oxidase type B inhibitor (see below), has also been useful in some patients with fluctuations.

Dyskinesias and vomiting are side-effects which may be lessened by decreasing the dose of L-dopa (for vomiting) by switching from the 10:1 to the 4:1 ratio in Sinemet. Dopamine-blocking drugs have also been used: haloperidol can decrease dyskinesia but may worsen the parkinsonism; the more selective agent tiapride (still being studied) can effectively decrease dyskinesia despite the probable increase in L-dopa required to bring the parkinsonism under control once more; metoclopramide in small doses can prevent vomiting without aggravating the parkinsonism.

Pyridoxine (vitamin B_6) antagonizes the effect of L-dopa. Some medicines used in the elderly may contain pyridoxine and could disturb the treatment of parkinsonism. but the antagonism does not occur if the L-dopa is combined with a decarboxylase inhibitor.

Dopaminergic derivatives

These are of current interest, mainly in endocrinology, but also in the treatment of parkinsonism.

Bromocriptine (*Parlodel*) can relieve akinesia, rigidity and tremor in parkinsonism: it has a longer duration of action than L-dopa (its plasma half-life is 3–4 times that of L-dopa) and it causes less dyskinesia, but it is unlikely to be of much value in elderly patients on account of its side-effects (postural hypotension, nausea, digital arterial spasm and a high incidence of mental disturbances including nightmares, hallucinations and paranoia—possibly related to the lysergic-acid-amide portion of the molecule). Mental side-effects may persist for up to 6 weeks after stopping the drug. The main value of bromocriptine in parkinsonism is when small doses are given together with L-dopa or Sinemet to reduce 'on-off' (see above); L-dopa or Sinemet dosage needs reduction when bromocriptine is added, as the toxic effects of the two agents are additive, and mental disturbances and hypotension are especially likely to occur. Introduction of bromocriptine should be extremely cautious: 1.25 mg is enough, increasing over a week or two to 2.5 mg t.i.d., then more if necessary with increments at 4- or 5-day intervals.

A dose of 3.75–10 mg daily of bromocriptine is roughly equivalent to 100 mg of L-dopa plus a decarboxylase inhibitor.

Recently it has been shown that a peripheral dopamine-blocking drug, domperidone, which does not cross the blood–brain barrier, was effective in reducing adverse effects of bromocriptine; by analogy with Sinemet this concomitant regimen may prove to be useful in the treatment of parkinsonism.

Other ergot derivatives

Lergotrile has been shown to be hepatotoxic. *Lisuride* and *pergolide* are showing some promise in parkinsonism.

Amantadine (Symmetrel)

This antiviral drug was found serendipitously to help patients with parkinsonism. It increases presynaptic dopamine release, and may be used alone or together with L-dopa. Although dyskinesias are rare after amantadine, mental confusion with hallucinations may occur; this may compound any mental changes due to concomitant L-dopa therapy. Livedo reticularis is another reported side-effect. The effects of amantadine on parkinsonism are not usually marked, but a worthwhile improvement may be obtained: it may take a week for improvement to begin. In a few patients benefit may be lost after 2–3 months, but more often any improvement persists.

Anticholinergic drugs

The balance between the cholinergic and dopaminergic systems is disturbed in parkinsonism, and an excess of cholinergic activity may be present. This is the basis for the time-honoured use of anticholinergic drugs, which were the mainstay of treatment for parkinsonism before L-dopa was introduced. They are indeed useful for milder cases at younger ages. Indeed, concern over the possibility of loss of effect of L-dopa in the long-term has caused some authorities to recommend that such patients should start on anticholinergics, keeping L-dopa in reserve for more severe cases. This is not a wise decision in elderly patients, in whom anticholinergic drugs are very likely to produce memory impairment, mental confusion and hallucinations, possibly because of the selective cholinergic failure which may already be present in the elderly, especially those with existing dementia. Other major side-effects include constipation, urinary retention, glaucoma.

Benzhexol is a popular choice but seems particularly likely to cause trouble in elderly patients with parkinsonism. Orphenadrine and the other anticholinergics may, however, do likewise, and there are individual variations between the response in different patients.

Deprenyl

This new drug is a potent and irreversible inhibitor of monoamine oxidase (type B). It has no effect on parkinsonism when given alone despite its presumed action in preventing or slowing dopamine breakdown in the brain; but it prolongs and enhances the action of L-dopa. As a result, the dose of L-dopa can be reduced, and the concomitant therapy is in effect like a sustained-release administration of L-dopa. Existing sustained-release formulations of L-dopa have not proved satisfactory, so the introduction of deprenyl may be a useful innovation. Such therapy would be particularly helpful for nocturnal or early morning immobility.

ANTIEPILEPTIC DRUGS

Epilepsy is not infrequent in old age; it is usually late-onset epilepsy due to cerebrovascular disease, or occasionally to cerebral tumours, or associated with dementia of unknown cause, or, if that is not feasible, to suppress the attacks (whether grand mal, focal, myoclonic or petit mal). The major drugs available are shown in Table 13.2.

Table 13.2 Antiepileptic drugs.

		Drug (Trade name)	
Type of epilepsy	Generic name	USA, Canada	UK, Europe
Grand mal or focal epilepsy	Phenobarbitone	Stental Eskabarb	Luminal Gardenal
	Primidone	Mysoline	Mysoline
	Phenytoin	Dilantin	Epanutin
	Carbamazepine	Tegretol	Tegretol
	Diazepam	Valium	Valium
	Clonazepam	Clonipin	Rivotril
	{Valproic acid/	Depakene	—
	Sodium valproate	—	Epilim
	Sulthiame	Ospolot	Ospolot, Trolone
Myoclonic	Clonazepam		
	{Valproic acid/ Sodium valproate		
Petit mal	Ethosuximide	Zarontin	Zarontin
	Clonazepam		
	{Valproic acid/ Sodium valproate		
Psychomotor	Primidone		
	Phenytoin		
	Ethosuximide		

When to treat

A single fit does not warrant long-term therapy, but therapy will be needed to terminate a train of fits or frank status epilepticus. Here the treatment of choice is a benzodiazepine: diazepam 5 mg by intramuscular or intravenous injection, repeated if necessary until control is attained; or by slow intravenous injection at the rate of 10 mg/min.

If fits recur and an underlying cause cannot be found or dealt with, maintenance therapy will be needed. An EEG should help in identifying the type of epilepsy, if other evaluations leave any doubt; the appropriate choice of therapy can then be made.

Choice of drug in maintenance therapy

Only one drug should be used, if possible.

Grand mal and focal epilepsy

Phenobarbitone should be avoided in the elderly, since it may cause drowsiness and confusion; high blood levels may result from impaired renal excretion of this drug in old age, but in any case the plasma half-life is 80 hours, so that accumulation is inevitable, even with once-daily dosage.

Primidone is metabolized to phenobarbitone in the body, and is therefore not recommended for the elderly. It should never be given with phenobarbitone.

Carbamazepine is as effective as phenytoin for grand mal and partial seizures; it is also useful for trigeminal neuralgia. It may cause drowsiness, dizziness and ataxia in higher doses. However, the metabolism of this drug is auto-inducible—i.e. carbamazepine stimulates its own metabolism—so that plasma levels gradually fall during the first few weeks of treatment; and plasma half-life is lower after chronic treatment than earlier on. Twice-daily dosage is usually feasible.

Carbamazepine may also induce enzymes affecting the metabolism of other drugs, e.g. clonazepam, phenytoin, warfarin and doxycycline.

Clonazepam, an analogue of nitrazepam, is best reserved for myoclonic epilepsy (see below), for patients in whom anxiety is marked, and for petit mal. It causes drowsiness and tolerance may develop with regular use. It may be used in status epilepticus but diazepam is preferable.

Valproic acid or sodium valproate

This important antiepileptic drug has a simple nitrogen-free chemical structure, quite different from other antiepileptic drugs. It may also differ in its mode of action, possibly acting via an increase in GABA levels in the brain. It is rapidly absorbed and distributed: peak plasma levels occur 1–4 hours after an oral dose, the drug is strongly protein-bound and its plasma half-life is 8–12 hours or a little less. Metabolism occurs in the liver and the metabolites are excreted in the urine; one of these may interfere with urine tests for ketone bodies.

Valproic acid is a versatile antiepileptic drug. In the USA it is approved for sole and adjunctive treatment of absence seizures (petit mal) and as adjunctive therapy for other types of epilepsy occurring in conjunction with absence seizures. In Europe it is used for most forms of epilepsy. Interactions with other antiepileptic drugs have been described.

Side-effects are usually mild; gastrointestinal irritations may be minimized or avoided by swallowing the tablet or capsule whole, during a meal, or by an enteric-coated tablet. Liver function tests may become abnormal but rarely require cessation of treatment; liver damage of clinical significance is rare. Acute pancreatitis has occurred. Haematological changes (inhibition of secondary platelet aggregation, occasional mild reversible thrombocytopenia) have been reported; disordered haemostasis is rare. A fine tremor may occur; other central nervous system side-effects are rarer. It is recommended that platelet counts and liver function tests be monitored at intervals in patients on valproic acid.

Dosage: Valproic acid is available as 250 mg capsules (or as a syrup) in the USA. Sodium valproate is available in the UK as 100 mg tablets, and 200 mg and 500 mg enteric-coated tablets of valproic acid and sodium valproate (1:1). Liquid preparations are also available.

Treatment may be started with one 250 mg capsule of vaporoic acid or one 200 mg tablet of sodium valproate 3 times daily; the dose may be increased gradually at 3–7 day intervals until control of the epilepsy is achieved or a maximum dose of 2500–2600 mg per day is reached. If control of seizures is not achieved by this dose, another antiepileptic drug may be added carefully, watching for possible drug interactions and oversedation. Patients on small doses may receive the drug twice a day.

Sulthiame

This drug has been used for grand mal, temporal lobe (psychomotor) epilepsy, focal seizures and myoclonic epilepsy, but in the elderly it has found particular use in the control of aggressive behaviour accompanying a confusional state. Dosage starts at 100 mg b.i.d., but 300–600 mg daily may be needed. Side-effects are few and mild (paraesthesiae of extremities and face are the most common side-effects).

Phenytoin

Phenytoin has been recommended as the treatment of choice for the elderly patient with grand mal, focal, partial or psychomotor epilepsy. However, it is a difficult drug to use well in clinical practice since:

(a) it has a narrow therapeutic ratio, which makes it more important than usual to individualize dosage;

(b) there is wide variation in serum levels between subjects (regardless of age);

(c) bioavailability and interaction problems are common;

(d) its metabolism follows saturation kinetics, which means that the relationship between dose and serum-level is not linear: slight changes in dose may lead to disproportionate changes in serum concentrations—especially when the latter are near the optimum range of 10–20 μg/ml (40–80 μmol/l);

(e) there is an age-related increase in serum levels for a fixed dose;

(f) reduced protein-binding in the elderly is associated with increased plasma clearance of phenytoin.

The practical outcome of these considerations is that the usual practice of gradually increasing the dose to achieve full control of fits or to the limit of toleration, followed by slight reduction in dose, is inappropriate and tends to give suboptimal serum concentrations. It is far better to adjust the dose so as to achieve the optimum serum level: in this way nearly all patients with grand mal can be effectively controlled on phenytoin as sole therapy.

There appears to be no need to give smaller doses to the old than to the young, but it then becomes even more important to monitor serum levels. While it is difficult to generalize, the dosage for the elderly will most often lie between 200 and 350 mg daily. Administration may be b.i.d., but the plasma half-life varies with many factors, and the drug may have to be given 3 or even 4 times a day, in certain individuals. Care must be taken with regard to possible drug interactions (see Table 13.3).

As will be seen, enzyme induction is a common result of phenytoin administration; long-term use may lead to osteomalacia or megaloblastic anaemia, both important in old age. Osteomalacia develops when enhanced metabolism of cholecalciferol produces hypocalcaemia. Another factor contributing to hypocalcaemia is phenytoin-induced inhibition of receptor sensitivity to parathormone. Occasionally fits have occurred due to hypocalcaemia, and if phenytoin is then increased the situation is worsened and a vicious circle develops; in these rare cases the correct approach is to treat the hypocalcaemia by giving vitamin D.

Folic acid deficiency due to antiepileptic drugs has long been recognized but never fully explained. Folate metabolism may be enhanced; but the demand for folate as a coenzyme may increase at the same time. Once folate deficiency has occurred, drug elimination is retarded (due to loss of

Table 13.3 Drug interactions with phenytoin.

Interacts with	To produce	Mechanism
Alcohol	(Chronic usage)—decreased anticonvulsant activity	Increased metabolism
	(Acute intoxication)—increased anticonvulsant activity	Decreased metabolism
Anticoagulants (oral)	Increased phenytoin toxicity	Enzyme inhibition
Antidepressants (tricyclic)	Increased phenytoin toxicity	Uncertain
Carbamazepine	Decreased phenytoin effect	Enzyme induction
Chloramphenicol	Increased phenytoin toxicity	Enzyme inhibition
Dexamethasone	Decreased steroid effect	Enzyme induction
Disulfiram ('Antabuse')	Increased anticonvulsant effect	Decreased metabolism
Dopamine	Hypotension (with i.v. phenytoin in intensive care)	Uncertain
Frusemide ('Lasix')	Decreased diuresis	Uncertain
L-dopa	Decreased L-dopa effect	Uncertain
Quinidine	Decreased quinidine effect	Enzyme induction
Sodium valproate	Increased phenytoin toxicity	Displacement from plasma protein

the coenzyme function); folate repletion may lead to loss of control of the epilepsy.

Other adverse effects of phenytoin include drowsiness and ataxia, gum hypertrophy (where the patient's own teeth are present), slowing of motor conduction in peripheral nerves, peripheral neuropathy, worsening of diabetes mellitus and gastrointestinal symptoms.

Many of these toxic effects and drug interactions due to enzyme induction are seen also with phenobarbitone and primidone.

Ethosuximide. This is succinimide with a half-life long enough to permit once-daily dosage; but it may induce nausea and vomiting and may, therefore, be better tolerated twice daily in divided doses. It may cause drowsiness and dizziness; leucopenia has been reported.

Myoclonic epilepsy

This form of epilepsy may be difficult to control with the more common drugs, but clonazepam or sodium valproate will probably be successful.

Psychomotor epilepsy

Phenytoin should be tried first; ethosuximide (see above) is an alternative.

Petit mal

This is relatively uncommon in old age: it may be confused with partial or focal epilepsy. Clonazepam or sodium valproate should be used in the elderly rather than ethosuximide, but if necessary the latter may be tried.

DRUGS IN THE TREATMENT OF STROKE

Acute cerebral infarction

Acute and ingravescent stroke

Vasoactive drugs

Reduction in cerebral blood flow after an acute stroke may be hemispheric or global, but a hyperaemic zone develops around the ischaemic area because metabolites accumulate. Normal cerebral autoregulation, by which the cerebral circulation is kept independent of changes in systemic blood pressure (within certain limits), is lost focally and generally; the patient is now at risk from changes in systemic blood pressure.

The use of vasoactive drugs may do harm in this situation: even a slight fall in systemic blood pressure may aggravate cerebral ischaemia and extend the infarcting area. Furthermore, they may produce an 'intracerebral steal' effect, by which the healthier cerebral arteries may dilate and so take much-needed blood flow from areas supplied by more rigid atherosclerotic vessels: this again may extend the infarction.

On the other hand, some potential for good may be seen in vasoactive drugs: e.g. an 'inverse steal' phenomenon has been described after intravenous infusion of low molecular weight dextran, with clinical improvement; and reduction of the swelling of capillary walls and of blood viscosity (increased after a stroke) may occur after administration of certain vasoactive drugs.

Individual reports of benefit to acute stroke patients have appeared and benefit has been claimed for intravenous papaverine, hexobendine and pyritinol; and some neurologists would welcome a more aggressive approach along these lines in the management of ingravescent cerebral infarction, although they are careful to emphasize the need for facilities for monitoring regional CBF. In the more usual clinical situation where such monitoring is not available, this type of therapy is of uncertain value and carrys considerable risk.

Drugs to reduce cerebral oedema

Corticosteroids (parenteral or oral) have their advocates in this situation, and have been used effectively for the reduction of cerebral oedema, particularly in patients with cerebral tumours. Some studies have reported benefit in acute cerebral infarction, but others have shown no useful result from this therapy and the subject remains controversial. The side-effects of steroids must be remembered, especially ulceration and/or bleeding from the gastrointestinal tract, impairment of glucose tolerance and intercurrent infections.

Glycerol (orally or intravenously in saline) has been reported to improve regional CBF in the early phase of brain softening; it may also aid in normalizing cerebral metabolism in the ischaemic brain. It seems to be relatively free of adverse effects and may be used when renal function is markedly impaired; it acts as a diuretic. Other osmotic diuretic agents, e.g. intravenous mannitol, have also been used to reduce cerebral oedema.

Anticoagulants

These are indicated for cerebral embolism, although studies have not always shown benefit and haemorrhagic complications may occur. Anticoagulants are not indicated for other forms of cerebral infarction. Doubt as to aetiology generally rules out anticoagulants in practice.

Thrombolytic agents, e.g. streptokinase, are contraindicated.

Drugs affecting blood pressure

As explained above, CBF responds passively to changes in systemic blood pressure when autoregulation is lost. The physician should aim at maintaining blood pressure within a normal range for the patient; the use of antihypertensive therapy in the hypertensive acute stroke patient could be catastrophic, especially since baroreceptor function often deteriorates after a stroke. Similarly, drugs which increase blood pressure may be difficult to control, and should only be used as a life-support measure if severe hypotension is present.

In elderly stroke patients the use of a tilt-table may be preferable to the use of drugs in the management of the blood pressure.

Completed strokes

Vasoactive drugs

These have been used in patients recovering from completed strokes, with some claims that neurological status was improved and rehabilitation facilitated. Many of the drugs already described have been the subject of such reports. The evidence is conflicting, and, in the present state of knowledge, no definitive statement is possible.

Anticoagulants are not indicated, except in cases of embolism.

Transient ischaemic attacks (TIAs)

Patients who have TIAs have a 30% risk of developing a florid cerebral infarction within 5 years, but this risk increases with age. Treatment is directed towards prevention of further episodes of the embolic phenomena which are believed to cause the TIAs.

Vasoactive drugs such as isoxsuprine and cyclandelate have been reported to decrease the incidence of TIAs (see discussion on these drugs in Chapter 12). Altered autoregulation has been improved in such patients when given papaverine.

Anticoagulants have been of value in preventing recurrence of TIAs; but anticoagulant therapy does not appear to increase overall survival after the onset of TIAs. Long-term anticoagulant therapy increases the risk of intracranial haemorrhage, and shorter courses (up to 1 year) are more often recommended.

Antiplatelet drugs are now becoming the main focus of medical treatment for patients with TIAs. Aspirin, dipyridamole and sulphinpyrazone are the drugs most often used for this indication. Aspirin has been shown to reduce the risks of stroke and death in normotensive men but not in hypertensive men or in women; but both sexes have shown a decreased incidence of TIAs on aspirin therapy. There is insufficient evidence to indicate that the other two drugs mentioned prevent the development of stroke in patients with TIAs. The subject is discussed further in the next section on prevention of stroke.

Prevention of stroke

Treatment of hypertension

Hypertension is a well-documented risk factor for stroke, and mortality from stroke is higher in hypertensive than in normotensive stroke patients.

Judicious control of hypertension is thus an important preventive measure; but in the elderly the whole question of antihypertensive therapy is often controversial, and if patient selection and management are carried out without scrupulous attention to detail and to balancing all possible risks against the potential benefits, more harm than good is very likely to result.

Treatment of patients with TIAs

This too is the subject of some controversy. Influencing factors include the following.
(1) *Territory of the TIAs*—the prognosis is said to be better for patients with vertebrobasilar TIAs than for those with TIAs in the carotid distribution; but this is not fully agreed. For suitable patients with carotid TIAs surgical treatment (carotid endarterectomy) may be possible; for non-operated patients with carotid TIAs and for most patients with vertebrobasilar TIAs drug treatment is needed.
(2) *Duration of history of TIAs*—patients with TIAs of recent onset are at greater risk of cerebral infarction, especially in the 2 months after the first attack. Some authorities withhold treatment if the last TIA was more than 1 year previously.

Choice of drug. Some authorities, after carefully evaluating a great deal of evidence, still recommend initial anticoagulant therapy (starting with heparin if the patient is within 2 months of the first TIA) for a period of 3 months, followed by aspirin until the patient has been free of TIAs for 1 year. Others start with aspirin therapy, or anticoagulants may be contra-indicated for other reasons. Small doses are considered to be sufficient.

REFERENCES AND FURTHER READING

Byer (1980) Therapy of ischaemic cerebro-vascular disease. *Annals of Internal Medicine* **93,** 742.

Isaacs B. (1984) Stroke. In Brocklehurst J.C. (Ed.) *Textbook of Geriatric Medicine and Gerontology*, 3rd edition Ch. 19. Churchill Livingstone, London.

Richens A. (1978) *Anti-epileptic Drugs in Recent Advances in Clinical Pharmacology*, vol. 1, pp. 147–62. Churchill Livingstone, London.

Chapter Fourteen
Urinary Bladder

J. C. BROCKLEHURST

OVERVIEW

In old age perhaps the greatest problem that stems from bladder disorders is incontinence of urine. Therefore, the main emphasis of this chapter is on the causes of urinary incontinence and the method of using drugs in its management. This requires first a consideration of the innervation of the bladder since much of the treatment is concerned with altering the effects of the autonomic nervous system as it relates to the bladder. Another important field is to consider the use of long-term indwelling catheters in old people who are incontinent, and the best way in which they may be managed. Finally, brief consideration will be given to the use of drugs in the management of carcinoma of the prostate. The whole question of infection of urine will not be considered here as it is dealt with in Chapter 17.

THE ANATOMY AND NEUROPHYSIOLOGY OF THE BLADDER

The urinary bladder is really a very simple organ which has 2 main functions. First it must be able to contain urine without absorbing either the urine or any of its constituents; second, it should be able to maintain a reasonable quantity of urine so that the interval between acts of micturition is not too frequent. These are its principal properties but in the human being and in a number of domestic animals we have to add the important corollary that voluntary postponement of the act of micturition, when it is inappropriate, must be possible. For most members of the animal kingdom this is not necessary although certain mammals use the bladder and its contents in special ways—perhaps the most obvious of which is the dog using small quantities of urine to mark out its territory.

Although the bladder is, on the face of it, a simple reservoir and although it is very accessible to investigation, nevertheless, even now a true understanding of its neurophysiology is not available. The long-held theory of the dual and reciprocal innervation between the sympathetic and parasympathetic nervous system has been found to be too simplistic and for a long time it has been upheld that the principal innervation of the bladder is entirely the parasympathetic outflow. However, more recent work has indicated α and β adrenergic nerve terminals in the bladder neck and urethra, and pharmacological studies have shown in particular that the α innervation may be important in maintaining smooth muscle contractions around the urethra. If this is so, the long-held theory of reciprocal innervation may not be so far from the truth.

The bladder consists essentially of 2 different muscle masses and these have different embryological origins. The main muscle, the *detrusor*, is formed in a number of different layers and provides the interwoven appearance which is particularly well seen when the muscle hypertrophies as a result of bladder outlet obstruction, a condition which is called trabeculation. The detrusor is the muscle of the fundus of the bladder and its fibres at the bladder neck are continued into the first part of the urethra (that is the whole of the female urethra, and the male urethra as far as the verumontanum). The detrusor is the principal muscle which causes bladder emptying and its innervation is cholinergic. Contractions of the detrusor muscle are, therefore, prevented by the use of anticholinergic/antimuscarine drugs (Table 14.1) and drugs with this quality will also have as a side-effect the possible causation of retention of urine. Any drug having as side-effects blurring of vision or dryness of the mouth may also cause retention of urine.

It seems, however, that the extension of the detrusor around the urethra is particularly affected by α-adrenergic stimulation and that in certain conditions in which the urethra maintains its contracture while the rest of the detrusor is also contracting, a condition called detrusor sphincter dyssynergia may arise. This may be improved by drugs which have an anti-α-adrenergic effect (see Table 14.1).

The second bladder muscle is the *trigone*. The trigone is an extension of the smooth muscle of the ureters and as this enters the bladder at the ureteric orifices, fibres pass horizontally to join each other in the interureteric bar (Mercier's bar) and they also form the small triangular muscle known as the trigone. The trigone lies superficial to the detrusor and it also extends into the proximal urethra. The trigone has a rich supply of adrenergic nerve endings and it is not entirely clear what the purpose of this muscle is. It is thought to have some function in ejaculation. It has also been suggested that contraction of the trigone by pulling open the internal urethral orifice may initiate micturition. However, this is not a generally accepted theory at the present time. The trigone is also more richly endowed in sensory nerve endings than most of the rest of the bladder.

A third muscle which is not part of the bladder itself but which surrounds the urethra is the external sphincter, and this is, of course, a striated muscle which is innervated by the pudendal nerve (arising from the first, second and third sacral nerve roots). A number of experiments have indicated that the external sphincter is not necessary for normal continence and that it can be removed without causing incontinence. Similarly incontinence does not follow pudendal neurectomy. The external sphincter is probably

Table 14.1 Drugs used in the management of urinary incontinence.

Type of drug	Drug name (Trade name)	Dosage
Anticholinergic	Methantheline USNF (Banthene)	15 mg p.o.
	Propantheline Bromide BP (Probanthine)	200 mg p.o.
	Emepronium bromide (Cetiprin)*	
	Imipramine hydrochloride (Tofranil)	25 mg p.o.
Antimuscarine	Dicyclomine hydrochloride USNF, BP (Merbentyl, Bentyl)	10–20 mg p.o.
	Orphenadrine hydrochloride (Disipal)	50 mg p.o.
Smooth muscle relaxant	Flavoxate (Urispas)	200 mg p.o.
Cholinergic (muscarine)	Bethanechol chloride (Urecholine chloride)	5 mg s.c. 5–10 mg p.o.
Anticholinesterase	Distigmine bromide (Ubretid)	5–10 mg p.o.
	Neostigmine bromide, BP, USP	5 mg p.o.
α-Adrenergic	Phenylpropapanolamine USNF (Propadrine hydrochloride) BPC	25–50 mg p.o.
	Ephedrine hydrochloride or sulphate BPC, USNF	15 mg p.o.
α-Adrenergic antagonist	Phentolamine mesylate USP, BP (Rogitine)	10 mg i.v.
	Phenoxybenzamine hydrochloride BP, USNF (Dibenaline, Dibenzyline)	10–100 mg p.o.
Skeletal muscle relaxant	Dantrolene (Dantrium)	25 mg p.o.

*Not available in North America.

an additional 'failsafe' device and it does allow the cessation of micturition in midstream. The main problems which arise with the external sphincter are in conditions where it is spastic, as in paraplegia. This is the one situation in which a skeletal-muscle-relaxing drug such as dantrolinium (Dantrolene) may have some effect in a bladder disorder.

We must also keep in mind the epithelial lining of the bladder and urethra. The bladder itself is lined by transitional epithelium, which allows a folding together of its cells as the bladder empties and a stretching of the sheet of epithelium as the bladder fills. The urethra, however, is lined with a form of stratified squamous epithelium and this is of the same origin (in the female) as the stratified squamous epithelium lining of the vagina and vulva. It is, therefore, oestrogen sensitive—an important fact to be considered in relation to certain forms of dysuria in aged females.

The bladder and urethra have connections to the spinal cord through the sympathetic outflow and through the sacral parasympathetic outflow (s2, 3 and 4). There are numerous levels of nerve relay and coordination in the midbrain but the most important level for the conscious control of micturition is a bladder centre in the forebrain situated within the cingulate gyrus.

To understand the way in which micturition is controlled (and thus the way in which control may be lost in old age), it is simplest to concentrate on 2 centres, the sacral bladder centre in the second, third and fourth sacral segments of the spinal cord and the cortical centre in the forebrain (see Fig. 14.1). The sacral bladder centre is the bridge for the simple reflex arc of micturition and by itself allows the bladder to fill and empty reflexively. In the young baby and other animals this is all that is necessary. As the bladder becomes distended with urine, stretch receptors in its wall are activated which discharge impulses to the sacral bladder centre. These build up by various physiological mechanisms and, in turn, discharge impulses to the bladder muscle causing small contractions to occur. As the bladder nears its capacity the contractions become larger until an emptying contraction causes a complete emptying of the bladder.

To acquire continence, control of this reflex arc must be achieved, and

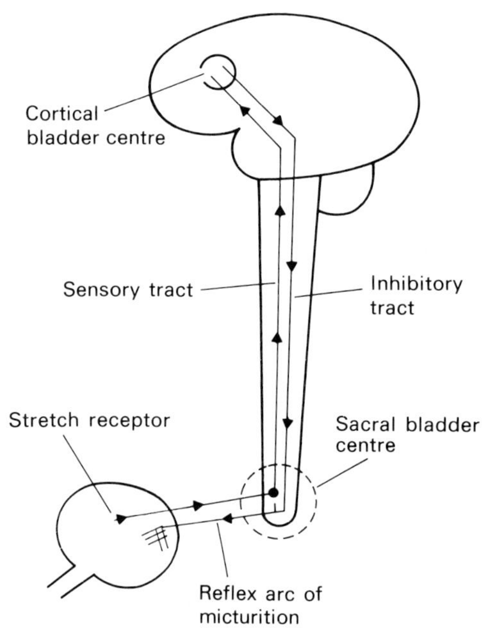

Fig. 14.1 Diagram of the bladder connections with the central nervous system.

this involves being able to block the transmission of impulses through it. However, before this can happen the young child has to develop an awareness of bladder sensation and also an awareness of the actual social necessity of postponing micturition until time and place are appropriate. The awareness of bladder filling results from the development of long tracts from the bladder sacral centre in the lateral parts of the spinal cord which convey the sensation of distension into consciousness. The awareness of the necessity to postpone micturition, of course, is part of the training which the young child receives from its mother. Once it appreciates the need to postpone micturition then it does this by developing long efferent tracts from the cortical bladder centre which block the sacral micturition reflex. This process is known as inhibition and once the young child has learned to inhibit the reflex arc completely then no intrinsic contractions will be seen in the bladder as it becomes distended.

Indeed, in a person with normal bladder control, distension may continue to the point of discomfort without any intrinsic contractions appearing as long as the subject is voluntarily attempting to prevent micturition and thus maintaining inhibition. If this cortical inhibitory ability is lost (as for instance, in some patients with stroke) then the bladder becomes uninhibited and in that case uninhibited intrinsic contractions appear which will cause a feeling of the need to empty the bladder earlier and, indeed, if this cannot be responded to quickly, then quite possibly it will lead to incontinence. This is sometimes called the *uninhibited neuropathic bladder*.

The uninhibited neuropathic bladder occurs in many pathological conditions affecting the frontal cortex (e.g. trauma, infection, dementia) and also occurs in some degree as a result of cortical neuronal aging itself. Thus many old people suffer from daytime urgency or nocturnal frequency, without being incontinent.

Other types of bladder disorders arising from interruption of the long tracts in the spinal cord (as in multiple sclerosis or paraplegia or, indeed, some cases of prolapsed intervertebral discs) may cause more or less loss of connection between the sacral bladder centre and the cortical bladder centre. If the loss is complete, the bladder is the same as that in the baby, it fills up without the subject having any awareness of distension; it develops uninhibited contractions and it empties reflexively from time to time. This is the case in many paraplegics.

If there is interruption in the sensory input to the cortical centre, the bladder may become overdistended and develop chronic retention with overflow incontinence. This was typically the condition seen in tabes dorsalis in which destruction of the posterior horn cells led to the tabetic bladder—an atonic bladder because of loss of sensation. Tabetic bladders are less common nowadays but it is becoming increasingly recognized that another form of atonic neuropathic bladder may result from autonomic neuropathies and particularly that associated with diabetes.

Diabetic autonomic neuropathy may include symptoms such as diarrhoea, postural hypotension, impotence, alterations in sweating patterns and chronic urinary retention.

Finally, in some neurological disorders (e.g. some forms of spina bifida or in the destruction of the cauda equina by metastases) the bladder becomes completely decentralized and so the sacral micturition reflex arc no longer exists. In these cases the bladder will fill and empty inefficiently in continual spurts, and of course there will be no sensation.

On the basis of this discussion it is now possible to classify in a simple way the different types of neurogenic bladder disorders—an essential preliminary to rational drug therapy (see Table 14.2).

Table 14.2 Classification of the neurogenic bladder.

Uninhibited	(cerebral disease: stroke, tumour dementia; partial spinal cord lesions)
Reflex	(complete spinal cord lesions: paraplegia)
Atonic	(sensory nerve or posterior horn cell lesions: tabes, diabetes)
Unstable	impairment of central inhibition without evidence of CNS disease

N.B. Some clinicians regard 'uninhibited neurogenics' and 'unstable' as direct alternatives.

With the information now available it might be considered that the following drugs could have some part to play in the management of various forms of neurogenic bladder disorder (see Table 14.1).

(a) The antimuscarine/anticholinergic drugs in the prevention of uninhibited bladder contractions.

(b) The cholinergic drugs in the prevention or management of the atonic bladder, with or without chronic retention.

(c) The α-blocking adrenergic drugs and skeletal-muscle-relaxing drugs in detrusor sphincter dyssynergia (detrusor urethral dyssynergia).

(d) The spasmolitic drugs in patients with uninhibited intrinsic bladder contractions.

Before considering these, however, it is important to consider the steps by which an accurate diagnosis of the true underlying condition may be made.

THE INVESTIGATION OF URINARY INCONTINENCE

Investigation first requires a knowledge of the differential diagnosis.

Neurogenic (or neuropathic) causes are high on the list because impairment of the efficiency of the cortical bladder centre is common in old age, not only because of cerebrovascular disease but also because of the effects of aging itself. The loss of functioning neurones which is a characteristic of aging has among its many other effects, a tendency to produce impairment of cortical inhibition of the sacral micturition reflex. For this reason many elderly people have bladders which are not working as they should. They tend to empty with urgency because of the proximity of the sensation of first desire to void and an emptying bladder contraction. They may also develop increasing nocturnal frequency. People of both sexes get up at night to empty their bladder increasingly often as they grow older. In addition, the bladder may not empty itself as well as usual and a degree of residual urine is increasingly common with advancing age.

The effect of these underlying changes in bladder control is that an old person is not incontinent as long as she has control of her own environment but loss of independence—and particularly admission to hospital—precipitates incontinence: that is, when she requires to go urgently in the daytime or to get up during the night no nurse is to hand to help her.

Therefore high on the list of causes of incontinence is simply the presence of an uninhibited neuropathic bladder due to aging, together with loss of physical independence.

Recovery from the acute illness possibly with the addition of rehabilitation and the restoration of independence will cure incontinence of this type. This is, therefore, a 'transient' form of incontinence, cured by restoring independence and mobility. Other causes of incontinence, both transient and established are shown in Table 14.3. These include both neurogenic and non-neurogenic causes. The former will be considered first, the others later (see p. 194).

The diagnosis of the neurogenic bladder may be made with confidence by a *cystometrogram* (see Fig. 14.2, p. 189). This procedure is generally available within departments of urology or gynaecology and in Europe in many departments of geriatric medicine. A cystometrogram in its simplest form is made by filling the bladder from a reservoir and observing its reaction to stretch. In the normal person the bladder will fill up to a capacity between 350 and 700 ml with a rise in intravesical pressure in the range of 10–15 cm of water but with no contractions being seen. The subject will register an awareness of bladder filling at about half the capacity and as the total capacity is reached, there will be increasing discomfort. Once the bladder has been filled up, empty it, refill it to about half capacity, and then apply a number of provocative tests. These involve changing the patient's posture from lying to standing and asking her to cough. In cases of the unstable bladder (see below) one or other of these stimuli will fire off an intrinsic bladder contraction.

The various forms of neurogenic bladder may be identified as follows. The uninhibited bladder—the most common in old age—will show a rather

Table 14.3 Causes of transient and established incontinence.

Transient (associated with acute illness)
Loss of mobility
Acute brain failure
Acute cystitis
Stroke
Retention
side-effects of drugs
constipation
Established (not associated with acute illness)
Cerebrovascular disease, cerebral tumour
Chronic brain failure
Spinal cord lesion (prolapsed disc, paraplegia, multiple scleroris, secondary carcinoma)
Atrophic urethritis (with atrophic vaginitis)
Retention
prostatic enlargment
atonic neuropathic bladder

more rapid rise in intravesical pressure with the presence of uninhibited contractions and an emptying contraction occurring below normal capacity. The sensation of bladder filling and desire to void may well precede the emptying contraction by only a very short interval.

If the spinal cord is affected (sometimes called the reflex neuropathic bladder), a similar tracing will be obtained without evidence of desire to void. If the bladder is atonic, the filling may continue to one or more litres of fluid and the rise of intravesical pressure will be much more gradual than in the normal bladder and there will be no sensation of bladder filling.

There are many forms of cystometer available. Traditionally they have filled the bladder with water or saline and more recently a number of instruments using carbon dioxide have been marketed and are fairly widely used. There is no general agreement as to which is superior. The gas-filled system will record contractions of smaller amplitude but it is questionable whether very low amplitude contractions are significant. A bladder contraction regarded as an uninhibited contraction is usually one which reaches 10 cm of water pressure. Cystometrograms may also be made in different ways: i.e. by rapidly filling at the rate of 100 ml per minute or more, filling gradually at a slower rate, or filling in increments of 50 ml at a time.

The second investigation which may be useful is to visualize the bladder

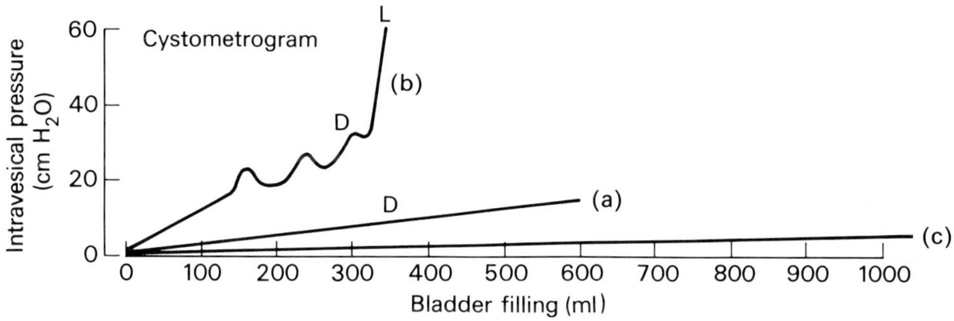

Fig. 14.2 Cystometrogram: (a) normal; (b) atonic; (c) uninhibited neurogenic. L = leakage; D = desire to void.

outlet radiologically by a *micturating cystogram.* This is particularly useful in trying to be sure of a diagnosis of stress incontinence (incontinence in which there is leakage of urine from the bladder following a rapid rise in intraabdominal pressure due to running, coughing or laughing or changing posture). In this case the leakage is due to weakness of the bladder outlet and will occur without any bladder contraction occurring. Therefore it is useful to combine both a micturating cystogram and a cystometrogram, and this has been done in the videocystourethrogram. Here both the form and the pressure within the bladder are obtained simultaneously and these are recorded on videotape.

The closing pressure within the urethra may be determined by carrying out a *urethral pressure profile.* To do this a catheter with an open eye is slowly drawn through the urethra with the eye moving from the bladder itself to the outside of the body. Through the catheter is leaked, at a very slow rate, water from a reservoir and the resistance which this encounters may be recorded as a pressure curve. The usual measurement in assessing the urethral closing pressure is that of the maximal pressure recorded.

A uroflowmeter measures the speed at which the subject is able to empty his bladder. This will give a useful indication if there is obstruction of the bladder outlet.

These are the main forms of investigation generally available in urodynamic assessment units, but of them all the cystometrogram is probably the most important. A simple cystometrogram may well be used as an office precedure and will certainly be helpful in indicating whether the bladder is neurologically normal or abnormal.

Other investigations include the culture of a midstream specimen of urine for infecting organisms; a smear of vaginal epithelium to measure its degree of maturation (or atrophy) and, of course, cystoscopy by a gynaecologist or a urologist.

The unstable bladder

In the last few years the concept of the unstable bladder (or detrusor instability) has become generally accepted. An unstable bladder is one occurring in a patient without evidence of central nervous system (CNS) disease, in whom uninhibited contractions may be demonstrated on a cystometrogram either on a straight run-through or as the result of provocation (change of posture, coughing, laughing, etc.).

Essentially the unstable bladder is one which escapes from cortical inhibition as the result of some sensory or emotional stimulus.

This stimulus is usually a sudden increase in intravesical pressure following a sudden rise in intra-abdominal pressure for one of the reasons indicated above. The unstable bladder may, thus, be a cause of incontinence and since the bladder contraction commonly follows change of posture or cough it may be difficult in women clinically to differentiate this from true stress incontinence. It is important to make this distinction since the treatment of each is different. The differentiation usually requires a cystometrogram.

Bladder instability probably occurs in many people at some time in their lives as a result of emotion (e.g. sitting examinations or performing a solo in a concert), when urgency and frequency of micturition may precede the event. Ideopathic detrusor instability has a strong functional element. Commonly, it is also associated with some pathological lesion affecting the bladder. In males this may be associated with prostatic hypertrophy and in females with disease of the pelvic organs or following surgery in that region. It may also occur with pathology in the bladder including particularly an acute infection.

THE DRUG TREATMENT OF INCONTINENCE

The unstable bladder and the uninhibited neuropathic bladder

In both of these cases the presence of uninhibited contractions leading to bladder leakage is the basic abnormality and the most straightforward method of trying to prevent this, therefore, is to block the reflex arc of micturition. Since the detrusor muscle is principally supplied with cholinergic (muscarine) nerve endings, the appropriate drugs are those with an antimuscarine effect or those which have a direct paralysing effect on the smooth muscle of the bladder itself. For a century belladonna and other solenaceous alkaloids have been used for this purpose, particularly in enuresis in children. The drugs commonly in use at the present time include:

Propantheline
Emepronium bromide } anticholinergic drugs
Imipramine

Orphenadrine	(an anticholinergic drug which also may have some effect in the spinal cord itself)
Flavoxate	(has a papaverine-like action directly on smooth muscle itself)

In North America emepronium bromide and flavoxate are not available and so the choice is more limited. Tablet size and maximum daily dose are shown in Table 14.1 (see p. 183).

Propantheline, orphenadrine and emepronium bromide are quarternary ammonium compounds and as a result of this their absorption is very much less than the natural alkaloid when given by mouth. For this reason the effectiveness of the quarternary ammonium antimuscarine compounds is often disappointing and it is useful to combine them with a drug having a direct spasmolytic effect, i.e. give flavoxate and either propantheline, imipramine or emepronium bromide. The alternative is to combine orphenadrine (with its internuncial neurone effect) with propantheline or dicyclo mine. In this case the possible side-effects will be additive.

Ideally it is useful to obtain immediate information as to whether these combinations will have an effect in an individual patient and this can be done by undertaking 3 repeat cystometrograms every hour after an oral dose of the drug for 3 hours. If the bladder capacity is increased and uninhibited contractions diminished, some clinical effect may be hoped for and a therapeutic trial should be started.

The amount and timing of the drug will depend on the nature of the incontinence and, therefore, the drug treatment should be used in combination with a chart of the incidence of incontinence throughout the 24 hours. If the patient is at home, she or her relatives should fill it in, if she is in hospital, the nurse should fill it in. The chart is also used as a reminder for the patient to empty her bladder since, of course, drugs used in the treatment of the uninhibited or unstable bladder will only increase its capacity and help to postpone incontinence but certainly provide no substitute for the regular emptying of the bladder. The chart should be filled in every 4 hours initially and if the patient is shown to be substantially wet during this time then it should be filled in every 2 hours. (Sometimes an alarm, reset each time, serves as a short-term reminder). A note should be made as to whether the patient is wet or dry and then she should go to empty her bladder and a note that this has been done should also be made.

Patients who are incontinent only at night should be given the medication before retiring to bed and a repeat dose when they waken during the night to empty their bladders. Patients who are wet throughout 24 hours should receive the drugs 6-hourly. A course should be given at an optimum therapeutic dose for 4 to 6 weeks. If there has been no effect at the end of this time, they should be withdrawn. If they have cured or ameliorated the condition, then over the course of time an attempt should be made gradually to wean the patient off them. This may or may not be successful.

Side-effects of drug treatment

In old people side-effects of the anticholinergic drugs are very important. They include, of course, blurring of vision and dryness of the mouth, which can be tiresome and sometimes lead the patient to abandon the drug altogether. They may also lead to gaseous distension of the bowel.

Emepronium bromide is irritant if maintained in contact with the mucosa and old people who tend to keep tablets in their mouths, may, therefore, develop buccal ulcers with it. Similarly, since aging affects oesophageal motility, tablets may be held up at the lower end of oesophagus for periods of up to three-quarters of an hour in some elderly people. If this occurs with emepronium bromide, then ulceration of the lower end of the oesophagus may occur. That drug in particular, therefore, should be given with a large draught of water and the attendant should pay particular attention to see that it has been swallowed.

Another side-effect, and one which is perhaps less obvious, is the development of chronic retention of urine. This may slowly convert incontinence due to an uninhibited neuropathic bladder to incontinence due to retention with overflow. This change may not be noticed unless the nurse or physician is alert to the possibility and examines the abdomen from time to time. If there is any suspicion of retention, the residual urine should be measured.

Many people have found the drug treatment of the uninhibited neuropathic bladder to be disappointing. In part this may have been because of imprecise diagnosis and using this form of treatment when, in fact, the patient's main problem was infection, viginitis, or even retention with overflow. Probably at least one-third of the patients with uninhibited neuropathic bladders will be helped or cured of their incontinence by the use of these drugs. This may be a relatively low proportion but nevertheless is extremely important for those in whom the results are positive, particularly since other therapeutic approaches to this condition are so limited.

Two main pharmacological approaches to treatment of the uninhibited reflex neurogenic bladders, and the unstable bladder, have recently been described. Prostaglandin F2α has been shown to occur in the contracting bladder and, therefore, prostaglandin synthetase inhibitors have been tried to prevent contractions. Flurbiprofen has been reported with some success.

The second approach has been with calcium antagonists. Both nifedipine and flunarazine have had good reports and further study of the place of these drugs in the management of incontinence is awaited with interest.

Another method of treatment not involving drugs which has been described is the use of biofeedback in attempting to increase cortical control over the sacral micturition reflex. The bladder is slowly filled up and the subject watches the tracing for the development of uninhibited contractions, and their development is also noted by a sound signal. As they develop the subject attempts to inhibit and some success has been claimed in reacquiring inhibition by this process.

Behavioural therapy involving bladder drill has been used with great success in the ideopathic unstable bladder, and in the neurogenic bladder associated with chronic brain failure. Hospital admission strengthens the effect of this procedure. Patients are told to empty their bladders at exact times—usually starting $1\frac{1}{2}$ hourly—neither earlier nor later. This interval is gradually increased until a 4-hour period is reached. Anticholinergic drugs may be used simultaneously.

The atonic bladder

In the treatment of patients with chronic retention with overflow incontinence, cholinergic (muscarine) drugs and anticholinesterases may have a place. Bethanechol (urecholine, available in 5, 10, 25 mg tablets and 5 mg per ml for subcutaneous injection) is a cholinergic drug. It should not be used by either intramuscular or intravenous injection. The anticholinesterases are prostigmine and distigmine (Ubretid).

Bethanechol is without doubt an effective drug when given parenterally, although its action when given by mouth is less certain. Side-effects may include gastrointestinal symptoms such as epigastric distress, abdominal cramps and belching, blurring of vision due to difficulty in accommodation, headaches, salivation, flushing and sweating. This drug must, therefore, be used with care in old people and since the regimen required is fairly intense, it needs close medical supervision.

In the patient with an atonic bladder in whom bladder outlet obstruction has been ruled out, the bladder should first be emptied by catheterization at a slow rate of 300 ml every 2 hours. The catheter should then be removed and the patient observed. There may be no need for further treatment. However, if the retention recurs or a residual urine of over 100 ml develops then treatment with bethanechol should be instigated. In this case 2.5 mg subcutaneously should be given 6-hourly. Residual urine is measured every second day. Once the residual comes down to 100 ml the drug may then be given by mouth—usually in a dosage of 50 mg 3 to 4 times daily. While response to a single dose of this level is poor, the drug accumulates, so that high doses may be hazardous and these should be monitored with care.

Neostigmine bromide (Prostigmine) is available in 15 mg tablets. In addition to its effects in causing bladder contraction, it will also tend to produce bradycardia, possibly hypotension and diminish the cardiac output. It will increase the propulsive waves in the colon and may cause cramp.

Distigmine bromide (Ubretid) is an anticholinesterase compound with a prolonged action over a period of 12–24 hours. Given parenterally it will cause a rapid rise in intravesical pressure together with the development of rhythmical bladder contractions, but its effect on retention when given by mouth is rather more doubtful. Both of these substances are quarternary ammonium compounds and for this reason their absorption by mouth is poor. They may be kept as reserve drugs either to add to the effect of bethanechol or to use on a longer term basis in the management of the atonic bladder. Their real usefulness in this regard has, so far, not been evaluated.

OTHER DRUGS IN THE MANAGEMENT OF URINARY INCONTINENCE

If the incontinence is associated with an *acute urinary infection* then this should be treated with the appropriate antibiotic. This subject is dealt with in detail on page 240. It may be associated with *atrophic vaginitis* (a diagnosis which can usually be made on clinical examination but can be confirmed by undertaking a vaginal smear). Clinically there may be blood-stained vaginal discharge, with or without pruritis, and small red spots together with excoriation of the vagina will be seen. The condition is a combination of epithelial atrophy and superadded infection. It responds well to treatment with oestrogens by mouth, either synthetic preparations such as ethinyl estradiol (tablets of 0.01 mg) or diethylstilboestrol (0.1 mg tablets) or so-called natural oestrogens such as conjugated equine oestrogen (Premarin) and oestradiol valerate (Progynova and Progynon) may be used. They should be given daily for 1 month and often the course has to be repeated 2 or 3 times a year. If the above-mentioned low doses are not sufficient, they may have to be increased somewhat.

Oestrogen cream has also been used for this purpose but it is difficult for old women to apply, sometimes inducing secondary infection from the anal area and may be more likely to cause postmenopausal bleeding due to rapid absorption.

In *genuine stress incontinence* treatment is intended to increase the tone and improve the condition of the pelvic muscles and this involves physiotherapy (providing special exercises) which may be combined with electrical treatment including faradism, anal and vaginal stimulators and interferential therapy. Biofeedback methods have also been used in this treatment, an intravaginal-pressure-recording balloon allowing the woman to see the extent to which the power of the pubococcygeus muscle is being developed. If true stress incontinence is associated with prolapse, then the use of either pessaries or gynaecological surgery will be necessary.

As an adjunct to physiotherapy in stress incontinence the α-adrenergic drugs phenylpropanolamine hydrochloride (Propadine hydrochloride) or ephedrine hydrochloride (or sulphate) may be used. Phenylpropanolamine has been shown to increase maximal urethral closing pressure (as seen on urethral pressure profile) by between 65 and 75% in patients with incontinence due to bladder outlet weakness (stress incontinence in females and post-prostatectomy incontinence other than that due to an underlying uninhibited neuropathic bladder in males). One trial showed 10 out of 20 patients becoming completely dry and 7 others being improved. Phenylpropanolamine must be used with great care in old people and is contraindicated in the presence of hypertension, hyperthyroidism and diabetes. It should not be used with (or within 7 days of) amino-oxidase inhibitors.

Ephedrine has been used in incontinence for decades on the basis of an adrenergic 'relaxing' effect on the detrusor. Such an effect now seems unlikely, but its α-stimulant action may increase urethral smooth muscle tone. Contraindications to its use are the same as for phenylpropanolamine.

Finally, blockage of adrenergic activity in the urethra has been attempted in the syndrome of detrusor sphincter dyssynergia. The α-adrenergic blocking agents phentolamine mesylate (Rogitine) and phenoxybenzamine hydrochloride (Dibenyline) have been used for this purpose. Phentolamine is given intravenously as a means of assessing the usefulness of the procedure. If results are encouraging, a course of phenoxybenzamine tablets is given. Side-effects include hypotensive effects, which contraindicate this drug in old people with postural hypotension and demand great care in patients with hypertension or coronary artery insufficiency. Oral dosage should be started low (10 mg daily) and cautiously increased.

Detrusor sphincter dyssynergia may also arise from spasticity of the striated external sphincter. In such cases a skeletal muscle relaxant such as dantrolene may be helpful.

THE INDWELLING FOLEY CATHETER AND ITS MANAGEMENT

The indwelling Foley catheter is a useful tool in the management of certain patients with urinary incontinence but is much overused at the present time. An indwelling catheter should be a last resort and never a first resort. It should only be used after an accurate diagnosis of the incontinence has been made and every attempt has been made to apply specific therapy. If this is unsuccessful, the choice lies between the use of a catheter, of external appliance or simply of pads and protective pants. External appliances are of some value in males and the sheath urinal (Texas catheter) or one of its many variations is useful in numbers of males who are able to cooperate. No appliance is available for successful use in females. In general, pads and pants are disappointing because the patient's skin tends to remain wet and very often her clothing also becomes wet. However, they do have an important place in protection against occasional wetting, particularly in patients with stress incontinence.

The indwelling catheter, therefore, has a place in patients with intractable incontinence, and in old age this is usually those with cerebrovascular disease or advanced dementia. It has been possible to prevent bladder infection from developing if the catheter is used only for 2 to 3 days but longer use has always been associated with infection.

The management of indwelling catheters

The 2 major problems with indwelling catheters for which drug treatment may be thought to be useful are:

(a) infection of the bladder urine and its extension into the urinary tract;

(b) the formation of crystals, leading to catheter blockage.

It has been noted above that infection of the bladder urine is inevitable when an indwelling catheter is used and no well-conducted study has been published which demonstrates any way of preventing this from happening. It can be prevented with closed systems for 2 or 3 days. The use of antibiotics will sterilize the urine in a small proportion of patients but only for a few days and the use of urinary antiseptics will not prevent urinary infection from developing. The important question, therefore, is whether this infection is of significance and has to be considered as a danger to the patient's health. Studies have shown that infection of the urine with indwelling catheters is associated with infection of the kidney, and in old people this may affect creatinine clearance. However, in the short-term (1–2 years) this is probably not of serious import. In young patients with chronic illness in whom life expectancy may reasonably be measured in 5 or 10 or more years there is a real danger associated with urinary infection of indwelling catheters. In these cases the renal infection which occurs will very probably have serious results and in many cases will lead eventually to the patient's death. In younger patients, therefore, every attempt should be made to avoid indwelling catheters.

In the old, although renal infection does occur, it does not appear to be life-threatening to the patient during the few years of life which remain to the average old person with intractable incontinence. This means that catheters can be used (on the evidence we have at present) with reasonable confidence for a period of 1 to 2 years at the end of a patient's life. Patients with intractable incontinence almost certainly suffer from multiple cerebrovascular disease or advancing dementia and it is unlikely that their prognosis will extend much beyond this period. Therefore, in such cases, catheters may be used. However, they should not be used in other old people in whom the cause of the incontinence will almost certainly be susceptible to specific treatment, as outlined above.

Infected urine, however, may provoke an acute symptomatic infection within the urinary tract. This 'catheter fever', often associated with septicaemia, certainly does require treatment when it occurs, and this treatment will be with the appropriate antibiotic.

To what extent may urinary antiseptics diminish the amount of renal infection, the frequency of episodes of acute infection and episodes of catheter blockage? There is no information about the usefulness of such drugs in relation to renal infection. Studies, however, have shown that episodes of acute symptomatic infection can be diminished by about two-thirds in patients on urinary antiseptics. Catheter blockage due to crystals can be diminished also by this means. It would seem, therefore, that there may be a useful place for urinary antiseptics in patients with indwelling catheters to diminish the frequency of catheter blockage and of episodes of acute urinary tract infection.

Urinary antiseptics for use with indwelling catheters

A commonly used urinary antiseptic is methenamine (see Table 14.4). This drug has its effects by releasing formaldehyde in urine which has an acid

Table 14.4 Urinary antiseptics.

Drug name (Trade name)	Dosage
Methenamine (hexamine) mandelate (Mandelamine, Mandurin)	500 mg, 4–8 tablets daily
Methenamine mandelate + d.l. methionine (G.500)	250 mg, 8–16 tablets daily
Methenamine hippurate (Hiprex)	1 g, 2–4 tablets daily
Nalidixic acid (Negram)	500 mg, 2–4 tablets daily
Nitrofurantoin (Furadantin, Furam, Berkfurin, Ceduran)	50 mg, 2–4 tablets daily
Conoxacin (Cinobac)	500 mg capsule, twice daily

reaction (see Fig. 14.3). Methenamine is effective against *E. coli* but not against *Proteus*. Formaldehyde is bactericidal at a pH between 5 and 8 but it is necessary to reduce the pH of the urine in order to have the formaldehyde released. It is generally accepted that the pH must be less than 5.5 for this to be effective and there is, therefore, no point in giving methenamine to patients whose urinary pH is above this figure. The 2 forms of methenamine in most common use are salts combined with acids—that is methenamine and mandelic acid (methenamine mandelate) and methenamine with hippuric acid (methenamine hippurate). These are Mandelamine and Hiprex. Of the two, methenamine mandelate is the more effective although its major drawback is the need to give a fairly high dose of rather unpalatable tablets. The dose has to be 4 g a day (4–8 tablets a day), although this dosage may be halved if an acidifying agent is given at the same time. These include ammonium chloride (1 g 4 times a day) and sodium acid phosphate (300 mg tablets 4 times a day), the former being more successful.

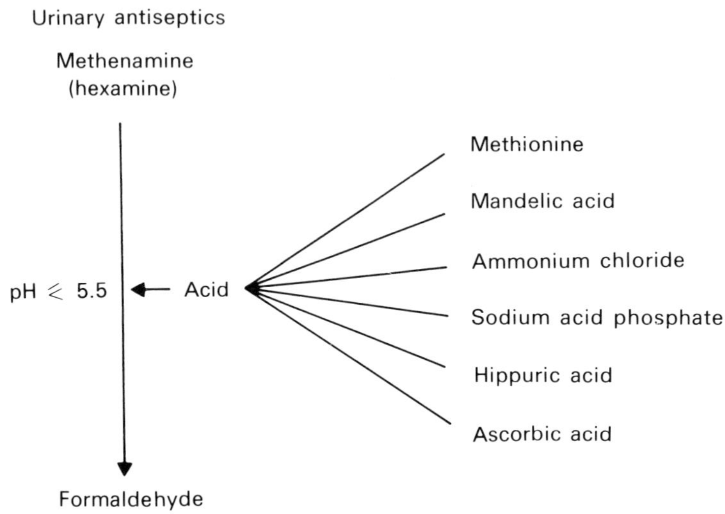

Fig. 14.3 The action of methenamine.

Ascorbic acid has also been used to acidify the urine but its effect is unpredictable and at least 2.5 g a day are required.

Methenamine is decomposed by gastric juice and the tablets are, therefore, given with an enteric coating. Since it forms formaldehyde and ammonia it is a drug which is contraindicated in patients with liver damage. Since it is effective only after it breaks down in the urine it is not contraindicated in patients with renal failure, although in such cases the acids required to change the pH of the urine would be contraindicated, and so, in effect, the regime itself is contraindicated.

Other drugs comparable to urinary antiseptics are nalidixic acid and nitrofurantoin.

Nalidixic acid

Nalidixic acid (Negram) inhibits the synthesis of DNA in bacteria and is effective against *E. coli*, *Proteus* and *Klebsiella*, although not against *Pseudomonas*. It is well absorbed when given by mouth and there is a high degree of plasma binding leading to a fairly prolonged half-life (this is 8 hours normally and may extent to 21 hours in patients with renal failure). Thus there is a likelihood of this drug accumulating and in long-term use this would require careful monitoring. It is usually given with a loading dose of 2 g a day for 2 weeks, followed then by a maintenance dose of 1 g daily. Because of the plasma binding, very little active drug is available in the body itself. It is excreted into the urine either unchanged or as hydroxynalidixic acid which is also actively bactericidal.

Side-effects include nausea, vomiting and abdominal pain; allergic reactions (skin rashes, oesinophilia and fever) occasionally occur. It also occasionally produces depression of bone marrow leading to thrombocytopenia and leukopenia and, very rarely, haemolytic anaemia. Headaches, drowsiness, vertigo, visual disturbances and muscle pains are also occasional side-effects.

The potential dangers of these side-effects mean that nalidixic acid for long-term use must be considered with reserve. If it is used in this way, regular liver function and haematology tests are required. Cinoxacin (Cinobac) is a recently introduced drug chemically similar to nalidixic acid requiring to be given only twice daily and with fewer side-effects.

Nitrofurantoin

Nitrofurantoin (Furadantin) is an effective bactericide against *E. coli*, *Klebsiella* and *Staphylococcus*, although *Proteus* and *Pseudomonas* are quite often resistant to it. It is more effective in an acid urine. It is rapidly and completely absorbed from the gastrointestinal system and has a relatively short half-life of up to 1 hour. Its excretion is diminished in renal failure and so side-effects increase in this condition. It may produce a brown-coloured urine.

Nitrofurantoin has a number of well-known and rather unusual side-effects. Interstitial pulmonary fibrosis is one of these—more commonly in old than in younger people. Polyneuropathy is another serious side-effect. It may also depress marrow function, producing leukopenia and, occasionally, a haemolytic anaemia. It also produces allergic effects, particularly rashes.

Nitrofurantoin is available both as 50 mg tablets and as an oral suspension. The usual adult dose is 200 mg a day although a better method of assessing dosage is to use a formula of 5–10 mg/kg. This latter dosage is particularly the case in the elderly. A number of recent reports have shown nitrofurantoin to be effective when taken in a dose of 100 mg at night only. The excretion of urine during the night is less than an equivalent time during the day and the urine is more concentrated so that the level of the drug is higher. It thus produces a period of antisepsis during the night, which seems to be effective in eradicating many infections and in maintaining sterility.

Conclusion

A comparison of the use of the urinary antiseptics and of mandelic acid and nitrofurantoin is necessary. In the management of indwelling catheters use will be long-term and for this period methenamine mandelate with the addition of ammonium chloride is probably the optimum. If this is not tolerated, then methenamine mandelate alone or methenamine hippurate with ammonium chloride is a possible, though largely untried, second approach. In patients with indwelling catheters these drugs will not maintain sterility of the urine but will help diminish episodes of acute infection and of catheter blockage.

Their use in urinary tract infection in the absence of indwelling catheters also needs some consideration. In episodes of acute infection the appropriate antibiotic, or cotrimoxazole, is almost certainly preferable and indeed methenamine in any of its forms is a very poor drug for the treatment of an acute infection. Either mandelic acid or nitrofurantoin, however, may be of use if the infection is resistant to the common antibiotics (and sensitive to either of these drugs).

The management of chronic urinary tract infection in the absence of an indwelling catheter in old people is a much more difficult problem on which it is harder to give clear guidance. Chronic bacteriuria probably occurs in about 20% of old people and this figure rises to 30% or more of those who are immobile. Thus chronic bacteriuria is a very common condition in old people in nursing homes and extended care homes. There is no doubt that the extent of chronic bacteriuria can be diminished by the use of urinary antiseptics and that they are more effective in the long-term in maintaining sterility than is the episodic use of antibiotics. In fact it is dangerous to continue using a series of antibiotics in old people with chronic bacteriuria since the number of resistant organisms so produced is a serious matter within a community of elderly people. The attendant risks of antibiotics (particularly allergic reactions) are also summated.

For this reason it is suggested that chronic bacteriuria should not be treated unless it is producing symptoms. Even if it is associated with urinary incontinence a chronic bacteriuria may not be the direct cause of the incontinence but rather a secondary effect associated with residual urine which in turn is caused by whatever is the cause of the incontinence itself. Thus sterilizing the urine will not remove the incontinence.

The distinction between an acute urinary tract infection and chronic bacteriuria in the elderly may be difficult to make. Urinary tract infection associated with acute symptoms of pain, dysuria and fever should always be treated and preferably with the appropriate antibiotic or sulphonamide preparation. In the absence of such symptoms but in the presence of incontinence the infection should be treated when it is first encountered. If the incontinence persists, repeated courses of treatment are not indicated.

If the patient is asymptomatic, urinary tract infection should be treated when it is first encountered but recurrences thereafter should not be treated as long as they continue to be symptomatic.

Catheter blockage

One of the difficulties in the use of an indwelling catheter is its encrustation with crystals. This results from the combination of protein (from shed epithelial cells and possibly from pus cells) with salts (especially of calcium and phosphorus). The degree of saturation of the salts is an important matter but more important probably is the individual reaction of different people. Some subjects are more prone to form crystals within the urinary tract than are others, and this seems to be a factor in the formation of calculi anywhere within the tract. Various attempts have been made to try and diminish the precipitation of crystals in such patients; one of these methods is to change the pH of the urine by acidifying it. However, successful reduction of the pH to 5.5 has not been shown to affect the formation of calcium, citric acid or ammonium salts (in at least 1 study). The alternative is to use specific inhibitors of crystal growth in urine and numbers of these are now being explored. Indeed, it is suggested that it is the absence of these inhibitors that allows the formation of large crystalline deposits of calcium oxalate which form the nucleus of many renal tract stones.

The alternative approach is an attempt to prevent crystalline deposits by the use of regular bladder washouts. These may be tap water, saline or antiseptic or dilute acid solutions. The use of tap water has recently been claimed to be as safe as 1/5000 chlorhexidine solution (Gerrie *et al.* 1979).

Antiseptic solutions which may be used for bladder irrigation (see Table 14.5) include neomycin, chlorhexidine (a quarternary ammonium compound) and solution of noxythioline (a substance which probably acts by a slow release of formaldehyde and which may produce an intense burning sensation). The proprietary preparation Noxyflex contains amethocaine hydrochloride 10 mg to 2.5 g of noxythioline to relieve this sensation and is therefore more suitable.

Acetic acid 0.25% solution has the advantage of both an antiseptic and an acidifying effect and may well be the most useful solution in the prevention of catheter encrustation. The addition of sodium acetate buffer (sodium

Table 14.5 Solutions used for bladder irrigation.

Tap water
Neomycin 0.2% (Polybactrin G.U.)
Chlorhexidine 1:5000 (Uro-Tainer)
Noxythioline 1–2.5% (Noxyflex)
Acetic acid 0.25%
Magnesium citrate (Uro-Tainer Suby-G)

Proprietary preparations ( )

acetate 2.1%, polysorbate '80' 0.5% and glacial acetic acid q.s. to yield a solution of pH 5) has been reported to have double the antiseptic effect. However, for present purposes the solution of acetic acid in water is satisfactory. A solution of magnesium citrate may also be used.

It must be noted that the use of irrigation in patients with long-standing indwelling catheters is regarded by some urologists as contraindicated. Their view is that the sudden, quite forceful distension of a bladder which has normally become contracted may lead to some rupture of the mucous membrane and so to the introduction of infection. The author does not accept this as a contraindication but it does underline the need for any bladder irrigation to be done gently without using any high head of pressure.

As indicated earlier, some patients show very little tendency to catheter encrustation and in them irrigation may be unnecessary. In others it may be carried out once a week or even 2 or 3 times a week. It may be possible to teach relatives to do this.

Sometimes leakage alongside the catheter is due to uninhibited bladder contractions expelling the small amount of urine which may be present, related to the Foley catheter balloon below the level of the catheter eye. The catheter balloon may precipitate such contractions in patients with unstable or uninhibited bladders. The use of an anticholinergic or antispasmodic drug may be helpful. Always be sure that the catheter is not kinked and that leakage is not due to the patient obstructing it by sitting on it or by the bag becoming overfilled.

REFERENCES AND FURTHER READING

Blaivas J.C., Labib K.B., Michalik S.J. & Zayed A.A.H. (1980) Cystometric response to propantheline in detrusor hyperreflexia: therapeutic implications. *Journal of Urology* **124,** 259–62.

Brocklehurst J.C. (1984) Genito-Urinary System—The bladder. In Brocklehurst J.C. (Ed.) *Textbook of Geriatric Medicine and Gerontology*, 3rd edition, Ch. 30. Churchill Livingstone, London.

Brocklehurst J.C. & Brocklehurst S. (1978) The management of indwelling catheters. *British Journal of Urology* **50,** 102–5.

Frewen W.K.F. (1982) A reassessment of bladder training in detrusor dysfunction in the female. *British Journal of Urology* **54,** 372–3.

Gerrie B.G., Glen E.S. & Hunter B. (1979) Long term urethral catheter drainage. *British medical Journal* **2,** 1046–7.

Jarvis G.J. (1982) The management of urinary incontinence due to primary vesical sensory urgency by bladder drill. *British Journal of Urology* **54,** 374–6.

Ritch A.E.S., George C.F., Castleden C.M. & Hall M.R.P. (1977) A second look at emepronium bromide in urinary incontinence. *Lancet* **i,** 504–6.

Shepherd A.M. (1980) Re-education of the muscles of the pelvic floor. In Mandelstam (Ed.), *Incontinence and its Management*. Croom Helm, London.

Sonda L.P., Gershon C., Biokno A.C. & Lapides J. (1979) Further observations on the cystometric and uroflowmetric effects of bethanechol chloride on the bladder. *Journal of Urology* **122,** 775–7.

Stanton S.L. (1973) A comparison of emepronium bromide and flavoxate hydrochloride in the treatment of urinary incontinence. *Journal of Urology* **110,** 529–32.

Willington F.L. (Ed.) (1976) *Incontinence in the Elderly*. Academic Press London.

Chapter Fifteen
Gastrointestinal System

J.C. BROCKLEHURST

OVERVIEW

Many conditions arising within the gastrointestinal system do not present special problems in the elderly distinguishing them from their management in younger people. This chapter therefore is concerned about 2 major areas of disease where special facts do apply in relation to old people. These are peptic ulceration and constipation. Both are common conditions and the latter in particular tends to be neglected by physicians to the extent that much faecal incontinence is found among old people, especially those in institutions. Much of this is evidence of medical and nursing neglect.

THE STOMACH

It is now well known that the secretion of hydrochloric acid in the stomach diminishes with age and this applies to both basal and maximal gastric secretion. The percentage of persons with achlorhydria also increases with age. It appears that diminished acid secretion is associated with evidence of atrophic gastritis. However, there are still large gaps in knowledge about the effects of aging on gastric secretion.

The prevalence of peptic ulceration does not diminish as people get older and indeed autopsy studies such as that of McKeown (1965) have shown a surprisingly high prevalence of peptic ulceration (e.g. 8.5% of the over 70s with gastric ulcer and 4% with duodenal ulcer).

This, of course, is a hospital series and in about a half of all these patients the ulcer was the principal cause of death. The figures cannot, therefore, be extrapolated to the total population of elderly people. They do, however, stress the great importance of considering the possibility of gastric or duodenal ulcer when any symptoms present pointing to the upper gastrointestinal tract. As with so many other illnesses in the elderly, presentation tends to be much less specific. Abdominal pain may be vague and epigastric tenderness less common that in the young. The availability of flexible gastroscopy now helps to meet this demand for careful investigation of the stomach in suspicious cases.

Both gastric and duodenal ulcers in the elderly are associated with increased acid secretion and the mainstay of treatment as in the young is to diminish the amount of gastric secretion and so raise the pH level within the stomach.

Gastric secretion is stimulated by an increase in the hormone gastrin which, in turn, is stimulated by activity in the vagus nerve and by entry of carbohydrate and protein into the stomach. The phases of gastric secretion are usually regarded as being the following 4:

(a) cephalic, arising from the sight and smell of food and effective through the action of the vagus;

(b) gastric, affected by the direct action of carbohydrate and protein on the secretion of gastrin;

(c) intestinal, stimulated by a rise of intestinal pH and inhibited by a drop of intestinal pH below 2.5 and mediated by the hormones secretin and enterogastrone;

(d) resting or interdigestion phase of basal secretion between meals.

Hydrochloric acid is produced from the parietal cells and its production is stimulated through the H_2 receptors.

The 3 major groups of drugs to consider in the treatment of peptic ulcer are:

(1) the traditional antacids;
(2) carbenoxolone;
(3) cimetidine and ranitidine.

Antacids

There is a difference in acid secretion in patients with duodenal and gastric ulcer. In the former (the great majority of whom are males) there is 2 to 6 times normal output of gastric juices both in the resting and stimulation phases. (The parietal cell mass is approximately twice normal.) In the latter there may be little difference from normal. Nevertheless, antacids relieve pain in both gastric and duodenal ulcers when the pH of the gastric contents is increased to 2 or over. All antacids increase the output of hydrochloric acid and volume of gastric juice; lowering the pH increases the half-life of gastrin which, in turn, leads to an increase in gastric motility and an increase in the pressure within the lower oesophageal sphincter. It is to be noted that there is a considerable placebo effect and, indeed, one study showed no significant difference between antacids and placebo in producing relief of pain. The effect of antacids in healing peptic ulcers is still uncertain.

The use of anticholinergic drugs (e.g. propantheline) as an adjunct to antacids is to delay gastric emptying, increase gastric secretion and thus increase the retention of antacids.

The antacids in most common use are shown in Table 15.1. These are chosen to represent alkali substances in which the cation is not absorbed from the gut and so they do not tend to produce metabolic alkalosis (the cation forms insoluble basic compounds in the intestine). In addition to

Table 15.1 Drugs in the treatment of peptic ulcer.

Drug name (Trade name)	Dosage
Aluminium hydroxide gel, BPC, USP	Suspension 15 ml
Magnesium trisilicate BPC, USP	Tablet 500 mg, suspension 15 ml (a mixture of equal parts of these is recommended)
(Dijex)—aluminium hydroxide, magnesium carbonate compound	Tablet 400 mg
(Gaviscon)-a combination of the above with alginates	To be chewed
Magnesium hydroxide	
(Magaldrate USP)—a hydroxy-magnesium aluminate	
(Riofan)	Tablet 400 mg, suspension 80 mg/ml
Tri-potassium di-citrate bismuthate (De-Nol)	5 ml in 15 ml water
Carbenoxolone sodium	
(Biogastrone)	50 mg tablet
(Duogastrone)	50 mg capsule
Cimetidine (Tagamet)	400 mg tablet
Ranitidine (Zantac)	150 mg tablet

the neutralizing effect, aluminium hydroxide also has an absorbent effect and this may slow the absorption of drugs given concurrently. There is an advantage in mixing aluminium and magnesium salts since magnesium tends to produce diarrhoea and aluminium constipation. It is worth noting that prolonged aluminium hydroxide administration can cause the binding of dietary phosphate and may tilt the balance into osteomalacia in old people who are already at risk. Long-term aluminium may, rarely, cause dementia; magnesium should be avoided in the presence of renal impairment.

The colloidial bismuth preparation tri-potassium di-citrato bismuthate which has recently been introduced appears to have been effective in healing gastric ulcers although its mode of action is not certain. It is at the present time a drug of choice in the treatment of gastric ulcers in the elderly.

Gaviscon (a combination of aluminium hydroxide and magnesium trisilicate with alginate and mannitol) is particularly recommended in the symptomatic treatment of hiatus hernia. These tablets should be thoroughly chewed and may be taken on retiring to bed and at other times when the pain is expected.

Other methods of treatment

Carbenoxolone sodium a liquorice derivative with associated mineralocorticoid effects has been shown to heal gastric ulcers in about 50% of those treated for 3 months and a large proportion of those treated for a year but recurrent ulceration following healing occurs in a significant number and this has not been prevented by a maintenance dose of the drug. The side-effects of carbenoxolone are particularly those of fluid retention and these are usually sufficient to contraindicate this drug in old people (hypokalaemia and an increase in blood pressure also occur). It is possible to prevent these effects by the concomitant use of diuretics and calcium supplements but such a complex regimen diminishes the value of this drug compared to others in the elderly.

Cimetidine and ranitidine

Histamine is the proximate chemical transmitter to the secretion of gastric juice. It is now known that there are 2 forms of histamine receptor—H_1 (in skin, lung, etc.) and H_2 on gastric parietal cells and in other organs including heart, uterus, skin and lymphocytes. The H_2 receptors in the gastric parietal cells are affected by acetylcholine, gastrin, food and drugs. Cimetidine inhibits the secretion of gastric acid mediated by H_2 receptors no matter what the stimulus is to the receptor. Cimetidine has a selective effect over a long period of use. It therefore seems to be a safe drug with one major proviso, that is the diagnosis is beyond doubt before treatment starts. The reason for this is that the symptoms of carcinoma of the stomach may also be relieved by cimetidine and malignancy has been masked in these cases during the treatment with cimetidine. Pre-treatment diagnosis, therefore, must be quite definite in excluding carcinoma. If there is any doubt, repeat gastroscopy during the course of treatment is indicated.

Cimetidine (200 mg 3 times daily and 200–400 mg at night) is more effective than placebo in the treatment of both duodenal ulcer and gastric ulcer and the majority of ulcers will be healed with 6 weeks of treatment. Pain relief is more striking in duodenal ulcer than in gastric ulcers. Unfortunately, once cimetidine is withdrawn relapse is common. Acid secretion returns to previous levels and about 25% of patients will relapse. Maintenance treatment is with 400 mg taken at night. Ranitidine, a more recently introduced H_2 antagonist is effective in lower dosage than cimetidine. It appears to cause fewer confusional episodes in the elderly and is probably to be preferred. Vagotomy is recommended if relapse occurs.

Treatment regimen

Initial treatment should be with antacids giving a combined suspension of aluminium hydroxide and magnesium trisilicate. A full dose should be taken whenever symptoms begin to appear or if this is impracticable, a dose of 15–30 ml should be taken 4–5 times daily. If this regimen is ineffective or unacceptable, De-nol should be substituted. If relief is still not obtained, the patient should be given a full course of cimetidine. Check gastroscopy for healing should be carried out in 6 weeks time and then treatment discontinued. If symptoms recur, a maintenance dose of 400 mg a day is safe to use for up to a year but for longer term use there is still insufficient knowledge about long-term effects. Symptoms continuing beyond this period of time, therefore, probably require surgical treatment.

Gastro-oesophageal reflux

Metoclopramide (Maxolon) (10 mg tablet), a drug which increases oesophageal sphincter tone, increases gastric motility (and so speeds up gastric emptying) and also has a central anti-emetic effect and is widely used in the management of oesophageal reflux. Results are variable. Side-effects must be looked for in elderly people and especially drowsiness and lassitude. Diarrhoea, constipation and extrapyramidal signs are less common, but the latter must be considered especially with patients who are also on phenothiazines. Anti-cholinergic drugs will block the effect of metoclopramide.

BOWEL FUNCTION AND AGING

A number of studies have shown that the general population in the UK and in the USA have a range of bowel motions between 3 times a week add 3 times a day. Almost 99% of the population falls within these limits. The elderly are no different although surveys have indicated that they are more prolific users of laxatives than younger people (e.g. 30% aged 60 and above took laxatives regularly once a week compared with 16% of those aged 10–59 years).

While it is possible that this reflects a tendency to constipation in the elderly, it is more probable that it is a cultural difference. People who are now old lived through the era of the medical fad of 'auto-intoxication from the colon' when this was thought to be the cause of many systemic diseases of otherwise unknown aetiology. The full list of diseases attributed to colonic stasis is quite horrific (Lane 1915) and includes the appearance of premature senility, round shoulders, flat feet and knock knees, asthma, imbecility, loss of teeth, rheumatoid arthritis and a necessary preliminary to tuberculosis. Those brought up believing that constipation could lead to such terrible complications will not unnaturally still include a large number of regular laxative takers.

There is, however, one group of old people who are particularly prone to become constipated and these are the immobile. However, in this case constipation is a reflection of immobility and not of age and also affects the immobile who are middle-aged and younger. Physical movement is one of the factors which leads to the onset of the gastrocolic reflex, usually in combination with a hot drink or the entry of food into the stomach and proximal intestine. These are the stimuli to the so-called gastrocolic reflex and in the immobile this reflex may not occur. In such a case the faeces tend to accumulate in the rectum and then build up more proximally until the whole descending colon becomes filled. Indeed distension of the whole colon may be demonstrated together with a bulky and easily palpable caecum. This condition may be associated with very hard faecal masses (faecoliths) in the descending colon and in the rectum. This is the condition of faecal impaction. This type of constipation has been called the 'terminal reservoir syndrome.'

The complications of constipation

The most common and unfortunate complication of constipation in the elderly (and particularly of the terminal reservoir syndrome) is faecal incontinence.

Among old people in institutional care the prevalence of faecal incontinence may be anything up to 50%. The unpleasantness of this condition both for patient and attendant needs no emphasizing and is apparent to all. Faecal incontinence is a condition which is preventable and those institutions which have a significant amount of it are therefore, guilty of medical and nursing neglect.

Not all faecal incontinence is secondary to constipation. In a minority of cases it is the presenting symptom of organic disease within the colon. Rectal and colonic carcinoma, diverticular disease, ischaemic colitis, Crohn's disease, ulcerative proctocolitis may all occur in old age, and in this age group commonly present with faecal incontinence. Impairment of anal sphincter function (as in rectal prolapse or damage following surgery) is another cause of faecal incontinence. The fact that faecal incontinence may be the first presenting symptom of these diseases indicates the need for physicians to take it very seriously. If it is not associated with constipation or, if it continues once constipation has been relieved, a full lower bowel investigation is mandatory.

A third cause of faecal incontinence is 'neurogenic'. In this case there is an absence of cerebral cortical inhibition so that when the gastrocolic reflex occurs and the faecal mass moves into the rectum (the rectum developing intrinsic contractions and the anal sphincter relaxing) the subject is unable to inhibit these effects. The result is that a formed stool is passed and if time and place are inappropriate the patient will be incontinent. This is a particular problem in patients with brain failure (e.g. senile and multi-infarct dementia) and a small proportion of patients with stroke.

Other complications of constipation include idiopathic megacolon which itself may lead to volvulus of the sigmoid and so to intestinal obstruction.

While immobility is the most common cause of constipation in old people other causes must also be kept in mind. These include hypothyroidism, hypercalcaemia, depression and the effects of various drugs including codeine and iron.

THE TREATMENT OF CONSTIPATION

Classification of laxatives

It has been customary for many years to classify the laxatives under four main headings—the lubricants, the irritants, the salines and the bulk laxatives. The lubricants, which include liquid paraffin (mineral oil), dioctyl sodium sulpha succinate (DSS) and dioctyl calcium sulpha succinate (DCS), have been thought to act by lowering surface tension on the stool and so increasing its permeability to water and fats (in the case of DSS and DCS) or by diminishing water reabsorption by the intestinal mucosa possibly by coating it with an inert oily substance (in the case of liquid paraffin). The irritant laxatives have been thought to have a direct stimulant effect on the myenteric plexuses and so to increase persistalsis. The osmotic laxatives are thought to have increased the osmolality of the gut content and so drawn water out of the tissues into the lumen (and so acting as a bulk laxative finally). The bulk laxatives are assumed to act by increasing peristalsis and so diminishing gut transit.

Recent thought (e.g. see Binder 1977) suggest that this traditional view of the method of action of various laxatives may be quite erroneous and that a rethinking of classification may therefore, be necessary; for instance, present understanding of large bowel motility suggest that the most common form of motility (shuttling movement between adjacent haustra) actually has a constipating effect by holding up the onward movement of the faecal mass and it is only the occasional mass peristalsis which sweeps the colonic contents onward into the rectum which actually causes defaecation. Moreover, an increase in motility is only one of a number of effects of the irritant laxatives; for instance, ricinoleic acid, bisacodil and phenolthalein may all reverse the nett fluid absorption from the bowel to a nett fluid accumulation within the bowel and the primary change underlying this may be an active ion secretion stimulated by the laxative. It may, therefore, be that the increase in the fluid bulk of the stool is the effective means of hastening defaecation and that whatever motility effects occur are secondary. It is known for instance that other substances which cause an active secretion of anions by the gut wall cause diarrhoea. These include bacterial enterotoxins and a number of enteric and non-enteric hormones (e.g. vasoactive intestinal polypeptide, gastric inhibitory polypeptide, cholecystokinin, secretin, prostaglandin E1, etc.).

Other laxatives which may act similarly (by stimulating active ion secretion) include the bile acids and stool softeners.

At the present time, therefore, a classification of laxatives based on their method of action is inappropriate and the classification given in Table 15.2 is based only on their chemical type.

Table 15.2 The laxatives.

Type of drug	Drug name (Trade name)	Dosage
Wetting agents	Dioctyl sodium sulphasuccinate BPC, USP (Dioctyl-Medo, Colace)	50 mg, 100 mg capsule and tablet
	Dioctyl calcium sulphasuccinate USNF (Surfak)	50 mg capsule
Diphenymethanes	Phenolphthalein USNF, BP	60 mg tablet
	Bisacodyl USP, BP	enteric coated tablet 5 mg, suppository 10 mg, dose 5–10 mg
Anthraquinones	Senna: standardised senna (Sennosides A & B)	
	(Senokot)	Syrup 1.4 mg/ml, tablets 7.5 mg, granules 5 mg/g, dose 10–15 mg.
	(Glysenid)	12 mg tablet
	Cascara: Aromatic cascara fluid extract USP	5 ml
	Cascara tablet USNF	300 mg
	Cascara elixir BP	2–5 ml
	Danthrin USNF	Tablet 75 mg
	Dorbane	150 mg
Saline	Magnesium sulphate BP, USP	
Bulk	Bran	
	Methyl cellulose USP, BP	1–4 g daily
	Methyl cellulose granules BPC (Celevac)	1.5–6.0 g
	Psyllium BPC, Plantage seed USNF (Isogel; metamucil)	5–15 g
	Sterculia BPC (Normacol—granules)	10 ml
Mineral oil	USP Liquid paraffin BP	10–50 ml
Synthetic disaccharide	Lactulose	
	(Duphalac)	Syrup 10–30 ml

Wetting agents

These are anionic surface-acting agents which reduce the surface tension and so allow increased penetration by water and fat into the stool. They are, in fact, detergents. They are particularly useful, therefore, in the treatment of faecal impaction and they may also have a place in the prevention of faecal impaction. Combinations of drugs of this type with an anthrocene (e.g. Dorbanex, Normax) have been found useful in preventing constipation in some old people. A comparative trial suggests that dioctyl calcium sulpha succonate is superior to the sodium salt. They may increase absorption of hepatotoxic agents and must, therefore, be used with care in the elderly.

Diphenyl methane group

Phenolthalein is a very commonly used laxative in people of all ages. It is effective 6 or more hours after being taken by mouth. Some is excreted in the urine and if the urine is alkaline it will colour it pink or red. It also has a propensity to produce skin rashes. Bisacodil is also a commonly used laxative. This preparation is largely unabsorbed and for this reason is particularly safe. It may be given either by mouth or by suppository (which acts in about 25 minutes). The suppositories may cause a burning sensation in the rectum.

Anthroquinones

A proportion of the anthroquinones pass unabsorbed through the bowel but much of the drug is absorbed and re-excreted into the intestine. Infusion of senna pods has been a popular home remedy for a century. Probably the best preparation now is the standardized form of senna (Senakot or Glysenit).

It is known that the long-continued use of anthracene purgatives may cause degeneration of the myenteric plexuses. The condition of cathartic colon characterized by pseudostrictures and hypokalaemia has been reported in patients who have taken proprietary vegetable laxatives over long periods of time, the major ingredient is colocynth. These laxatives are not now recommended for use but may still be used in self-medication.

Salines

Magnesium sulphate has a brisk and rapid action and there is little place for it in medicine in old age except possibly where a rapid clearing of the bowel is needed on one occasion only, for instance as preparation for investigation.

Bulk laxatives

Bran and the bulk laxatives are useful in old people who are mobile but should be avoided in the immobile. They will diminish intestinal motility in patients with diverticular disease and so relieve pain which is due to spasm. They should not be used in immobile old people because they may produce intestinal obstruction and faecal impaction and in any case will not be helpful in the 'terminal reservoir syndrome'. Another danger is that they may obstruct at the lower end of the oesophagus if they are taken dry in tablet form. It is well known that a proportion of people in the 80s and 90s have presbyoesophagus in which there may be a delay of anything up to three-quarters of an hour at the lower end of the oesophagus. This may allow the tablets to swell and cause obstruction. All medications in the elderly should be taken with liberal drafts of water and this applies particularly to bulk laxatives.

The bulk laxatives have a particular place in the management of colostomies and illiostomies and in the symptomatic treatment of diarrhoea. Bran has been shown to normalize the intestinal transit in that it increases transit time in those in whom it is below normal and slows transit time in those in whom it is too rapid.

Mineral oil (liquid paraffin)

Mineral oil has many disadvantages in the elderly and is best avoided. It will dissolve fat-soluble vitamins and so may precipitate osteomalacia, it may produce lipid pneumonias and this is particularly a risk in elderly people with a degree of presbyoesophagus who have difficulty in swallowing and it may seep from the anus and produce faecal incontinence.

Synthetic disaccharide

The synthetic disaccharide lactulose (galactose and fructose) has no corresponding disaccharidase available in the small bowel and so it reaches the colon unchanged. Here it is broken down by bacteria to form non-absorbable organic anions which have an osmotic and possibly other effects. Some trials have shown a diminution of faecal incontinence in long-term patients treated with lactulose.

Whole-gut irrigation

Recently the process of whole-gut irrigation has been introduced in the treatment of the terminal reservoir syndrome (Smith *et al.* 1978). In this case a wetting agent is given daily for 5 days and then the whole colon is emptied by irrigation from above in a matter of 2 to 4 hours. Isotonic saline at body temperature is run into the stomach through a nasogastric tube at the rate of 2.5–3 l per h. This is preceded by 40 mg of frusemide and 10 mg of metoclopramide intravenously. It is continued until the effulent starts to clear, a mean time of about 3½ hours. During all this time the subject is seated comfortably on a padded commode. Although the procedure sounds somewhat heroic, in fact it is well tolerated by quite frail elderly people and has the advantage of getting the whole empyting process over at once.

A less dramatic alternative is for the patient to drink 1 litre of 10% mannitol (cooled and flavoured) and up to 2 litres of normal saline (or other clear fluid) within 1 to 2 hours.

Enemas

Probably the most commonly used enema in the elderly nowadays is the phosphate enema (Fleet enema, Fletcher's enema). This is an aqueous solution of sodium acid phosphate and sodium phosphate in hypertonic form in a plastic bag containing 130 ml. The bag is fitted with a rectal tube. The enema works by attracting water into the rectum and so producing rectal distension. These enemas are effective but the nozzle must be inserted with care. A number of cases in which trauma to the anus or rectum occurring during insertion from the nozzle, followed by necrosis, have been reported.

Constipation due to the terminal reservoir syndrome

In this common condition the laxatives are of little use and the bulk laxatives in particular are contraindicated. The usual method of treatment is to empty the bowel from below either by suppositories or by enemas. Enemas are probably most satisfactory because of the very considerable content of faeces. One enema will empty the rectum and produce a very large and bulky result. Sometimes, however, this has to be preceded by wetting agents or by an oily enema, (e.g. olive oil). One enema in itself, however, will by no means simply move round and fill the rectum. Generally, 7 to 10 enemas given at a rate of 1 per day are required for the total emptying of the bowel of an immobile old person with the terminal reservoir syndrome.

Prevention of constipation

Once the treatment of constipation (and so of its accompanying faecal incontinence) has been successfully accomplished, it is equally important then to prevent the condition from recurring. In the permanently immobile this is only too likely to happen. Every effort should be made to promote mobility even if it is only standing with support, several times up and down from the chair, first thing in the morning. If it can be more than that, then better still. Nurses must be particularly diligent to respond to the needs of dependant old people. They must ensure that a commode or access to the lavatory is available as soon as the old person experiences the desire to defaecate. If this is not so, then the desire to defaecate will pass off and when the old person is eventually offered the facilities she may no longer be able to empty the bowel.

Faecal incontinence of neurogenic cause

In cases of this type where the patient is not constipated the treatment originally suggested by Garrett and Exton-Smith may be found helpful: that is, to provide assisted purgation first thing in the morning by giving standardized senna at night and then preventing further gastrocolic reflexes by giving a constipating agent such as chalk and opium or Lomotil. This is in effect exaggerating the normal timing of the morning stool and then preventing further stools during the day. Another method is to constipate the patient by the above means for 2 to 3 days and then secure a total planned evacuation by giving enemas.

THE SYMPTOMATIC TREATMENT OF DIARRHOEA

As with faecal incontinence, so diarrhoea in the elderly may be a presenting symptom of a whole range of diseases of the lower bowel. It may also be the result of certain drugs (and laxative-taking unknown to the physician must always be considered) or due to intestinal malabsorption or a gastrocolic fistula. All of these have to be considered and excluded. The symptomatic treatment of diarrhoea may be required while investigations are taking place or, very occasionally, on a longer-term basis. One of the chief reasons for this is the irritable colon syndrome; another is in postvagotomy diarrhoea. The drugs available are those with a morphine-like effect.

Morphine increases colonic shuttling motility and so tends to promote constipation. It is not used alone for this purpose other than in the dying but is used in combination with light kaolin, BP, and calcium carbonate for their absorbent effects and increase in the bulk of the intestinal contents. Available mixtures include kaolin and morphine, BPC (dose 10 ml), and aromatic chalk with opium mixture, BPC (dose 10–20 ml). These mixtures are not available in the USA. Preparation of kaolin without morphine include kaolin mixture, BPC (dose 10 ml) and kaolin mixture with pectin, USNF, (dose 30 ml). Codeine is a derivitive of morphine which may be used for its constipating effect in short-term treatment–codeine, USNF and BPC (5–10 mg)–but in view of its addictive qualities it is not recommended for this purpose except with terminal illness.

Diphenoxylate hydrochloride, BP, USNF, Lomotil, is derived from the synthetic analgesic drug meperidine which is chemically different to morphine although clinically it has very similar effects including sedation, analgesia and euphoria. Diphenoxylate may also produce dependency and therefore cannot be recommended for long term use. Lomotil is a mixture of diphenoxylate and atropine sulphate in a tablet of 2.5 mg or a syrup containing 2.5 mg per 5 ml of diphenoxylate.

While the above preparations are all effective in treating diarrhoea they all have to be used with care in elderly people, particularly where the indication is ongoing. Sometimes the bulk laxatives (see above) may have an adequate constipating effect in certain diarrhoeal states.

REFERENCES AND FURTHER READING

Binder H.J. (1977) Pharmacology of laxatives. *Annual Review of Pharmacological Toxicology* **17**, 355–67.

Boyes B.E., Woolf I.L., Wilson R.Y., Cocley A.J. & Dymock I.W. (1975) Treatment of gastric ulceration with bismuth preparation. *Postgraduate medical Journal* **51**, 29–33.

Castell D.O. (1980) Medical therapy of reflux oesophagitis. *Annals of Internal Medicine* **93,** 926–7.

Connell A.M., Hilton C., Irvin G., Lennard-Jones J.E. & Misiewicz J.J. (1965) Variations in bowel habit in two population samples. *British medical Journal* **ii**, 1095–9.

Gear M.W.L. (1983) Proximal gastric vagotomy versus long term maintenance treatment with cimetidine for chronic duodenal ulcer: a prospective randomised trial. *British medical Journal* **286**, 98–9.

Jarratt A.S. & Exton-Smith A.N. (1960) Treatment of faecal incontinence. *Lancet* **i**, 925.

Lane W.A. (1915) *The Operative Treatment of Chronic Intestinal Stasis*. James Nisbet & Co. Ltd., London.

Peterson W.L. *et al* (1977) Healing of duodenal ulcer with an antacid regime. *New England Journal of Medicine* **297**, 341–5.

McKeown F. (1965) *Pathology of the Aged.* Butterworths, London.

Smith R.G., Curry A.E.J., & Walls A.D.F. (1978) Whole gut irrigation new treatment for constipation. *British medical Journal* **3,** 396–7.

Sturdevant R.A.L., Isenberg J.I., Secrist D. & Ansfield J. (1977) Antacid and placebo produced similar pain relief in duodenal ulcer patients. *Gastroenterology 1*, **72**, 1–5.

Zeldis J.B., Friedman L.S. & Isselbacher K.J. (1983) Ranitidine: a new H_2-receptor antagonist. *New England Journal of Medicine* **309**, 1368–73.

Chapter Sixteen
Analgesics

C.M. CASTLEDEN

OVERVIEW

Painful conditions are common in the elderly although, in general, they are more resistant to pain than younger adults, and many classically painful conditions such as myocardial infarction are painless. A careful search is required to define the cause, as analgesics may be inappropriate. If analgesics are indicated, dosage must be adequate and sufficiently frequent to prevent pain occurring, especially in patients after operation or with cancer. Such regimens require a knowledge of the pharmacokinetic properties of analgesics; they need careful tailoring to suit each individual. The selection of analgesics is wide but the pharmacological properties of most drugs differ sufficiently to make the clinical indications for prescription clear.

SPECIFIC POINTS TO REMEMBER IN THE ELDERLY

Pain is a symptom, and analgesics are inappropriate until the cause has been defined; for example, abdominal pain may be caused by many conditions such as constipation, urinary tract infection or surgical emergencies for which analgesics alone would be entirely wrong. Always ask the patient to point to the site of pain and to map out on himself any radiation so as to reduce errors due to the use of misleading terms.

The elderly are most resistant to pain and many conditions which are classically described in younger patients as painful are apparently painless in older patients; for example, myocardial infarction is frequently silent and presents more usually as congestive cardiac failure, falls or with some lesion of the central nervous system. Many old patients with acute perforation or obstruction to the bowel have only minimal pain or none at all.

The elderly are most susceptible to adverse drug reactions including those following analgesics. However, drugs should not be withheld for this reason but selection of the type of drug may be altered; for example, women over 65 years are 4 times more likely to suffer from aplastic anaemia following phenylbutazone and related drugs than younger adults. Since there is no clear-cut indication for prescribing phenylbutazone rather than other anti-inflammatory analgesic drugs, this drug is best avoided in the elderly, or, at least, serious consideration given before it is used.

Since over 90% of analgesics are taken at home and thus without supervision, many are not taken as the doctor prescribes and the dose fluctuates according to the patient's symptoms. Patients need instruction as to when this is a correct procedure and when it is harmful; for example, paracetamol for occasional pain from an osteoarthritic hip could be taken entirely at the discretion of the patient, whereas allopurinol for the prevention of gout needs to be taken regularly when the patient is asymptomatic.

Finally, it should be remembered that analgesics are only one part of the treatment of any patient with pain. Reorganization of the lifestyle and aids, such as a walking stick or a wheelchair, may be necessary. General measures such as reduction in weight, and the use of physiotherapy, exercise and local heat are frequently as important as analgesics.

SELECTION OF AN ANALGESIC

Steroids are not generally recommended for treating elderly patients with arthritis. Although they quickly relieve symptoms side-effects are common even with small doses and outweigh such short-term therapeutic gains. Their use should be restricted to intra-articular injections, or to treating painful conditions known to respond lastingly to steroids such as temporal arteritis or polymyalgia rheumatica.

Analgesics and anti-inflammatory drugs are given solely for symptomatic relief. They usually act rapidly and, therefore, a drug that has no effect in a few days should be changed. Since many analgesics are required on a long-term basis it is wise to start regular therapy with the simplest and the safest which are probably the proprionic acid derivatives (see Table 16.1, p. 221). There are now many different mild analgesic anti-inflammatory drugs, and there is little difference between them in efficacy but often a lot in patient acceptance. It is therefore wise to try several of a single group before changing to another more potent group. Even if the major anti-inflammatory drugs such as indomethacin, flurbiprofen or large doses of aspirin (acetyl salicylic acid) are used, supplementation by the simpler analgesics is advisable to keep the dose of the major anti-inflammatory drugs as low as possible.

In the treatment of rheumatoid arthritis, extension of therapy beyond the major anti-inflammatory drugs to gold, penicillamine and cytotoxic drugs requires the cooperation of a specialist and access to laboratory facilities.

Dextropropoxyphene and pentazocine are mild analgesics but are not usually recommended for the elderly. Dextropropoxyphene can be prescribed alone or in combination with compounds such as paracetamol. However, it has not been shown to be more effective in pain relief than other mild analgesics, and yet dependancy and withdrawal symptoms occur. Furthermore, the drug is dangerous on its own in overdosage causing convulsions, pulmonary oedema and depression of respiration and blood pressure. Pentazocine is also not recommended for the elderly since it produces a high incidence of gastro-intestinal side-effects, dizziness and hallucinations, and is not a superior analgesic to others in this group.

THE TREATMENT OF PAINFUL CONDITIONS IN ELDERLY PATIENTS

Pain in joints

Osteoarthrosis

Analgesics should initially be given on demand but subsequently in an effective regular dose. Initially drugs such as proprionic acid derivatives (see Table 16.1) or paracetamol (Acetaminophen USP) should be used but later more potent drugs such as indomethacin may be needed. If there is pain during the night or pain and stiffness on arising in the morning, indomethacin capsules or suppositories should be given at night in a dose of 50–100 mg. Intra-articular injections of 10–15 mg of hydrocortisone are sometimes surprisingly effective but should not be repeated more than 3 times in a weight-bearing joint.

Osteoarthritis may not only cause pain and limitation of joint movement when walking but lead to loss of ability to get out of bed or rise from a chair and so aids may be necessary. However, many previously independent patients have been made dependent by the provision of a wheelchair or hoist unnecessarily and these should only be used as a last resort. If there is leg shortening, raised shoes may help. Special aids for picking up articles are available, as are elastic shoe laces and so on. Physiotherapy to strengthen muscles and (with local heat) to ease stiffness should not be forgotten.

Finally, it may be necessary to resort to surgery. This should always be considered in an otherwise fit elderly patient especially if there is mono-articular disease.

Rheumatoid arthritis

The incidence of this disease is about one-tenth that of osteoarthritis, but the condition may present for the first time in old age. Of all rheumatoid patients referred to hospital 80% manage to lead independent lives throughout the course of their disease; 20% pursue, a relentless downhill course despite all medical skills.

The main aim of drugs in rheumatoid arthritis is solely for symptomatic relief. Thus they should be selected with discretion and continually and regularly reviewed. When the joints are acutely swollen they should be rested and splinted in a position of function. This period must be kept as short as possible in the elderly, and physiotherapy and occupational therapy instituted as soon as possible to maintain function.

Special therapeutic problems

(a) Iron, folic acid and vitamin D deficiency are common in chronic rheumatoid arthritis.
(b) Septic arthritis should be suspected if there is acute inflammation in a single joint regardless of whether that joint is involved in the rheumatoid condition. Culture of blood and synovial fluid followed by appropriate antibiotics and splintage are necessary if this condition is diagnosed.
(c) Popliteal cysts are bursae which communicate with the knee joint. Rupture of these cysts may cause synovial fluid to tract into the calf muscles mimicking a deep venous thrombosis. Diagnosis of this condition requires arthrography.
(d) The anti-inflammatory effect of most drugs takes a few days to reach a maximum.

Drug therapy

A classification of the anti-rheumatic drugs commonly prescribed is given in Table 16.1.

Simple analgesics. These drugs relieve the pain without any effect on inflammation and thus are not suitable alone for the treatment of acute rheumatoid arthritis. They are, however, useful adjuncts to anti-inflammatory drugs. Examples of single analgesics are aspirin (ASA in low doses) 600 mg, dextropropoxyphene either in combination with paracetamol or alone, and paracetamol. Simple analgesics in combination formulae should be avoided in the elderly since they may contain certain drugs such as caffeine and phenacetin. Numerous epidemological studies have suggested a temporal and dose relationship between phenacetin ingestion and renal dysfunction. Prolonged use of phenacetin—containing analgesics has also been associated with cancer of the renal pelvis and urinary bladder. The value of caffeine in analgesics is questionable except in the treatment of vascular headache. Its use is especially contraindicated in cardiovascular, psychological and renal disease.

Proprionic acid derivatives and equivalent drugs. These drugs are particularly suitable for disorders in which inflammation is not marked, such as all but the most active cases of rheumatoid arthritis. They have comparable analgesic potency to aspirin (ASA) but the anti-inflammatory effect of many of them is less. They are, however, first-line drugs and the choice depends on patient preference. It is beneficial to the physician to have this wide choice since patient acceptability often varies between 2 of the same class

Table 16.1 Classification of analgesics.

Drug	Dose	Frequency	Common side-effects of conventional doses
SIMPLE ANALGESICS			
Paracetamol (BP) Acetaminophen (USP)	1 g	6–8 hourly	None
Codeine	30 mg	6–8 hourly	Constipation, nausea, vomiting, dizziness
Dihydrocodeine	30 mg	6–8 hourly	Same as codeine but less constipating
Aspirin (acetyl salicylic acid)	600 mg	6–8 hourly	Gastrointestinal
ANALGESICS WITH MINOR ANTI-INFLAMMATORY PROPERTIES			
Propionic acid			
Fenbrufen	300–600 mg	12–24 hourly	Mild gastrointestinal, dizziness, drowsiness
Fenoprofen	600 mg	6–8 hourly	
Ibuprofen	400 mg	8 hourly	
Ketoprofen	50 mg	8 hourly	
Naproxen	250 mg	12 hourly	
Anthranilic acids			
Flufenamic acid	200 mg	8–12 hourly	Mild gastrointestinal, dizziness, drowsiness
Meclofenamine acid	250 mg	8 hourly	
Arylacetic acid			
Alclofenac	1 g	8 hourly	Mild gastrointestinal, dizziness, drowsiness
Diclofenac	25.50 mg	8 hourly	
Others			
Azapropazone	300 mg	6 hourly	Mild gastrointestinal, dizziness, drowsiness
Salindac*	100 mg	12 hourly	
Salaslate*	500–1000 mg	8 hourly	
Tolmetin	200 mg	8 hourly	
ANALGESICS WITH MAJOR ANTI-INFLAMMATORY PROPERTIES			
Indomethacin	25 mg 75 mg	8 hourly nocte	Gastrointestinal upsets, headaches and unpleasant cerebral sensations, fluid retention
Aspirin (acetyl salicylic acid)	900 mg	6 hourly	Tinnitus, nausea, gastric irritation and bleeding, asthma
OTHER ANALGESICS WITH MARKED ANTI-INFLAMMATORY PROPERTIES			
Flurbiprofen	50 mg	6–8 hourly	Gastrointestinal symptoms
Piroxicam	20 mg	24 hourly	

* Not available in North America.

of drugs and it is possible to avoid progression to the more potent anti-inflammatory drugs by changing several times within this class.

Major inflammatory analgesic drugs. These drugs are only indicated in conditions in which inflammation is prominent, and should not be used for non-specific minor aches and pains.

Aspirin (ASA). This drug is only anti-inflammatory in very high doses, at least 3.6 g per day. At such doses there is a high incidence of side-effects, particularly gastrointestinal, such as epigastric pain, nausea and vomiting, and auditory, such as tinnitus and deafness. Although anaemia and overt gastrointestinal are less common, ASA should never be given to any patient with a tendency to bleed due to a local or clotting disorder. It may also precipitate or aggravate asthma or allergic rhinitis. Patients should be warned that aspirin (ASA) is contained in many combination products.

Benorylate is broken down in the blood stream and liver to aspirin and paracetamol and thus suffers the same drawbacks as these drugs. It is given as a solution—an advantage for those who cannot swallow tablets.

The non-steroidal anti-inflammatory drugs are widely and effectively used in the elderly but side-effects are common. Long-continued use of a single agent should be avoided whenever possible.

Indomethacin. A dose of 25 mg t.d.s. is usual. It is particularly effective for night pain and morning stiffness, for which an additional 75–100 mg at night can be used. If adverse symptoms occur, then the daytime dose of indomethacin can be replaced with a proprionic acid derivative whilst the nocturnal dose is maintained. A particular problem in the elderly is that indomethacin causes sodium retention and may precipitate heart failure.

Phenylbutazone. The usual dose is 100 mg t.d.s. but the drug has little advantage over indomethacin and can cause marrow aplasia which is completely unpredictable and often irreversible. It also causes cardiac failure, and, in general, phenylbutazone should not be used. It has now been withdrawn by the manufacturer.

Other drugs. Flurbiprofen, although a proprionic acid derivative, is a potent prostaglandin inhibitor. The recommended dosage is 150–200 mg in 3 to 4 divided doses, but a total daily dosage of 300 mg can be used. Piroxicam is a new drug in this class and thus has the advantage of unsubstantiated claims. Its one distinct advantage is a long half-life of about 37 hours, so that a single daily dose can produce analgesia lasting for 24 hours.

Gold, D-penicillamine and chloroquine. These drugs (see Table 16.2) should only be considered if there is objective evidence of persistent disease activity despite correct use of the above drugs. Objective evidence constitutes persistent joint swelling, radiological changes, a high plasma viscosity or low haemoglobin. The benefit of these drugs is not apparent for about 3 months.

Table 16.2 Other drugs referred to in the text.

Gold
Sodium aurothiomalate
Penicillamine
Chloroquine
Hydroxychloroquine
Prednisolone
Cytotoxic drugs
Azothioprim
Cyclophosphamide
Methyl-textrate
Colchicine
Allopurinol
Carbamazepine
Phenytoin
Idoxurodine
Amantadine

Gold. About two-thirds of patients obtain benefit from gold. The mode of action is uncertain and there is no close correlation beween serum gold concentration and either clinical benefit or the presence of toxicity. A small test dose should be given first and thereafter 50 mg intramuscularly of sodium aurothiomalate weekly. Up to a total dose of 1 g can be given but if there is no improvement by 750 mg it is wise to stop. Those patients who respond well to a first course can be maintained on 20 mg weekly for many months or even years.

However, it is necessary to keep a constant watch for toxicity, which may be more common in the elderly. The most common toxic reactions are rashes and mouth ulcers of which less than 5% are serious. Proteinuria may occur and be severe enough to lead to the nephrotic syndrome. It is never irreversible if the drug is stopped as soon as proteinuria is noted. Suppression of the marrow (of which a reduced platelet count is often the first indication) is usually also reversible.

Penicillamine. The usual dose is 125 mg per day increasing by 125 mg every 2 weeks until the daily dose is 500 mg. If no improvement is evident after a further 6 weeks, the dose can be slowly increased to 1 g of penicillamine a day. Maintenance dose thereafter is half the maximum.

Toxic manifestations to penicillamine almost always disppear when the drug is stopped. Rashes and mouth ulcers often respond to transient withdrawal of the drug, whilst gastrointestinal symptoms such as loss of taste or a bitter taste are usually transitory. Proteinuria up to 100 mg per 100 ml is very common and is not necessarily an indication for stopping the drug, although heavy proteinuria or the nephrotic syndrome occurs in 10–20% of patients. Nevertheless, provided the drug is withdrawn there is no permanent renal damage even though the abnormality may persist for months. Heavy proteinuria rarely occurs during the first 6 months of treatment, and is usually not seen after the first year. Marrow depression is usually manifested by thrombocytopenia. Myasthenia gravis is a very rare complication and once again responds to withdrawal of the drug.

Chloroquine. The drug has minimal toxicity but a minor place in the treatment of rheumatoid arthritis. Any long-term effect takes many months to become apparent. Chloroquine phosphate 250 mg should be given once or twice a day, or hydroxychloroquine 200 mg twice or thrice a day.

The major unwanted effect is due to selective deposition of the antimalarial drug in the uveal tract. This causes coloured haloes around lights and can progress to serious retinopathy with macular degeneration if the drug is used for 2 years or more in high doses. Thus if long-term therapy is instigated, regular ophthalmic checks are necessary after the first year and the dosage may need to be decreased.

Steroids. These drugs produce an immediate effect and therefore patient acceptability is high. However, there is no long-term suppression of the disease and considerable unwanted effects occur. The dose should never exceed 10 mg of prednisolone per day. There is evidence that therapy on alternate days allows normal secretion of the pituitary adrenal axis. It is wise to avoid splitting the doses during the day but if morning stiffness is a special problem 5–7.5 mg can be given only at night. The major advantage of intramuscular corticotrophin is that it is short acting and allows prescription to be under the doctor's control. Toxicity is a particular problem in the elderly who already have a high incidence of osteoporosis, fluid retention, hypertension, peptic ulceration and thin, friable skin. Steroid therapy should therefore be restricted to specific aims which preferably should be short-term and explained to the patient (see also pp. 261 and 263). Once started withdrawal should be slow.

Cytotoxic. Azothioprine, cyclophosphamide and methyltrexate have been used in severe progressive rheumatoid arthritis and to spare steroids. They have considerable side-effects and are not indicated without expert advice.

Gout

Gout is common in the elderly and may be precipitated by diuretic therapy. It may also be secondary to blood dyschrasias such as leukaemia and polycythaemia rubra vera, in which case a family history is absent and attacks tend to be prolonged and atypical in site.

Acute attacks respond rapidly to indomethacin 50–100 mg initially then 25–50 mg t.i.d. If indomethacin is contraindicated, ibuprofen or colchicine can be used. A dose of 100–250 mg of indomethazine on day 1 is necessary but this should quickly be reduced to 75 mg daily. Colchicine is given as a single 1 mg dose initially and then 0.5 mg hourly up to 8 mg.

When the acute attack is completely better long-term treatment with allopurinol can be considered. It should not be started after a single or infrequent attacks. Serum uric acid greater than 9 mg (Meq.)/100 ml, tophi or renal stones are strong indications for allopurinol. The drug should be started at a dose of 50 mg twice daily increasing slowly over 1 month to 100 mg three times a day. If allopurinol is contraindicated, uricosuric drugs such as probenecid are alternatives. Any prophylactic treatment may precipitate an acute attack especially if it is given in large doses. Thus it is wise to cover the initial therapy with indomethacin or colchicine.

Pain in soft tissues

Muscular and ligamentous pain especially in the back

These conditions are usually self limiting and respond to rest. Prolonged treatment, especially of backache, is not indicated without adequate investigations. It is important to provide adequate analgesia especially after the initial period of rest and it is wise to start with one of the simple analgesics or a proprionic acid derivative (see Table 16.1). Local heat from a hot water bottle, an infra-red lamp or rubefacients especially if accompanied by deep massage will almost cause relief of 'fibrositis'. A single steroid injection is useful in tenosynovitis, although the pain may be worse on the day of injection, when treating tennis elbow; the steroid should be combined with a local anaesthetic and given at the point of maximum tenderness. Carpal tunnel syndrome may also respond to a steroid injection, with or without rest in splints, but if there is not immediate relief surgery should be contemplated.

Polymyalgia rheumatica and temporal arteritis

These conditions respond immediately to prednisolone. Initially 40–60 mg a day may be necessary which should be rapidly reduced when symptoms have been relieved and titrated according to the clinical response and the plasma viscosity. Treatment may be necessary for up to 2 years.

Cancer pain

Mental stress is often related to physical discomfort which should be tackled first. The principles of treating a dying patient in pain are as follows.

(1) A thorough examination to find the cause of pain. Is it for example

due to bedsores or constipation, or to primary or secondary neoplastic growth?

(2) Pain should be prevented from occurring and not treated only when present. It is most important to ensure that the patient completely loses fear of having pain. Thus analgesics should be given frequently; at intervals based on knowledge of their rates of elimination and in adequate dosage. The regimen depends on the pharmacokinetics of the drugs used but usually means dosing throughout the night. Once the patient is relieved of pain, smaller doses are often sufficient for maintenance.

(3) Analgesics must be continued until death even when the patients' need for these has apparently disappeared.

(4) Look for, and if necessary treat, co-existing depression.

Type of analgesic

Whilst the simple analgesics such as paracetamol and codeine are useful, narcotics are the most effective and are usually necessary. The majority of patients can be maintained on oral morphine or diamorphine up to 48 hours before death. Thereafter subcutaneous may be kinder than intramuscular injections in emaciated patients. There is no single optimal dose or maximum effective dose. Each patient requires treatment as an individual and fear of using high doses such as 30 mg of morphine 4-hourly are groundless if this is the level required to relieve pain. Frequently, high doses are tolerated without loss of mental facilities. Tolerance is not a practical problem, and physical dependency may develop but does not prevent the downward adjustment of dose when it is clinically feasible.

Brompton mixture (containing diamorphine or morphine with cocaine in a sweetened alcoholic basis) has become unjustifiably popular amongst clinicians, but is not recommended for elderly patients. The euphorant effect of cocaine is often unpleasant, unnecessary and may lead to confusion, while some patients find that the intoxicating effect of alcohol is objectionable.

Prostaglandin inhibitors such as aspirin (ASA), indomethacin and flurbiprofen are indicated if the pain is secondary to bony deposits. In such a case the pain is thought to be due to local prostaglandin release.

Chlorpromazine is a useful drug if there is vomiting and nausea and can also be used to increase the effect of analgesics.

Hypnotics are not substitutes for diagnosing the underlying cause of insomnia; for example, they are inappropriate treatments for cough or shortness of breath which have their own specific treatments.

Occasionally drug therapy is not enough and treatment such as nerve blocks should be given by a specialist. Chemotherapy of cancer is not described here since it is a specialized field nowadays requiring advice, in most cases, from an oncologist. Chemotherapy of course may have a role in pain prevention in addition to that of prolongation of life. In old people, where the latter may be seen as less relevant, the former may be an important justification for the use of antimitotic chemotherapy.

Steroids may also have an important analgesic effect particularly in intracranial neoplasm.

Post-operative pain

This is largely the province of the surgeon and anaesthetist, but it frequently ranks second to concern for the pulse rate, blood pressure, presence of hypoxia and fluid and electrolyte balance. Treatment frequently depends on how demanding the patient is and on the attitude of the nursing staff. Like cancer pain it may be due either to anxiety about the condition, which may be relieved simply by a chat, or secondary to other sources of major discomfort, such as flatulence and bladder distension. Not infrequently analgesia may be withheld because of hypotension that is in fact due to pain, or as a result of exaggerated fear of inducing dangerous complications such as respiratory depression or drug dependency. Analgesia must be adequate and given sufficiently often to prevent pain occurring. This means an intramuscular or subcutaneous injection every 4–6 hours over the first 24–48 hours, and then regular oral therapy up to at least the fifth to the seventh post-operative day. Analgesia must be tailed off slowly and through decreasingly powerful analgesic drugs. It is wise to avoid pentazocine in the elderly as it frequently gives rise to hallucinations and confusion.

Neuralgias

Trigeminal neuralgia

This pain can always be relieved by numbing the face and abolishing the sensory impulses that precipitate the pain. However, such numbness may cause discomfort and inconvenience and should be resorted to only as a final measure. The most effective drug is carbamazepine (orally in either tablet or syrup form). The individual dosage varies considerably. The initial dose should be small (100 mg) in the frail and elderly. This may then be gradually increased until a satisfactory clinical response is obtained, which may mean 1600 mg of carbamazepine daily. The majority of patients, however, are well controlled on 200 mg 3 or 4 times a day. Carbamazepine should be taken only during the acute phase and not as a prophylactic measure. The drug frequently causes dizziness and drowsiness but both are less if the dose is increased slowly. If carbamazepine is unsuccessful, phenytoin can be tried. A dose of 150–300 mg is usually required and can be given as a single nocturnal dose. Should drug therapy be ineffective, an injection of alcohol around the nerve should be considered. This will usually abolish the pain but allow the nerve to regenerate and function to return; sometimes, however, the pain recurs with function.

Post-herpetic neuralgia

The use of idoxurodine cream on the skin lesions decreases the incidence of this disabling condition. However, once established it is usually resistant to treatment with simple analgesics. Local transcutaneous electrical stimulation and local skin cooling with ethyline chloride spray can be tried. Local nerve block, deep X-ray radiation or surgical operations are sometimes resorted to in intractable cases but are usually ineffective. Section of the nerve or nerve roots is never successful but section of the spinothalamic tract may be carried out with benefit. Amantadine during the acute attack may also reduce the incidence of post-herpetic neuralgia.

Post-herpetic neuralgia may be prevented by painting the area affected with herpes with 5% iodox-uridine in demethylsulphoxide (Idoxurodine). This should be done 4 hourly for 4 days and may be followed by povidone iodine alcoholic paint, twice daily. The application of Idoxurodine may itself produce some transient pain. An alternative treatment is by glucocorticoids—Prednisolone 40 mg daily for one week, then reduced over a month to a total dose of about 600 mg.

REFERENCES AND FURTHER READING

Dubach U.C., Rosner B. & Pfister E. (1983) Epidemiological study of the abuse of analgesics containing phenacetin: Renal morbidity and mortality (1968–1979). *New England Journal of Medicine* **308**, 357–62.

Keczes K. & Basheer A.M. (1980) Do cortico-steroids prevent postoperative neuralgia? *British Journal of Dermatology* **102**, 551–5.

Chapter Seventeen
Treatment of Infections

C.M. CASTLEDEN

OVERVIEW

The diagnosis and treatment of bacterial infection in the elderly is not always straightforward. The classical signs of infection are frequently absent, and concomitant disease distorts presentation, complicates management and occasionally mitigates against the use of antibiotic therapy. Furthermore, confirmation of infection by investigation of blood, urine or secretions may be difficult due to problems with collections or alterations in the usual haematological changes. Finally, the rate of drug elimination is almost always slower, and thus plasma and tissue concentrations of drugs higher, so that toxic reactions are more common.

The choice of an antibiotic depends on the patient, his attendant diseases, knowledge of the likely infecting organisms and their sensitivity to antibiotics. Each physician should use a few well-known drugs, and not experiment with newer preparations, which are frequently no more effective but always more expensive. Rapid changes in antibiotics are not indicated until a drug has been prescribed for 48 hours, unless the patient has a toxic reaction. In such cases the advice of the local microbiologist should be sought.

SPECIAL PROBLEMS OF BACTERIAL INFECTIONS IN ELDERLY PATIENTS

Clinical features of infections in elderly patients

Although the classical signs of infection may be present in elderly patients, they are usually less dramatic and arise more insidiously. Presentation is frequently a non-specific deterioration of health and pyrexia is absent. Central nervous system signs may predominate, mimicking progression of a previous neurological lesion, or a toxic confusional state. The latter is common and must be differentiated from an infection in a patient with dementia. Whether the latter is present or not fluid intake is frequently insufficient so that the old person is also dehydrated and possibly has pre-renal uraemia.

Pathological investigations

Often the plasma viscosity or erythrocyte sedimentation rate is not raised and leucocytosis is absent. Specimens of sputum or urine for bacteriological culture may be difficult to obtain, but a blood culture is usually possible and helpful.

Renal function

Renal function falls with aging but because muscle mass also decreases, the blood urea and serum creatinine concentration may be within normal limits. Thus a patient of 80 years with a normal blood urea and serum creatinine may have a creatinine clearance of about 50 ml per minute, and his will be considerably lower in any patient in whom the blood urea or serum creatinine is raised. Drugs which rely on renal function for their elimination from the body are therefore particularly hazardous in the elderly unless allowances are made for this decrease in renal function. For this reason it is wise not to use aminoglycosides or nitrofurantoin if alternative antibiotics are available.

Pre-disposition to resistant organisms

There are 2 situations in elderly patients in which prophylactic or inappropriate antibiotic therapy can lead to serious major infection with resistant organisms. The first is treatment of the unconscious patient before any suspicion of infection arises or can be confirmed pathologically, and the second arises in patients with permanent indwelling catheters. As a general rule prophylactic antibiotics should only be given before amputation surgery, or such procedures as dental extraction in patients with damaged heart valves (see Table 17.1). The presence of an indwelling urinary catheter is always associated with bacteriuria and white cells in the urine. If the patient has no systemic or urinary manifestations of infection, it is unwise to treat this bacteriuria, since overgrowth with another organism resistant to the current antibiotic therapy is sure to occur (see Chapter 14). It is frequently found that a patient with a long-term catheter has been treated with 3 or 4 different antibiotics and that the infecting organism has become progressively more resistant to such therapy. Finally, if a septicaemia occurs the choice of antibiotic is severely limited.

Table 17.1 Alternatives in the prophylaxis of subacute bacterial endocarditis.

Drug	Dosage
Penicillin	1 mega unit plus
Streptomycin	0.5 g i.m.
Vancomycin	1 g i.v.
Phenoxylmethyl penicillin	6 hourly o. for 48 hours

Concomitent disease

It should be remembered that the elderly frequently have more than one pathological process. An infection may therefore unmask latent diabetes or precipitate heart failure. Finally, bronchopneumonia is often a terminal event in many chronic debilitating diseases. It has long been known in this situation as 'the friend of the aged' and may not therefore require antibiotic therapy. Such a decision requires intimate knowledge of the patient and his illness.

GENERAL PRINCIPLES OF ANTIMICROBIAL THERAPY

Antibiotics are now one of the most commonly prescribed drugs. Most have originated from a small number of drug families, the prototypes of which have been in existence for 25 years. The newer antibiotics derived by chemical and biological manipulation of core-molecules may possess pharmacological, antimicrobial or toxicological advantages but many new products have little advantage to those already available. It is clearly unwise to rely on advertisements from the pharmaceutical industry to identify major therapeutic advances in this field. The latest is not necessarily the best but is probably the most expensive. A practising physician should therefore know how to use a few antibiotics well. He will then be able to balance the risk-versus-benefit equation, recognize adverse reactions and alter dosage if he suspects impairment of elimination. He will also know how to vary his choice with the site of infection knowing which achieve adequate concentrations in CSF, bile or urine.

Collaboration with the microbiologist

The choice of which drug to use involves collaboration with a microbiologist. This does not necessitate sending samples in every case for culture and sensitivity tests, but at least discussion of local patterns of infection and antibiotic sensitivity; for example, the sensitivity of *Streptococcus pyogenes* to penicillin has remained unchanged over 30 years but a survey in Boston in 1976 showed that 33 antibiotics plus co-trimoxazole (trimethoprim-sulfamethoxazole) were used against this group of organisms; conversely *Pneumococci* and haemolytic *Streptococcus* are commonly resistant to tetracycline now.

Route of administration

In severe infections do not rely on the variable absorption of antibiotics from the gastrointestinal tract. Parenteral administration is mandatory in septicaemia, meningitis and infective endocarditis. Other routes such as intrathecal injections and occasionally topical antibiotics may have to be considered in relevant cases.

Factors influencing the choice of antibiotics

Toxicity

Preference should be given to the less toxic of 2 drugs if both will serve the purpose. Always base the choice on personal experience, local bacterial sensitivity patterns, and if possible laboratory diagnosis from adequate specimens looked at by an expert. It should be remembered that the only antibiotics which are directly fatal are penicillin given to highly sensitive individuals and in big doses intrathecally, and chloramphenicol. The former reactions should be entirely preventable and if they occur result from medical negligence; the latter reaction may be a necessary therapeutic risk.

Combinations

Combinations may be necessary first to give a greater range of action as, for example, in the treatment of *Streptococcus faecalis*; here a combination of penicillin and streptomycin is usually totally bacteriocidal, whereas either alone might leave survivors. Second, a combination may be indicated to prevent bacterial resistance as, for example, in the treatment of tuberculosis and perhaps *Staphylococcus aureus* infections. The most frequent combination used to prevent or overcome resistance is trimethoprim-sulfamethoxazole (co-trimoxazole). In general, a bacteriocidal drug should not be given with a bacteriostatic agent.

Concomitant therapy

Always consider the effect of present therapy on antibiotic treatment. Absorption, metabolism, distribution and elimination can all be affected by concomitant drugs at any age. In the elderly there is a particular danger of renal damage when cephalosporins are used concurrently with diuretics (the latter are commonly prescribed to the elderly). As a rule the cephalosporins are expensive and many indications for their use are amply covered by amoxycillin or ampicillin.

Hepatic dysfunction

Tetracyclines apart from doxycycline are best avoided in the elderly due to their effect on protein catabolism. Tetracyclines and erythromycin are also hepatotoxic in excessive doses, and both should be avoided if hepatic function is compromised.

Lack of response

If there is no apparent response to present therapy, it should be changed; however, rarely sooner than 48 hours unless the patient's condition is deteriorating. It may be better practice to add a further antibiotic rather than to change from one to another.

Plasma drug concentrations

These are not normally necessary but are mandatory when aminoglycosides are used. In such cases, it is important that the plasma concentration is measured immediately before the next dose.

Prevention of bacterial lung infections

Bacterial lung infections may be primary but frequently follow a viral illness. Vaccines are now available which offer some protection against pneumococcal pneumonia and influenza, and should be considered in any patient over 65 years.

Influenza vaccines. These contain a mixture of influenza *a* and *b* viruses. They are effective if given approximately 2–3 weeks before exposure provided the vaccine antigens are reasonably closely related to the epidemic strain. A routine yearly immunization with polyvalant influenza vaccine is recommended for all patients over 65 years regardless of their previous state of health. It is advisable to administer the vaccine subcutaneously in 2 doses a month apart for the initial immunization, and subsequently as a single subcutaneous booster once a year in September. Side-effects are unusual but it is unwise to vaccinate patients with a history of allergy especially if this is to egg protein.

Pneumococcal vaccines. These vaccines are highly effective in protecting against pneumococcal pneumonia and may also prevent pneumococcal meningitis of bacteraemic origin. Antibody concentrations can remain elevated for 5 years. Thus vaccination is not necessary in a patient with a recent pneumococcal infection and no patient should be revaccinated within 3 years. The vaccine must be given subcutaneously or intramuscularly, but, even so, local erythema and soreness at the injection site is common.

CHOICE OF SPECIFIC ANTIBIOTIC FOR COMMON PATHOGENS

Although the choice of an antibiotic may be altered on subsequent bacteriological advice, it is useful to have some idea of the sensitivities of the common pathogens. The list is by no means comprehensive and readers are referred to the many books on clinical pharmacology and bacteriology. This list is summarized in Table 17.2.

Streptococcus pyogenes

This organism is usually resistant to sulphonamides but not to penicillin and only if the patient is sensitive to this drug should erythromycin or cephalexin be used. For infections of the upper respiratory tract a 7-day course is advisable since a relapse may occur with shorter courses.

Streptococcus viridans

This organism is usually very penicillin sensitive. However, if there is any doubt the addition of streptomycin will produce a consistent success.

Streptococcus faecalis

This is a common cause of urinary tract infections and endocarditis. Most organisms are sensitive to penicillin or ampicillin plus streptomycin although if resistant to the latter, kanamycin or gentamicin can be used. It is wise to test the bacteriocidal action of combinations in vitro.

Staphylococcus

Many of these organisms produce penicillinase and thus are resistant to penicillin, streptomycin, tetracycline and often to chloramphenicol, erythromycin, novobiocin and kanamycin. The drug of choice is flucloxacillin although cephaloridine, cephalothin and cephalexin can be used. Co-trimoxazole (trimethoprim-sulfamethoxazole) may be successful for treatment of staphylococcal osteomyelitis.

Haemophilus influenzae

Ampicillin or amoxycillin is the antibiotic of choice. Tetracycline or a cephalosporin are suitable second-line drugs.

Table 17.2 Rating of antibiotics according to the organism to be treated.

Organism	1st choice	2nd choice	Usually resistant
Streptococcus pyogenes	Penicillin	Erythromycin Cephalosporins	Sulphonamides
Streptococcus viridans	Penicillin/ Streptomycin	Cephalosporins	
Streptococcus faecalis	Penicillin/ Streptomycin	Ampicillin Gentamicin Kanamycin	
Staphylococcus	Flucloxicillin	Cephalosporins Co-trimoxazole	Penicillin Streptomycin Tetracycline
Haemophilus influenzae	Ampicillin	Tetracycline Co-trimoxazole	
Pneumococcus	Ampicillin	Co-trimoxazole Cephalosporins Tetracycline	
Meningococcus	Benzyl penicillin	Chloramphenicol	
Gonococcus	Benzyl penicillin Amoxycillin + Probenocid	Tetracycline	
Anaerobes	Metronidazole	Chloramphenicol Clindamycin	Cephalosporins
Salmonella + *Shigella*	Co-trimoxazole	Chloramphenicol	
Enterobacteria			
E. coli			
Non-penicillinase	Ampicillin	Co-trimoxazole Cephalosporins	
Penicillinase	Flucloxicillin		
Pseudomonas aeruginosa and proteus	Uticillin Ticarcillin Tobramycin	Mexocillin Carbenicillin Cephalosporins Gentamycin Kanamycin	Co-trimoxazole Ampicillin Penicillin
Klebsiella	Gentamicin	Cephalosporins Streptomycin	Penicillin

Amoxycillin and Ampicillin are interchangeable in this table.
Cephalosporins are referred to generally as there are many preparations available and they are regarded as second-line drugs.
Co-trimoxazole is Trimethoprim-sulphamethoxazole.

Pneumococcus

Ampicillin or amoxycillin is recommended. Tetracycline is an alternative but some strains of pneumococci are now resistant. A cephalosporin is thus a better second choice if the patient is hypersensitive to penicillin.

Meningococcus

This organism remains very sensitive to benzylpenicillin, which is the drug of choice in patients not hypersensitive to it. Sulphonamides such as sulphadimidine may be given in addition but are not recommended for use alone as sulphonamide-resistant organisms are emerging. Chloramphenical is a second-line drug.

Gonococcus

This organism is less sensitive than previously to penicillin and therefore high doses, and preferably more than one are required. It is wise to prolong the action of penicillin with probenecid unless compliance for a therapeutic regimen can be assured. If only a single dose is to be given, then 2.5–3.5 g of ampicillin or amoxycillin plus probenocid should be used.

Anaerobes

The common anaerobes are almost always sensitive to chloramphenicol. However metronidazole is the drug of choice being safer and usually as effective. Actinomyces are almost always resistant to metronidazole but are sensitive to penicillin.

Salmonella and *Shigella*

Although chloramphenicol remains the best treatment for typhoid fever, some resistance has developed and the drug can occasionally produce aplastic anaemia or a shock-like state. It is also a bacteriostatic drug and therefore does not prevent the carrier state. Ampicillin in high doses (6–8 g) is less effective than chloramphenicol and should only be used in combination with chloramphenicol to eliminate the carrier state. Co-trimoxazole will relieve symptoms quickly but will not eradicate infection in all cases.

It is unwise to use antibiotics to treat paratyphoid enteritis even though this carries a particular risk in old and debilitated patients. Antibiotics tend to prolong the carrier state but if thought necessary the same should be used as for typhoid. Similar arguments are true for the treatment of *Shigella* infections, but in these cases co-trimoxazole is probably the drug of choice if antibiotics are felt to be necessary.

Enterobacteria and *Pseudomonas*

These organisms are naturally more resistant than most others and can acquire resistance from simple contact with resistant species.

E. coli. Ampicillin and amoxycillin are the drugs of first choice if the organism is non-penicillinase producing. Otherwise a similar line of treatment should be followed as for *Staphylococcus aureus.*

Pseudomonas aeruginosa and *Proteus* species. Until recently these organisms were difficult to treat and required antibiotics with low therapeutic indices. As a group these species tend to be resistant to co-trimoxazole. However there are now 2 new antibiotics, uticillin and ticarcillin which are expensive but effective. A drawback to the latter is that it has to be given parenterally. Alternatively, carbenicillin in large doses or the aminoglyco sides, gentamicin and kanamycin can be used; tobramycin appears to be particularly active against pseudomonas.

Fungal infections

Griseofulvin (See Table 17.3) is standard treatment for the dermatomycoses. Nystatin has a low solubility and is suitable for treatment of *Candida albicans* on mucous and cutaneous surfaces. It can also be given by inhalation for infection of the bronchi with candida. However, it has a most unpleasant taste and oral candida is better treated with amphotericin B lozenges. This drug should also be used for all systemic fungal infections. It is, however, one of the most toxic of antibiotics and may cause vomiting, fever, thrombophlebitis, and hypokalaemia. Some degree of permanent renal damage may result from a full course. For cryptococcal meningitis, 5-fluorocytosine should be used and a high concentration in the CSF occurs

Table 17.3 Drugs used for other infections referred to in the text.

Complaint	Drug used
Fungal infections	Griseofulvin
	Nystatin
	Amphoteracin B lozenges
	5-fluorocytosine
	Clotrimazole
	Miconazole
	Notamycin
Tuberculosis	Isoniazid
	Rifampicin
	Ethambutol
Herpes zoster	Idoxuridine

after oral therapy. Clotrimazole has been advocated for systemic candida and pulmonary aspergilosis, but there are conflicting reports on its efficacy.

TREATMENT OF INFECTIONS IN DIFFERENT SYSTEMS

Respiratory tract

Upper respiratory tract

A high proportion of infections in this area are viral and require only supportive therapy. Antibiotics are not indicated for the treatment of colds and undiagnosed upper respiratory tract symptoms. When a bacterial infection is likely, the causative organisms are frequently *Pneumococcus* and *Streptococcus* in acute sinusitis and acute otitis media, but may be *Haemophilus influenzae*. All these bacteria together with B-haemolytic *Streptococcus* causing pharyngitis are sensitive to amoxycillin or ampicillin.

Lower respiratory tract infections

Bronchitis. Again the principle pathogens are viral and thus only symptomatic therapy is necessary unless the sputum becomes purulent. Occasionally the infections are due to *Rickettsia* or *Mycoplasma* in which cases doxycycline is the drug of choice.

Chronic bronchitis. This is associated with permanent damage and pathological changes in the bronchial tree. Emphysema is frequently also present. General advice is necessary such as to avoid irritants, especially smoking. The use of corticosteroids is discussed elsewhere (p. 262). Infection is usually due to *Pneumococcus* and *Haemophilus influenzae* which inhabits the bronchial tree even between acute exacerbations. Thus when acute purulent bronchitis occurs it is often due to an overgrowth of these organisms which are sensitive to amoxycillin or co-trimoxazole. If the infecting organism is *Staphylococcus aureus*, then flucloxacillin may be necessary. When *Klebsiella* bacteria are present gentamicin is advised. Some patients have frequent acute exacerbations during the winter; these can be treated by short courses of antibiotics preferably initiated by the patient as soon as an exacerbation begins and continued until 2 days after the sputum becomes non-purulent. The alternative, long-term antibiotics, may lead to an overgrowth of resistant organisms.

Pneumonia. If this occurs in previously healthy lungs, the most common organism is *Pneumococcus*; less frequently it is *Streptococcus pyogenes* or *Klebsiella*. Since antibiotics have to be given before confirmation of the organism by the laboratory, ampicillin or amoxycillin are the drugs of choice. If a *Staphylococcus* is suspected it is wise to give amoxycillin and flucloxycillin in combination. This is because the *Staphylococcus* may produce penicillinase and flucloxycillin is relatively ineffective against non-staphylococcus penicillinase producing organisms. If the pneumonia is due to *Mycoplasma* or *Rickettsia*, then doxicycline should be used.

When pneumonia occurs secondary to chronic lung disease it is wise to assume that local organisms are responsible and thus treatment should be on the lines suggested above in acute exacerbations of chronic bronchitis. If no improvement has occurred in 48 hours, the antibiotic agent should be changed or an addition made on advice from the bacteriologist. If repeated pneumonias occur, it is wise to rule out upper respiratory tract sepsis or such lesions as achalasia of the cardia or deformities of the bronchial tree.

Any patient anticipating a planned non-emergency operation should stop smoking at least 2 weeks before the operation and if suffering from chronic lung disease requires vigorous pre- and post-operative physiotherapy.

Pulmonary Tuberculosis. Pulmonary tuberculosis should be suspected whenever there is unexplained fever and weight loss in an elderly patient. It may be impossible to obtain infected sputum but frequently gastric washings produce positive identification. The physician should not be deterred from diagnosing the condition by negative Mantoux tests. The principle cause of treatment failure is lack of patient cooperation since adequate regimens are otherwise 100% effective. On diagnosis, treatment should be started with isoniazid, rifampicin and ethambutol, the latter 2 drugs have replaced paraminosalicyclic acid and streptomycin as first-line drugs.

It is necessary to initiate treatment with 3 drugs because 5% of new cases are resistant to 1, and resistance to 1 drug given alone soon arises. All 3 drugs should be continued for 2 months until the sputum is negative and the sensitivity of the organism has been established. In most studies ethambutol has been stopped after 2 months and treatment continued with rifampicin and isoniazid. However, ethambutol and isoniazid make an acceptable alternative combination. Both regimens are available as combined tablets, which improves compliance and prevents resistance occurring to 1 drug taken alone. It is usual to start treatment in hospital for social reasons and because the patient is ill and it is easier to detect adverse reactions to drugs. Therapy should then be continued for a further 6–9 months with close supervision. If the patient is likely to default and supervision is intermittent, it is possible to give the treatment on a 2–3 times a week basis when larger doses are given.

It is wise to trace contacts and to initiate treatment if infection on clinical grounds is suspected or if a positive reaction to tuberculin develops.

Rifampicin may cause mild gastrointestinal and hepatic upsets and rarely purpura. The urine and body secretions turn red or orange with therapy.

Ethambutol is used with care in the elderly. Retrobulbar neuritis may occur and, although reversible if detected early, may be difficult to spot in old patients. The earliest sign is an alteration in colour vision.

Isoniazid rarely causes side-effects if the dose is less than 350 mg per day but can lead to restlessness, insomnia, muscle twitching and peripheral neuropathy especially in slow acetylators. This complication can be prevented by giving pyridoxine 10–20 mg daily.

Urinary system

A high fluid output is usually recommended with these infections and although such advice does not seem to improve outcome, it is still advocated on commonsense grounds. Until recently, a 7–10 day course of antibiotics used to be given routinely but there is recent evidence that 3-day treatments are as effective and possibly even a single dose may have the desired therapeutic effect. At present it is probably wise not to give less than 3 days of treatment. A 5–7 day course is advised in an elderly patient who has an uncomplicated urinary tract infection. If there are anatomical abnormalities in the urinary tract and these are associated with recurrent infections, then a trial of 6–12 months of antibiotics is justified. It should be remembered that early relapse may indicate that the wrong antibiotic was given initially or that compliance is absent. The most common organism is *E. coli* and amoxycillin, ampicillin or cotrimoxazole (trimethoprim–sulfamethoxazole) are usually effective. Other organisms are *Proteus*, *Streptococcus* and *Pseudomonas*.

If a patient has a long-term indwelling catheter, then the urine will almost inevitably become infected and unless there are signs of systemic infection such as fevers, rigors, and hypotension, antibiotics are not indicated. They will only eradicate the infection for a short time and lead to an overgrowth of more resistant organisms, so that when systemic infection occurs the choice of antibiotics will be limited. With systemic infections in these conditions the aminoglycosides are nearly always indicated (see also pp. 196–200).

Skin infection

Impetigo

This is caused by *Staphylococcus* with or without the addition of *Streptococcus*. The drug of choice is flucloxacillin, but ampicillin or amoxycillin may also be necessary. Alternative therapy is erythromycin or co-trimoxazole. This should be given for 7 to 10 days and can be accompanied by topical application, because treatment is required for such a short time and therefore contact dermatitis is not a problem. A suitable ointment would be 0.1% gentamycin. It is important to exclude underlying infection with scabies, lice or herpes simplex.

Erysipelas

The organism is *Streptococcus pyogenes* which is penicillin sensitive.

Recurrent boils

These result from infection with *Staphylococcus* spp., which are frequently penicillinase producing. It is important to exclude underlying diabetes mellitus, an immunological disorder or uraemia. The role of antiseptics such as chlorhexidine soap is unproven and their use may lead to contact dermatitis.

Viral infections

Warts. Most undergo spontaneous regression with time. The indications for treatment are:

(1) pain;
(2) uncertainty of the diagnosis;
(3) cosmetic.

The choice of treatment varies between local destruction with heat, cold, acid or curretage or weekly painting with podophyllin.

Herpes simplex. 5% idoxuridine cream should be applied 3–4 times a day for about 5 days. This drug competes with the virus for thymidic acid which is needed for DNA formation. If there is infection of the eye, the patient should be sent to the local ophthalmologist.

Herpes zoster. Similar treatment to herpes simplex should be given. It is important to watch out for secondary infection but antibiotics are not indicated until this occurs.

Candidiasis

This fungus rarely invades the skin of normal individuals. It is associated with intertrigo, chronic paronychia, immunosuppressant drugs, diabetes mellitus, antibiotic therapy and hypoparathyroidism. Treatment therefore necessitates a search for the underlying condition. Nystatin and amphotericin B can be used for mucocutaneous infestations since both are very poorly absorbed. Alternatives are natamycin, clotrimazole and miconazole.

Ringworm

For topical application there is no proprietary preparation with any advantage over Whitfield's ointment (Ung benzoic acid compound). Other preparations may cause contact sensitivity and are always more expensive than Whitfield's. If toe nails or the scalp are infected, prolonged treatment with griseofulvin is necessary. Treatment should be continued until all the infected keratin is shed, or until there is no fluorescence under Wood's light from scalp scrapings. Care is necessary with patients on anticoagulants since griseofulvin may decrease the absorption of warfarin.

Central nervous system infections

Bacterial meningitis has its greatest incidence in childhood but occurs in the elderly too. The most common organisms are *Haemophilus influenzae*, *Meningocossus* and *Pneumococcus*, in that order. Treatment should be continued until the patient is afebrile for at least 5–10 days and the CSF cell counts are normal. In theory the dosage of antibiotics should be increased as the meninges become less inflamed and therefore less penetrable to antibiotics. Most antibiotics penetrate to the CSF if adequate doses are given, which may require parenteral therapy. If there is any doubt, intrathecal therapy is necessary, but collaboration with the local microbiologist is essential. If no bacteriology service is available, ampicillin or amoxycillin will treat the 3 most common organisms. Tuberculous meningitis is uniformly fatal unless treated. Fungal infections require amphotericin B intravenously and intrathecally although an alternative in cryptococcal infections is 5 fluorocytosine. In syphilitic infections penicillin in high doses is effective but erythromycin and tetracycline can be given if the patient is sensitive to penicillin. The diagnosis of latent neurosyphilis is entirely a laboratory procedure and the treatment is procaine penicillin 1 Mu for 10 to 15 days, provided the patient is not sensitive to this drug. Follow up is necessary until the tests become negative.

Infective endocarditis

The diagnosis should be suspected if the patient has fever, emboli and changing murmurs. However, the clinical features are most unimpressive early on and a high index of clinical suspicion is required. The mortality of the condition is still high, approximately 30%, but this is not an indication for antibiotic therapy without a bacteriological diagnosis.

In elderly patients with valvular abnormalities, prophylactic therapy with antibiotics is indicated even for minor surgical operations and dental extraction. It is unnecessary to start such therapy 48 hours before an operation and indeed this is unwise as oral flora may become resistant. A single dose of penicillin is usually insufficient and 1 Mu of penicillin with streptomycin 0.5 g intramuscularly or vancomycin 1 g intravenously, or phenoxymethyl penicillin orally 6-hourly for 48 hours are advised.

The most common organism is still *Streptococcus viridans* which accounts for 50% of infections. This organism is sensitive to penicillin but it must be given in large doses; 1 Mu 6-hourly can be given intramuscularly but higher doses need to be given intravenously. It should be rembered that very large doses may lead to fits if renal function is impaired. In old people especially with bedsores, *Streptococcus faecalis* is a common organism and is usually penicillin resistant. A combination of penicillin and streptomycin is required. Other infective organisms such as *Streptococcus pyogenes*, *Staphylococcus aureus*, *Candida* and *Rickettsia* will require appropriate therapy. Bacteriostatic antibiotics such as sulphonamide, tetracycline and chloramphenicol suppress the infection but do not cure it and are not advised.

The duration of therapy should be 6 weeks and its effect should be judged by resolution of fever, settling of the ESR, rising Hb and the subsidence of the finger clubbing.

Gastrointestinal tract infections

Biliary

Many antibiotics are not excreted in sufficiently high concentrations to have an effect on organisms in the biliary tract. This is not a problem with ampicillin, amoxycillin, cephalexin and rifamide, all of which achieve adequate concentrations in bile. This is also true for cephaloridine, gentamicin and some of the newer antibiotics such as mecillinam and mazlocillin, which are useful second-line drugs for these infections.

PRESSURE SORES

It is usually easier to prevent pressure ulcers than to treat them. The skin over bony prominences should be examined twice every day by a responsible person (usually the nurse in charge of the ward). Additional inspection should be made every 2 hours when the patient is turned. Any sign of redness, irritation or abrasion is an indication to remove pressure immediately. It is important to keep the skin clean and dry at all times even if this means catheterization. Gentle massage of vulnerable skin may be beneficial but excessive rubbing or application of lotions should be avoided. Clothing should not be pleated and as far as possible be wrinkle free; tight, synthetic (non-porous) garments with prominent zips or studs are best avoided.

Non-operative management of pressure ulcers aims to establish a clean wound and improve the patient's general condition. A wound will usually become clean following debridement of necrotic tissue, and soaking with saline gauze, moistened every 4 hours and changed 8-hourly. Topical medications are rarely necessary, are always more expensive, and produce allergic reactions in some patients. They may be relied upon to such an extent that a false sense of security is instilled and simple measures are forgotten. No topical substances have been shown to promote faster healing than the technique of sharp debridement and wet-to-dry dressings; for example, enzymatic agents do debride the superficial layers of an ulcer but their use on deep devitalized tissue has not been proven. A few seconds with forceps and scissors can accomplish more than the application of these medications over many weeks.

Systemic antibiotic therapy usually has no place in the treatment of bedsores which are universally infected with mutiple organisms. An exception is before surgery where the chances of success are significantly lower if the wound is highly infected. Topical antibiotics do not penetrate the depths of wounds or affect bacterial growth in granulation sensitivity. Reduction of bacteria is more easily achieved by removal of devitalized tissue. Systemic antibiotics may have a place in decreasing the odour from particularly offensive pressure ulcers. This may be especially important for the patient and relatives.

The general nutritional state of the patient is important and if he is unable to swallow a nasogastric tube or even intravenous hyperalimentation may be needed. Diets should be high in protein, calories and have added vitamin C and zinc.

REFERENCES AND FURTHER READING

Clemens J.D., Horwitz R.I., Jaffe C.C. et al (1982) A controlled evaluation of the risk of bacterial endocarditis in persons with mitral valve prolapse. *New England Journal of Neurology* **307**, 776–81.

Fox R.F. (Ed.) (1984) *Infection in Old Age*. Churchill Livingstone, London. Longman, New York.

Freeman E. (1984) The Respiratory System. In Brocklehurst J.C. (Ed.) *Textbook of Geriatric Medicine and Gerontology* 3rd edition, Ch. 36. Churchill Livingstone, London. Longman, New York.

Willems J.S., Snaders C.R., Raddiough M.A. & Bell J.C. (1980) Cost effectiveness of vaccination against pneumococcal pneumonia. *New England Journal of Medicine* **303**, 553–9.

Chapter Eighteen
Anticlotting Therapy

J.E.F. POHL

OVERVIEW

The need for active interference in blood clotting arises usually in relation to other illness, is commonly circumscribed in time and a significant proportion of such therapy is prophylactic in nature. The provision of objective laboratory control, whilst often regarded as inconvenient and as a source of unwelcome additional expense, introduces the major benefit of furthering patient compliance. It is particularly valuable during the early stages of therapy when it will also be an important factor in risk reduction.

Clotting disorders are a considerable risk in old age for the following reasons.

(1) The lower cardiac output and frequent presence of mild congestive cardiac failure lend a general background to the production of stasis which is locally enhanced on the venous and cardiac side by pressure-induced dilatation.

(2) Structural damage in the large arteries in the form of ulcerated and degenerating atheroma plaques is responsible for platelet emboli with the production of transient ischaemic attacks particularly in the cerebral territory.

(3) The ultimate occurrence of critical reduction in lumen size may reduce flow and culminate in an occlusive thrombotic episode (myocardial infarction, massive mesenteric infarction or a gangrenous leg).

(4) Past episodes of venous thrombosis, particularly in women with a history of complicated pregnancies and the additive effects of long years of venous incompetence in sufferers from varicose veins, load the scales in favour of deep vein thrombosis and possible pulmonary embolism.

(5) The evils of immobility are also more clear-cut and prolonged in the elderly.

(6) The aging heart is liable to the development of atrial fibrillation which both in its intermittent and in its constant variety must rank as an important source of peripheral arterial embolism from a dilated non-contractile left atrium.

(7) Oestrogen substitution therapy in postmenopausal women (see pp. 260 and 264) may increase clotting tendency.

(8) Dehydration may develop during prolonged travel and during illness—perhaps equally based on diminished intake and the failure of the aging kidney to achieve adequate urinary concentration.

A good case can therefore be made for the frequent use of short-term prophylactic anticoagulant therapy to cover periods of high clotting risk in elderly patients and there are many possible indications for long-term anticlotting therapy. A careful analysis of risk factors and benefits in individual patients is therefore required.

Beyond the usual risks of haemorrhage inherent in this form of treatment, the elderly exhibit an excess risk in regard to hypertension—associated cerebral haemorrhage. They are also liable to wider fluctuations of anticoagulant activity because of uncertain compliance and variable liver function in consequence of variable degrees of liver congestion. Outright dementia would certainly militate strongly against any form of anticoagulation just as it would dissuade the doctor from most forms of active treatment.

Parenteral treatment

Prophylaxis

Prophylaxis may be considered in the following situations:

(a) elective surgery (e.g. hip replacement, herniorrhaphy);

(b) prolonged medical illness with more than a few days' bed rest, or with associated cardiac failure.

Two regimens are available, depending on the magnitude of the risk:

(1) low or ultra-low dose subcutaneous heparin regimens with daily heparin doses of 5000 to 10 000 i.u.

(2) continuous therapy of 20–40 000 i.u. per day i.v. by constant infusion pump.

In low-dose heparin therapy laboratory control by the determination of activated partial thromboplastin time on venous blood samples collected 3 hours after heparin injection is not mandatory, although desirable, and local haematoma formation can be minimized by a correct injection at a right angle to the plane of the skin from a CO_2 cartridge-driven jet gun.

Laboratory surveillance of high-dose heparin therapy is currently unsatisfactory. A two to fourfold prolongation of the thrombin time ratio would be considered a satisfactory standard, but its precise meaning is less certain than in the control of oral anticoagulant therapy and the degree of risk reduction is unknown. The resumption of adequate mobility by the patient should be the signal for discontinuation of low-dose therapy and rapid tailing off of high-dose therapy. Conversely, progression to chronic anticoagulant therapy preferably of the oral kind may have to be considered in a minority of patients.

Emergency therapy

The strong suspicion of even minor (and possibly premonitory) pulmonary embolism or the development of acute cardiac failure (either post-myocardial infarction or related to chest infection not responding to aggressive therapy within 12 hours of onset) are clear-cut indications for high-dose heparinization unless one of the conventional contraindications (e.g. an active peptic ulcer, a bleeding tendency) is present. Deep leg vein thromboses are more difficult to classify because the risk of embolization is inversely related to the local venous inflammatory response so that easily diagnosed cases are almost harmless, whilst the most treacherous cases develop their leg signs either not at all or a few days after massive pulmonary embolism has occurred. The standard therapy is by continuous heparin infusion for 1 to 2 weeks followed by oral anticoagulant therapy for 6 weeks to 6 months, depending on the initial degree of swelling of the leg and the rapidity of resolution of pain and swelling after the heparin infusion has been commenced. If there is good evidence of pulmonary embolism or if the leg symptoms recur, 6 months of oral anti-coagulant therapy becomes a mandatory minimum. There is no conclusive evidence in favour of treating acute retinal artery or vein thrombosis with heparin. The use of fibrinolytic therapy is controversial and a description of its application is outside the scope of this book. In cases of acute arterial embolism to the legs, venesection of 750 ml followed by dextran infusion is a risky but often worthwhile emergency measure. In favourable cases this will obviate surgical interference and in less successful cases may yet save the limb if endarterectomy has been unduly delayed.

The use of this method of treatment depends on the rapidity with which the diagnosis of acute arterial obstruction has been made, the availability of competent surgical help without delay and the fitness of the patient. If

Table 18.1 Anticoagulant and anti-platelet aggregator drugs.

Type of drug	Drug name (Trade Name)	Method of dosage
Anticoagulants	Heparin	i.v., s.c.
	Warfarin	o.
	Phenindione	o.
	Tromexan	o.
Anti-platelet aggregators	Aspirin—actyl salicylic acid—ultra-low dose	o.
	Phenylpyrasone (Sulphinpirazone, Anturan)	o.
	Dipyridamole	o.

these factors are favourable, surgery without delay is preferable, particularly since a Fogarty catheter can be passed under local anaesthesia, and this procedure may be well tolerated even shortly after acute myocardial infarction.

Oral long-term anticoagulants

This is indicated for at least 6 weeks, but commonly for much longer, after deep vein thrombosis or pulmonary embolism. Another indication is atrial fibrillation associated with a dilated left atrium, particularly if there is structural mitral valve disease. Because of the protective effects of prolonged pulmonary hypertension many patients with rheumatic valve disease lead good quality lives into extreme old age and it is a great pity to see good health catastrophically terminated by preventable cerebral, mesenteric or leg embolism.

The use of anticoagulants in chronic heart failure with dilatation of one or both ventricular cavities is more uncertain, not because anyone could doubt the much increased risk of peripheral arterial embolism, but because it is of limited efficacy and is supplementary to other methods of augmenting cardiac function.

The use of warfarin in old people is, at least initially, attended by enough uncertainty to make hospitalization mandatory. The loading dose should be as low as 10 mg in most cases, especially if there are doubts about the nutritional status of the patient or if a tender, distended and pulsatile liver indicates the presence of functional tricuspid incompetence. The occasional patient will justify a higher dose for suspected microsomal enzyme induction, especially if phenobarbitone has been prescribed as an anticonvulsant agent. The preliminary prothrombin-time ratio, or an equivalent estimation result, should preferably be available at the time of initial dosing. Daily laboratory tests are carried out but the warfarin dose is only adjusted every third day. Remember that preceding heparin therapy renders the first laboratory result uninterpretable. The aim must be to achieve and maintain a prothrombin-time ratio as close as possible to 2.5 and in any case not under 2.0. There is absolutely no merit in half-hearted therapy based on half-hearted indications because it is felt that the full risk of correctly applied therapy is not justifiable.

Once adequate control has been established the patient can be discharged from hospital provided adequate supervision of his medicine taking and a reliable scheme for blood monitoring can be instituted. Many patients eventually reach a high degree of stability and may only require a blood test every eight weeks and the warfarin dose may remain unaltered for years.

Remember that drugs including clofibrate and cimetidine have an effect on warfarin dosage because of competition for protein binding sites or effects mediated via liver enzymes. Episodes of overdosage will present with either haematuria or haemoptysis, or, rarely, with bleeding into the skin. Microscopic haematuria occurs within the desired therapeutic range and minor degrees of overt haematuria may be missed because of the patient's poor powers of observation or because the urine is discoloured by other drugs. Significant warfarin-induced bleeding is a medical emergency. The patient should be immediately hospitalized and given i.v. vitamin K, and fresh frozen human plasma. Once haemostasis has been restored, the indications for resumption of anticoagulation should be carefully evaluated, especially if the physician feels that some of the circumstances surrounding the bleeding episode suggest that a repetition of such a mishap is not unlikely. Once anticoagulation has been re-established, laboratory surveillance should be temporarily stepped up to reduce the risk of recurrence of either venous thrombosis or drug-induced bleeding. There is never any justification for aiming at a lower level of anticoagulant control since the risk of further thrombosis is actually enhanced after a bleeding episode which required temporary reversal of anticoagulation.

The decision to discontinue uncomplicated therapy should be implemented by a tailing off procedure extending over 1–2 weeks since rebound thrombosis is a distinct possibility. Other oral anticoagulant agents such as pheninidone or tromexan are subject to the same principles of administration, although details may differ.

Anti-platelet aggregation therapy

The presence of extensive intimal damage in the atheromatous large arteries of elderly people lends itself to a possible blanket argument in favour of anti-platelet-stickiness therapy. This may be reinforced by more specific considerations in those patients who have sustained a myocardial infarction or have other evidence of ischaemic heart disease. It becomes almost irresistible in the presence of transient cerebral ischaemic attacks (TIAs) which have not responded to hypertension control or are surgically uncorrectable. Drugs available are ultra-low dose aspirin (ASA), phenylpyrasone (sulphinpyrazone—anturan) or dipyridamole with the possibility of combining any 2 of these drugs. The arguments in favour of 75–150 mg of aspirin per day are largely theoretical and relate to the differential sensitivity to aspirin of archidonic acid metabolic enzymes productive of platelet aggregating prostaglandins (Thromboxane A + B) and prostacycline which is a powerful deaggregating factor.

Although trial evidence of the effectiveness of anti-platelet therapy in TIAs or after myocardial infarction is contradictory, the present consensus is in favour of such therapy. The risk to the patient is very low and certainly lower than that of anticoagulant therapy, however carefully controlled. The author has a personal preference for low-dose aspirin which has the additional attraction that the occasionally missed dose may actually be a boon.

REFERENCES AND FURTHER READING

Anturan Reinfarction Trial Research Group (1980) Sulfinpyrazone in the prevention of sudden death after myocardial infarction. *New England Journal of Medicine* **302**, 250–6.

Gruber U.F., Soldeen T. & Brokup T. (1980) Incidence of fatal postoperative pulmonary embolism after prophylaxis with Dextran 70 and low dose heparin: An international multi-centre study. *British Medical Journal* **1**, 69–72.

Hedlund P.O. & Blomback M. (1979) The effect of prophylaxis with low dose heparin on blood coagulation parameters. *Thromb. Haemost* **41**, 337–45.

Hirsh J. & Gallus A.S. (1977) Heparin. In: *Recent Advances in Haematology*, pp. 453–66. Churchill Livingstone, London. Longman, New York.

Kurec A.S. et al (1979) Clotting, activated partial thromboplastin and coagulation times in monitoring heparin therapy. *Annals. of clinical and laboratory Science* **9**, 494–500.

O'Reilly R.A. (1980) Anticoagulant Antithrombotic and Thrombolytic Drugs. In Goodman & Gilman (Eds.) *The Pharmacological Basis of Therapeutics*, 6th edition, pp. 1347–66. Macmillan Publishing Co Inc, New York.

Wintrobe M.M. (1981) Thrombosis and Antithrombotic Therapy. In Clinical Hematology, 8th edition, Ch. 52, pp. 1247–72.

Chapter Nineteen
Hormones

J.E.F. POHL

OVERVIEW

This chapter is concerned with the application of a large number of hormones and other potent pharmacological agents to a miscellany of conditions few of which are the particular province of old age. There is a clear distinction, however, between the use of various forms of hormonal replacement therapy which will occupy the main part of this discussion and the application of drugs for the production of pharmacological effects. Because of the limited life-expectancy and the presence of a multiplicity of degenerative conditions in old bodies, the aim of replacement therapy is permissive rather than curative and to aim for complete restoration of normality is often inappropriate. The many limiting factors also include difficulty with compliance especially if this involves variable dosage in response to surveillance criteria and a dependence on intact sensory perception and the acquisition and practice of new manual skills, e.g. the giving of injections.

HORMONE REPLACEMENT THERAPIES

Diabetes mellitus

Because of the association between age of onset of symptoms and obesity, non-insulin-dependent diabetes (type 2 DM) is common in the overfed Western World and is becoming increasingly common in aging populations. The establishment of insulin therapy almost half a century ago, has transformed the life-expectancy of primary insulin-dependent diabetics so that many now survive to reach the geriatric age groups. Added to their number is the yield of secondary failure of non-insulin therapy the occurrence of which has a linearly increasing probability with the passage of years on successful sulphonylurea or metformin therapy.

The immediate aim of therapy on first discovering the presence of diabetes in an elderly person is to induce a remission in the manifestations of carbohydrate intolerance. Unless the patient is already underweight this can be achieved in at least 80% of patients by weight reduction. Even though the aim should be the attainment of ideal weight for height and age, insulin-resistance usually diminishes after the first few kilograms are lost so that normal ambulant blood sugars but not normal glucose tolerance on formal testing returns long before the target weight has been reached. Since remissions commonly last for several years it is well worthwhile to cajole the patient into compliance with a permanent alteration of dietary intake and not just to induce acquiescence in a temporary crash diet which is bound to be followed by an inevitable relapse.

Dieting

It used to be customary to regard the prescription of severe carbohydrate intake limitations as the centrepiece of any diabetic diet. More recently we have come to realize that overall calorie intake is the more important variable and that an adequate organic fibre content of the food consumed not only ensures adequate roughage for stool formation and thus combats the evils of chronic constipation but actually improves the patients carbohydrate tolerance and lowers blood sugars. Ideally, the selection of cereals, trunky vegetables, fruits, substitution of whole-grain bread should suffice but if necessary bran can either be eaten as a breakfast cereal, sprinkled over other food or, in the last resort, consumed by the tablespoonful. Common misconceptions in the mind of the patient about the nature of progress during a weight-reducing regimen must be actively dispelled by repeated discussion between the doctor and the patient. The most serious error is to attribute early loss of fluid to the achievement of bulk reduction or, even worse, to enhance such fluid losses by deliberate fluid restriction. Body fluid re-expansion will eventually occur and the will of the patient to continue to diet founders on what the patient regards as incontrovertable evidence of failure when, despite the most rigid persistence in irksome dietary restrictions, the weight gradually edges upwards.

The aim of inducing a permanent reduction in dietary calorie intake is best achieved by a reduction in saturated fat intake although the evidence in favour of a wholesale substitution of polyunsaturated fats is insufficient and, in any case, they have the same calorific value. The strategy of slow weight reduction over a period of many months is not compatible with daily weighing on the patient's bathroom scales. Whilst it may be advantageous to induce mildly obsessional attitudes to the details of dietary adherence, a frequency of weighing in excess of once a week should be strongly discouraged. Patients not infrequently expect a pat on the back for the omission of food items allowed by the diet and are particularly prone to omit breakfast from their dietary programme. This tendency should be discouraged. It confers the characteristics of a punishment and reward system on the diet so that occasional dietary excesses are offset in the patient's mind by the imaginary merits accumulated. In time this will destroy the whole basis of the dietary regimen. In addition, the human metabolic machine was originally designed for intermittent food intake with long intervals of fasting interrupted by spells of high food intake at the time of successful kills achieved by our hunting ancestors. As a consequence, weight gain on a constant daily calorific intake is a function of the number of meals taken and is actually minimized, contrary to widespread popular belief, by the practice of snacking. Six to eight small meals would be ideal but to fit in with established civilized dietary customs and also because it helps to keep the total number of calories consumed within the set limits, a reasonable compromise would be three main meals and three minor meals a day.

It should not be beneath the physician's dignity nor an abuse of his medical skills to supervise the diet personally and also to take a direct part in the repeated dietary instruction of the patient.

The dietician's skill in planning the details of a balanced diet which is also acceptable to the patient's palate and fits in with his social and cultural background should not be taken as an excuse for the doctor's lack of personal involvement. The *complete* delegation of dietary management to ancillary personnel must engender in the patient the attitude that this aspect of his treatment is relatively unimportant, leading to an adverse effect on motivation and compliance.

Oral hypoglycaemic therapy

The scope of *sulphonylurea* therapy is properly limited to a small percentage of diabetic patients, who, after achieving adequate weight reduction, are still found to remain hyperglycaemic and yet do not manifest a tendency to develop ketoacidosis spontaneously. Whilst there is no doubt that such drugs are successful in lowering the blood sugars of many obese diabetics, obesity is likely to be enhanced, with possible acceleration of atheromatous disease. Provided then that the patient falls into the small group who are likely to benefit from sulphonylurea therapy the choice of drug should provide no difficulty. Short-acting tolbutamide 0.5–1.0 G t.d.s. is the drug with the lowest incidence of side-effects, the least risk of producing hypoglycaemia and is most unlikely to cause serious damage to the patient even in the event of inadvertent overdosage (a possibility to be borne in mind particularly with elderly or occasionally confused patients). The manufacturers claims for the increased potency of drugs such as chlorpropamide and glibenclamide are largely irrelevant in the context of the treatment of diabetes. The long duration of action makes chlorpropamide, which is heavily protein bound, particularly hazardous. Hypoglycaemic attacks produced by this drug must be treated by i.v. drip, and glucose may have to be administered by this route for 3 days after the cessation of therapy to allow the chlopropamide blood level to fall to half its initial value.

Biguanide treatment is only of limited hypoglycaemic efficacy but has the advantage that obesity is no contraindication. Weight loss is commonly induced and metformin, 500 mg t.d.s. has been successfully used for this purpose alone in non-diabetics. Cynics might maintain, however, that substantial weight loss only occurs in the 20% of patients who are markedly nauseated by this drug. The development of lactic acidosis which was the most serious side-effect of phenformin therapy appears to be extremely rare after metformin therapy.

The most serious limitation of oral hypoglycaemic therapy is that even successful treatment has almost always to be changed for insulin at times of medical crises and in anticipation of surgery.

Insulin therapy

With the acceptance of uncontrolled hyperglycaemia as the chief culprit in the development of diabetic small vessel disease and of the consequences of rampant atherosclerosis the development of ketoacidosis is no longer the only, or even the main, indication for changing a patient to insulin injections. The development of blindness, renal failure or peripheral gangrene are such dire complications and the excess mortality attributable to accelerated coronary artery disease looms so large that no apology is needed for the elective imposition of so unpopular a treatment even in the elderly patient. The treatment of a patient admitted to hospital as an acute case in the throes of an episode of diabetic ketoacidosis falls outside the scope of this book and will not be described.

The understandable fear of self-injection can be much alleviated by firm and sympathetic teaching if the patient can be admitted to hospital for this purpose. Provided the task of instruction is not delegated to the most junior nurse, and an atmosphere of optimism bolsters the patient's at first shaky confidence, most patients can learn to inject themselves competently within a few days. Even partially sighted patients can master a suitably modified technique provided the identification of the correct volume to be injected is changed into a tactile task or prefilled syringes are dispensed. Advances in making the daily insulin injection(s) as comfortable and easy as possible include plastic syringes with tight plungers and clear markings supplied together with plastic-hubbed needles. These disposable combinations are suitable for repeated re-use if kept in 70% ethyl alcohol, whilst refrigeration alone suffices for the syringes. Swab sterilization of the skin has been shown to be ineffective and provided the tenets of ordinary domestic hygiene are adhered to, no special preparation of the skin prior to injection is required.

Since absorption of insulin from subcutaneous sites of injection is subject to many variables in the same patient (as well as within patients) there is a need for standardization of technique. Although information contained in standard textbooks and manufacturers' literature about the duration of action of various insulin preparations forms a good starting point in designing an insulin injection regimen for a particular patient (see Table 19.1), the detailed characteristics of a particular preparation in an individual patient can only be discovered by trial and error. If this injunction is taken seriously, there is usually no need for the time-honoured induction of a deliberate hypoglycaemic attack to acquaint the patient with his own range of hypoglycaemic symptoms. The introduction of highly purified insulins and of monocomponent insulins has reduced the incidence of disfiguring lipoatrophy and thus extended the skin area available for injection. Human insulins, although of great theoretical interest, do not constitute a clear advance in patient management at the present time. Account must be taken of the increased absorption from the exercising limb at rest. These differences, which are related to subcutaneous vascularity, are clinically important. The absorption of insulin is faster from the anterior abdominal wall followed in that order by the arm and the leg and is slowest from the thigh. Otherwise inexplicable hypoglycaemic attacks may well be due to changing the anatomical site of injection.

Table 19.1 Types of insulin (dosage: 100 i.u./ml).

	Onset	Peak activity	Duration (h)
Short acting			
Soluble (Wellcome: Beef)	1	2–6	8
Neutral (Novo: Pork)	½	2–5	7
Quicksol (Boots: Beef)	0–2	2–6	6–8
Velosulin (Nordisk: Pork)	0	1–3	8
Intermediate acting			
Initard (Nordisk: Pork)	0	4–8	24
Rapitard MC (Novo: Beef 75%, Pork 25%)	1	4–12	22
Semitard (Novo: Pork)	2	5–10	16
Insulatard (Nordisk: Pork)	1	4–12	24
Long acting			
Lente (Boots, CP Pharm, Evans: Beef)	2–4	8–12	24–30
Lentard MC (Novo: Beef 70%, Pork 30%)	2	7–14	24
Monotard MC (Novo: Pork)	2	7–14	22
Ultratard MC (Novo: Beef)	4–6	10–30	32–36

Particularly with insulin therapy but also with the less exacting treatments of diabetes an efficient system of blood sugar level surveillance must be introduced. The traditional method of assuming that all is well if excess urinary glucose cannot be detected will still suffice provided the patient's threshold for urinary glucose excretion is checked at the onset by accurately timed blood glucose estimations. High renal thresholds are unusual in the absence of renal failure or acute dehydration, but low thresholds can be a great pitfall. The repeated occurrence of hypoglycaemia in a setting of persistent glucosuria should alert the physician to the possibility of low renal threshold. This is often overlooked or misunderstood by nurses. The remedy lies in switching to control by blood glucose estimations which are timed in relation to meals. Adopting this method for every diabetic would appreciatively improve the level of diabetic control because the average renal threshold for glucose excretion lies above the upper limit of normal of the ambulant blood glucose concentration (7 mmols/l 130 mg/100 ml). However, practical considerations argue against extending this counsel of perfection to all elderly diabetic patients. Refinements such as the estimation of glycosylated haemoglobin have not so far been proved to be of value in the practical management of diabetes in geriatric patients.

General care of the diabetic patient

The first duty of the physician is to instruct his patient on the facts about diabetes. Many dialogues are needed between patient and doctor and neither the comforting assumption that the patient will pick up spontaneously what he needs to know nor the wholesale dismissal of elderly patients as incapable of new learning are justified. The self-centred attitude of many old people with their pronounced interest in their own bodily functions provides sufficient motivation to overcome the expected losses of intellectual efficiency of normal aging. It is a mistake to expect a patient to cope with the demands of his condition if all instruction and discussion is directed towards his relatives. Such tuition, although necessary, is complementary to the time spent in teaching the patient. Nor must the initially regressed behaviour of the patient when first confronted with the realization of what the diagnosis of diabetes entails, be assumed to represent the sum total of his personality resources.

Detailed aspects of personal care must include the provision of well-fitting shoes, the application of chiropody (podiatry) to any areas of hard skin on the feet and jagged edges on the toe nails. This becomes particularly important if diabetic peripheral neuropathy has blunted the warning normally provided by pain and discomfort. Attention to general hygiene and keeping skin creases dry and ventilated will diminish the development of troublesome intertrigo. Established moniliasis will respond to topical antifungal remedies.

All bacterial infections have to be taken seriously whether they are symptomatic or not. This applies particularly to *E. coli* urinary tract infections which in diabetes even in the absence of previous urinary tract abnormality can convert a normal kidney into a bag of pus within a few days. Papillary necrosis with secondary renal pelvic obstruction should be suspected if a diabetic patients' renal infection is associated with a fall in urine output. Frank haematuria, although commonly an associated feature, need not be present. Investigation should include sieving the urine for papillary fragments and an intravenous pyelogram. Uni- or bi-lateral obstructive features should lead to the passage of retrograde catheters, which, if done in time, stands a good chance of saving such kidneys. The development of cataracts is a remediable cause of deteriorating vision which should be corrected by surgical extraction before major disability has ensured.

The recent advances in laser destruction of new vessels formed near the retinal macula have given fresh impetus to the prevention of blindness in elderly diabetics. To ensure the discovery of lesions at a stage when they are still treatable it is necessary to arrange for regular retinal inspections by an ophthalmologist. At each visit questions about vision should be directed at the patient and if there is any doubt, a crude test of visual acuity with Snellen test types should be performed for each eye separately. Regular blood pressure measurements should facilitate the early detection of hypertension, another important risk factor in accelerated atherosclerosis. Its meticulous control is particularly important in diabetic patients because independent risk factors are multiplicative.

Hypothyroidism

The insiduous nature of this complaint leads to its late recognition at any age and the possibility of its being overlooked altogether in the elderly. The patient and his relatives by sharing the same pessimistic view concerning the inevitable decline of all faculties with advancing years are prone to attribute mental and physical slowness, depression, frequent falls and cold extremities to the natural history of the human condition. Since inability to keep appointments and general inefficiency in communication are added to this difficulty it is not surprising that the diagnosis of hypothyroidism owes much to chance. In older people it occurs so late that major atheromatous vascular damage has often already occurred although symptomatically concealed by the metabolic turpitude of the patient. Treatment with L. Thyroxine must, therefore, be moderated by the possible emergence of angina pectoris and cardiac arrythmias. In severe myxoedema sudden death constitutes a real danger during the early stages of therapy and hospitalization should be seriously considered. The starting dose of L. Thyroxine should be small (of the order of 0.05 mg) and even when a patient presents with hypothermia during the winter months it is a mistake to yield to therapeutic impatience. It is arguable whether the substitution of triiodothyronine should be preferred in the latter case but the dose should be small and the major therapeutic expedient should consist of efficient re-warming.

After two weeks the dose of L. Thyroxine can be doubled provided no cardiac symptoms have emerged. The general policy is to judge the patient's progress clinically, to advance to the next higher dose only if 2–6 weeks of the previous dose level have been well tolerated or anginal symptoms have been adequately controlled. The ideal of complete restoration of a normal metabolic rate is often not reached. However, when the substitution dose is not limited by unwelcome symptoms, the question of reaching the optimum dose arises. There is some room for experimentation here but few elderly patients require a dose above L. Thyroxine 0.2 mg/day unless concurrent propranolol therapy raises the required dose by interfering with the conversion of thyroxine to triiodothyronine.

Since the main evil of incomplete correction of hypothyroidism—the accelerated course of atherosclerosis—is mediated by unrelieved secondary hyperlipidaemia, a restoration to normal of the patients lipoprotein profile is a useful endpoint. Alternatively, an estimation of plasma T_4 level may be helpful. It must be remembered that the normal thyroid gland secretes a mixture of T_3 and T_4 so that in the construction of normal ranges by laboratories the latter is counted in its own right and also serves as a marker for the former. During substitution therapy no T_3 is administered with the T_4 and hence the measured plasma T_4 levels should be at the upper end of the specified normal range. It is common for patients to be systematically undertreated because this important point is not appreciated.

Another use of laboratory tests is to check that the patient takes his thyroxine tablets. The result of thyroxine substitution therapy should be obvious within a few weeks and is usually highly gratifying to the patient. Falls related to cerebellar dysfunction may take a few months to clear and falls may get worse if related to the sick cardiac sinus node syndrome thus necessitating artificial pacemaker insertion. The increase in physical well-being and energy may cause problems if the patient suffers from irrecoverable organic dementia or if psychiatric symptoms originally hopefully attributed to the hypothyroidism are unresolved or even aggravated. It requires fine judgement to decide how far such a patient should be allowed to sink back into partial hypothyroidism.

Addison's disease and hypopituitarism

Deficiency of pituitary hormones is rarely acquired in old age. Indeed at any age the effects are usually mild apart from categorical effects on gonadal function. In older people presentation as hypothyroidism without fluid retention and the usual telltale coarsening of the features is most common. Replacement therapy with thyroxine may have the important consequence of uncovering a lack of adrenal cortical reserve manifesting itself in vomiting and collapse when the patient is exposed to physical stress, and possibly endangering his life when he is exposed to trivial accidents or illnesses or subjected to minor surgery. The prescription of adrenocortical replacement therapy is subject to the same rules and precautions as in Addison's disease and will be discussed in detail later in this section. Sex hormones are almost never required when panhypopituitarism occurs in this age group.

Addison's disease, which can occur at any age and should not curtail life expectancy, is nevertheless not so often encountered in the geriatric age group. This must raise the strong suspicion that the wages of suboptimal management are premature death of the patient. The trap lies in the well-established formulation of average daily requirements of cortisone acetate as 37.5 mg usually administered as two unequal doses. This eminently true statement leaves out of account the most important fact of variation of glucocorticoid requirement with circumstance. The range of this variation is very wide and when neither the physician nor the patient are willing to depart from the well-learned formula, a trivial illness like a cold becomes serious and anything worse is likely to have a lethal outcome. The first rule of treatment must, therefore, be variability of therapy, with doubling of the basic dose of cortisone acetate even on suspicion of trivial illness and doubling the dose again for anything more significant.

The second rule is to instruct the patient in such variation of dosage and the absolute need for seeking immediate medical consultation if an illness threatens free food and fluid intake or is accompanied by any feature of systemic upset. Mental stress such as experienced in bereavements, re-housing or arguments with relatives also qualifies for increased cortisone dosage.

The management of mineralocorticoid substitution is much simpler. Some patients have become habituated to a high salt intake prior to diagnosis and the persistence of this after cortisone therapy has been started may obviate the need for mineralocortoid substitution therapy. In others a fixed dose of 0.05 to 0.15 mg of 9α fludrocortisone per day is required. The only drawback of overdosage is the gradual development of mild hypertension which will be discovered at the mandatory periodic routine medical examinations. In very elderly patients the compromise between a degree of hypertension with its risk of precipitating a stroke and the diminished general well-being of the normotensive patient will have to be struck in favour of hypertension.

Gonadal support

In a world struggling to subdue the burden of human fertility the procreative function of sexual activity has receded somewhat in importance in favour of valuing the continuance of satisfactory sexual relations in marriage as an important pair-bonding mechanism. This attitude has freed physical love from its age barriers and we have reliable evidence that there exists a widespread expectation of significant conjugal relations into the eighth decade of both male and female life. It is very likely that this expectation is commonly disappointed for a wide variety of reasons.

Neither the fortunately rare autonomic causes of impotence nor the deleterious effects of general ill-health are relevant to this account but we are here concerned with remedying specific endocrine components which commonly interact with otherwise minor physical and psychological factors to lead to the premature breakdown of sexual function in an elderly couple. The very low oestrogen production by the post-menopausal ovaries is for many years supplemented by the secretion of oestrogen byproducts of steroid synthesis. At some stage during normal aging this will no longer suffice to prevent atrophy of vulval and vaginal tissues. At the same time the increasing vaginal alkalinity leads to the replacement of the protective lactobacilli by a mixed flora. The reduction in natural lubrication coupled with the thinness and friability of the vaginal epithelium leads to painful, difficult intercourse which will soon act as a permanent discouragement unless the condition is relieved.

Apart from commonsense remedies such as the provision of artificial lubrication and the specific eradication of monilial infection by nystatin pessaries and cream, the choice lies between local application of oestrogen creams and the full impact of oestrogen replacement therapy. Creams are only partial in their continued effectivensss.

If the patient has undergone a total hysterectomy and bilateral oophorectomy before the menopause, oestrogen replacement therapy is likely to have been established early. Despite the minimal risk of an increased tendency to venous thrombosis, it is appropriate to continue such therapy into old age although the dosage requirements may diminish with increasing years. The situation is less clear if the uterus is still *in situ*, because perpetual oestrogen replacement therapy is in these circumstances associated with an enhanced risk of developing carcinoma of the body of the uterus. It is unfortunate that the earliest symptom of such a carcinoma is postmenopausal bleeding which also commonly occurs as a functional symptom of oestrogen replacement therapy. After repeated curettage with negative results, the development of a false sense of security by either the patient or the doctor may mean that an early diagnosis is not made because curettage may have been omitted. Attempts to resolve the dilemma by the prescription of oestrogen/progestin mixtures have reduced the amount of oestrogen prescribed and this possibly diminishes the risk of carcinoma development but perhaps an even greater advance lies in the reduction of the incidence of functional uterine bleeding. Nonetheless, the complete safety of perpetual replacement therapy cannot be guaranteed and this must be clearly pointed out to the patient, who may well opt for local therapy after a number of years of successful replacement therapy. We will return to this subject when the topic of osteoporosis and its postmenopausal acceleration is discussed.

If one looks for a sudden cessation of male fertility on the basis of insufficient endogenous testosterone secretion, the much publicized male climacteric is a myth.

There is a wide range of testosterone level decline rates, however, which must at times make such decline the direct reason for failure of sexual function. The reason for the commonly observed failure of androgenic substances to relieve established impotence in males of all ages does not lie in a negation of this principle. The explanation of this paradox relates to the direct relationship between male libido and androgenic activity, so that those who complain of impotence and therefore seek medical advice are unlikely to suffer from endocrine failure, whilst the possibly equally large number who do so suffer are unlikely to present at all. The ethical questions raised by the need actively to seek out the diagnosis of androgenic failure, perhaps based on an oblique and perceptive interpretation of the wife's complaints, has to be solved by each practicing doctor individually. To surmount such difficulties is part of the essence of medical family practice.

HORMONES IN DISEASE

Adrenal steroid therapy

Introduction

The recognition of the enormous anti-inflammatory potency of adrenal cortical hormones applied in apparently unlimited doses (at least in the short term) led in succession to phases of irresponsible therapeutic euphoria and considerable revulsion occasioned by the creation of a vast array of undesirable side-effects. Forty years later we occupy an intermediate position having defined by prolonged trial and error the indications for long-term and short-term administration of glucocorticoids. The massive doses of prednisolone needed for the containment of otherwise fatal disease such as pemphigus vulgaris, rampant disseminated lupus erythematosis (DLE) or polyarteritis nodosa will not be considered, nor will the controversial use of steroids in the various shock syndromes. Those topics fall into the province of specialized hospital practice and are outside the scope of this book.

The more commonly encountered uses of steroids in allergic and chronic inflammatory conditions are based on the recognition that benefits are maximal early whilst the deleterious effects gradually accumulate with prolonged use. From these considerations a hit-and-run technique has been developed so that a short sharp course does not usually lead to maintenance therapy and a principle of extreme parsimony of dosage has also been formulated for those conditions were long-term or even lifelong therapy is contemplated. The dividing line between acute and chronic steroid therapy hinges on the production of suppression of the pituitary adrenocortical axis which appears to correlate rather better with the duration than the magnitude of the dose of the initial course of therapy. Discussion will be limited to two groups of conditions but the principles enunciated are more widely applicable.

Asthma and obstructive airways disease

By the time a patient seeks medical advice during an acute exacerbation of chronic asthma there is usually proof of the failure of his usual bronchodilator remedies since the prescribed dosage has already been exceeded. In elderly patients bronchiolar constriction and mucus plugging with consequent air trapping occurs against a background of considerable established lung damage; even between attacks respiratory reserve is usually much diminished. Although psychological mechanisms may loom as large as in younger patients and panic is not always confined to the relatives, sedation of any kind is strongly contraindicated because a degree of arterial anoxia and, less commonly, mild hypercapnia indicates in most elderly asthmatics that all exacerbations are accompanied by at least incipient respiratory failure.

From these considerations one can easily deduce the need for energetic action which will usually include a course of steroids. It is essential to aim for control of the reversible element of bronchospasm within 24–48 hours so that the whole course does not need to exceed 5–7 days in duration. This avoids the major evil of chronic steroid therapy which is the usual consequence of failing to get the patient off steroids before depression of the pituitary-adrenal axis necessitates the institution of a prolonged tailing off regimen. Such tailing off regimens are not only tedious but potentially dangerous since during the tailing off programme the patient is commonly overtaken by further attacks which require increases in steroid dosage. Thus he may end up on permanent steroid therapy with all its attendant horrors.

The disadvantages of permanent steroid therapy include unexpected death due to adrenal failure in crises, chronic steroid toxicity to the skin, skeleton and cardiovascular system, the premature precipitation of diabetes mellitus, the activation of peptic ulcers and quiescent pulmonary tuberculosis and finally asthmatic attacks becoming less responsive to increases in steroid therapy. The key to avoiding such a therapeutic disaster lies in choosing an initial steroid dosage equivalent to 60 mg prednisolone and being prepared to raise the dose to 100 mg/day if there is no clear response within 24 hours.

Once a response has occurred, even very high doses of steroids can be halved on successive days without inducing relapse. The remission does not have to be complete before dose-cutting is commenced and it is the rule to see further objective improvement in the degree of bronchospasm as the dose is rapidly reduced to zero over the next few days. It is perhaps ironical that the most common reason for inadvertently producing a steroid-dependent asthmatic is the prescription of an inadequate steroid starting dose, based on the fear of producing steroid addiction. Unfortunately, if unnecessary deaths are to be avoided no physician can altogether avoid the prescription of steroids in acute asthma.

The prominence accorded to the details of steroid management is not intended to convey the idea that other measures such as hydration, antibiotics and oxygen therapy are unimportant. The last, even when a 24% oxygen Venturi type mask is used, is sufficiently complicated to be often a sufficient reason for hospitalization in its own right. The most important rules are, first, that oxygen therapy must be uninterrupted to prevent a staircase-type progressive accumulation of CO_2, and, second, that a recently confused elderly asthmatic cannot be managed at home.

Since oxygen therapy may be fatal in patients with an hypoxic respiratory drive by allowing the accumulation of CO_2 due to its suppression, it is essential to carry out serial blood gas analyses in such patients. If even modest improvements in arterial oxygen tension cannot be achieved without producing prohibitive rises in arterial CO_2 tension, the patient becomes a candidate for ventilation therapy in a respiratory care unit.

A final word about the futility of achieving a clear diagnostic distinction between cardiac and bronchial asthma. In many elderly patients the two conditions coexist and may be mutually re-enforcing. A trial of a loop diuretic such as frusemide will not harm a bronchial asthmatic and even in acute pulmonary oedema short-term steroids are safe.

The administration of beta adrenergic therapy. e.g. salbutamol orally or intravenously, is more problematic since the bronchodilator and cardiac stimulatory advantages have to be set against the increased risk of producing cardiac arrhythmias, including fatal ventricular fibrillation if the diagnosis should have been acute left ventricular failure perhaps precipitated by acute myocardial infarction.

Rheumatoid arthritis and other rheumatic disorders

There are major contrasts between this and the preceding section. The only rheumatic disorder which provides a mandatory indication for steroid therapy is giant cell arteritis presenting as headache because of the risk of blindness but even in this condition high doses are only rarely needed. The other difference concerns the aim of providing long-term relief by the chronic prescription of very small doses of steroids. In rheumatoid arthritis the relief of incapacitating morning stiffness can be achieved by the exhibition of 5.0–7.5 mg of prednisolone in a single dose on retiring to bed at night. The benefits of such therapy would commonly, even in retired elderly persons, outweigh the disadvantages of the mild cushingoid syndrome that is inevitably produced. It is a mistake, however, to increase this dose to combat a general increase in the activity of the disease.

Troublesome individual joints not subdued by systemic background non-steroid anti-inflammatory therapy may yield to selective local steroid injections. Tendinitis and ligamentous pain may be similarly treated provided it is remembered that all injected steroids are finally absorbed into the bloodstream so that the previously stated limits to overall dosage must still be applied.

The provision of local steroid therapy to cases of degenerative (osteo) arthritis should not include injection of weight-bearing joints unless early joint replacement is envisaged or the general or specific locomotor incapacity of the patient renders the distinction between weight-bearing and non-weight-bearing joints meaningless.

The use of higher doses of steroids on alternate days has been shown to result in less suppression of the pituitary adrenal axis and arguably a reduced incidence of other steroid side-effects. This technique is at its most advantageous in the treatment of life-threatening disease with high dose steroids, where it may at times prevent the production of steroid psychosis.

Whenever adrenal glucocorticoids have to be exhibited in courses which last too long for complete cessation of therapy to be achieved within one week of its commencement it becomes mandatory to taper the steroids off slowly in an effort to prevent a sudden re-emergence of the original disease treated and also to reduce the risk of adrenal failure. During the final stages of tailing-off steroids, a reduction of as little as 1 mg per day each month may be appropriate. Since the symptoms of the underlying disease commonly recrudesce during prolonged steroid therapy, it proves often impossible to take steroid tapering to its logical conclusion.

OSTEOPOROSIS AND OSTEOMALACIA

Osteoporosis means decreased bone mass but the bone remains normally mineralized. Since the mass of remaining bone is clearly directly related to its tensile strength there exists an inverse relationship to the frequency of fracture occurrence. There is age-related bone loss, a normal physiological phenomenon which, however, shows a marked preponderence in females because of a sharp acceleration of this rate of net bone loss at the menopause. Adrenal steroids and disuse, both local and general, produce acceleration of this process in both sexes. Both the prevention and reversal of female osteoporosis after the menopause are possible by treatment with relatively low doses of oestrogen such as 20–50 μg per day of ethinyl oestradiol thus reducing the incidence of femoral and vertebral fractures. It is estimated that untreated white American women have a 26% incidence of vertebral fractures by 65 years which rises to 50% by the age of 75. Hip fractures double in frequency in white women every 5 years after age 60, causing considerable morbidity and mortality. This emphasizes the importance of tackling the serious public health problem posed by preventable fractures. Other avoidance measures include an insistence on maintaining mobility in old age and an attitude of extreme parsimony towards long-term steroid therapy. If higher doses of steroids have to be employed for life-saving purposes, the amount of osteoporosis produced can be reduced by alternate-day therapy. An alternative treatment of osteoporosis with porcine calcitonin must either avoid high enough doses to activate the parathyroid glands which would aggravate the osteoporosis, or the treatment must be covered by the prescription of 3 g calcium carbonate per day. On the whole, this treatment of oesteoporosis is inferior to oestrogens but calcitonin is the treatment of choice for Pagets disease producing pain or deafness by either direct involvement of the ossicles or compression of the auditory nerve by petrous pagetic bone. Repeated courses may be required however.

The advantages and disadvantages of oestrogen therapy have already been discussed under the heading of gonadal support, but in the author's opinion the case for minimal perpetual oestrogen replacement therapy, perhaps in combination with progestins, is appreciably strengthened by its undoubted effectiveness in arresting the progression of osteoporosis.

The term osteomalacia, which is often confused with osteoporosis although the two conditions quite commonly coexist in the same patient, refers to poor bone mineralization related basically to poor calcium absorption. This may either be secondary to small intestinal malabsorption perhaps against the background of a borderline dietary calcium intake or due to a deficiency of the active renal vitamin D metabolite 1:25 dihydroxycholecalciferol which, in turn, may either point to low dietary vitamin D intake, insufficient exposure to sunshine or renal failure. In elderly patients not uncommonly several of these factors combine to produce either a proximal myopathy which may lead to an easily missed cause of inability to walk or may precipitate a fracture. Always consider osteomalacia if a fracture occurs, particularly in men in the 7th decade. Osteomalacia can be diagnosed by a therapeutic trial of vitamin D thus obviating the need for expensive, time consuming and often inconclusive investigations. High doses by injection of expensive synthetic vitamin D analogues or metabolites are not required. A three week course of 1.25 mg of oral calciferol daily followed by the prescription of a physiological vitamin D dose (900 i.u. or 23 μg per day) will suffice.

Cancer therapy

Hormone therapy may be useful either in the temporary control of relatively well-differentiated, disseminated hormone-dependent cancers or in the control of symptoms produced by perimetastatic oedema in brain tissue. Disseminated prostatic carcinoma associated with painful spinal and pelvic metastases will usually show a symptomatic response to oral stilboestrol, although urethral obstruction will require a transurethral resection for its relief. Although the so-called prostatic serum acid phosphatase level is an insensitive indicator of the presence of metastases its suppression is an adequate index of sufficient stilboestrol dosage. Successful treatment will relieve bone pain, allow fractures to heal and even lead to recovery from the leucoerythroblastic anaemia of bone marrow infiltration. Once a response has occurred the dose of stilboestrol should be reduced to the lowest dose that still controls the acid phosphatase levels. This will abolish nausea and vomiting in most cases, reduce the risk of venous thrombosis and myocardial infarction but will not eliminate the development of nipple pigmentation and gynaecomastia nor restore sexual potency. It is the inevitability of occurrence of such side-effects which renders oestrogens unsuitable for the treatment of potentially curable undisseminated prostatic carcinoma often diagnosed by needle biopsy. It would be reasonable to arrange for regular urological check ups in otherwise fit elderly males to allow the diagnosis of prostatic carcinoma to be made at any early stage.

Carcinoma of the breast in very elderly women is often slow growing and although bony metastases occur, local ulceration of the lesion is commonly the most troublesome feature to the patient. This may respond better to oestrogen than to X-ray therapy, although high doses capable of inducing transient nausea and fluid retention may be required. The decision to use oestrogens or the antioestrogenic drug tamoxifen is often based on the presence of oestrogen receptors on carcinoma cells derived from the patient, but the prediction value of such receptor studies is only statistical and in the individual case it may still be permissible to try out hormone therapy in the face of negative oestrogen receptor augury.

Local excision of the lesion or simple mastectomy are alternative methods of treatment provided the malignant mass is not fixed to the rib cage. Once metastases to the liver have occurred, oestrogens lose their palliative value and death is not usually long delayed.

The immediate response of cerebral secondaries to high dose adrenal steroid therapy is often dramatic with cessation of headache and vomiting, clearing of the sensorium and regression of neurological localizing signs. Although relapse is inevitable it may be delayed for several months and good quality life may be possible in the interim. During a rather prolonged remission of symptoms it is worthwhile to protect the patient from secondary epilepsy by the institution of prophylactic anticonvulsant therapy.

Postural hypotension

This rather non-specific complaint is a common cause of decreasing confidence in the elderly leading to falls, fractures and immobility. Milder cases require an early morning consultation for diagnosis since the physiological overnight shrinkage of the plasma volume may then reveal postural hypotension as the cause of the patients unsteadiness. The first line of treatment is to review the patient's medication for items which might produce or aggravate the symptoms by reducing the plasma volume, limiting the cardiac output or by interfering with the postural reflexes. Such drugs include all diuretics, non-vasodilator hypotensive agents especially methyldopa and adrenergic neurone blockers, beta blockers and some psycholeptics such as chlorpromazine. Failure to provide relief by rationalizing the patient's medication must be followed by active measures. The aim to achieve a gentle positive salt and water balance can often be achieved by the combination of enhancing the patient's salt intake, if necessary by the prescription of salt tablets, and the exhibition of doses of 9 α fludrocortisone in excess of replacement requirements. Indomethacin has been suggested by some authors because of its antidiuretic action, but it may lead to bleeding from an asymptomatic and therefore unsuspected peptic ulcer and there also exists evidence that it may worsen myocardial ischaemia due to coronary artery disease. Pindolol (a beta blocker with strong partial agonist activity) and a small dose of hydralazine are often useful in younger patients with postural hypotension by provoking tachycardia and hence an increase in cardiac output but cannot be unreservedly recommended in the elderly because of the ubiquity of ischaemic heart disease, whether it is symptomatic or not.

When none of these measures is of avail because the retained fluid will not stay in the vascular compartment, elastic full length two-way stretch stockings and attention to nutritional hypoalbumenaemia may yet win the battle. Only in the very small minority of patients where autonomic neuropathy is the major cause of postural hypotension, such as occurs in some diabetics and a minority of Parkinsonian patients, need fitting of a pressure suit be contemplated. Because of the devastating psychological effects of postural hypotension it is important to make the diagnosis as early as possible so that effective remedies can be found before the patient's view of life has been permanently constricted.

Dermatological disorders

No physician can be in practice long before a series of successful dermatological cures achieved by adrenal steroid-containing creams convinces him of his omnipotence as a dermatological therapeutician and of the futility of seeking after dermatological diagnostic labels. This picture of medical bliss is commonly completed by the patients gratitude which is not often withheld from the successful doctor. Two notes of caution must be sounded here: first, all topically applied steroids are eventually absorbed into the bloodstream so that all protracted or repeated steroid cream applications have systemic consequences. Second, steroid toxicity to the skin itself may prematurely precipitate or enhance senile atrophy and cannot be reversed. Apart from avoiding the obvious pitfalls of disseminating infective disorders or setting the stage for a major psoriatic rebound by the actual misapplication of topical steroids, the practitioner should dilute his steroid-containing applications as much as possible and set himself a time limit both for the achievement of initial amelioration and for the duration of maintenance therapy. Lack of initial success or the need for prolonged steroid suppressive therapy are equally good reasons for dermatological referral.

REFERENCES AND FURTHER READING

Amis Kingsley. (1978) *Jake's Thing* Hutchinson, London.

Felig P. (1980) Disorders of Carbohydrate Metabolism. In Bondy & Rosenberg (eds) *Metabolic Control and Disease*, 8th edn, pp. 276–392. W.B. Saunders, New York.

Gregerman R.I. & Bierman E.L. (1981) Aging and Hormones. In Williams R.H. (ed.) *Textbook of Endocrinology*, Ch. 29, pp. 1192–212. W.B. Sauinders, New York.

Hodkinson H.M. & Irvine R.E. (1984) Thyroid Disease in Old Age. In Brocklehurst J.C. (ed.) *Textbook of Geriatric Medicine and Gerontology*, 3rd edn. Churchill Livingstone, London.

Ireland J.T., Thomson W.St., & Williamson J. (1980) *Diabetes Today*, HM&M Publishers, Alesbury.

Mortimer B.L. & Lippman M.E. (1981) Endocrine Responsive Cancers in Man. In Williams R.H. (ed.) *Textbook of Endocrinology*, 6th edn, Ch. 30, pp. 1213–27. W.B. Saunders, New York.

Oakley, W.G., Pyke D.A. & Taylor K.W. (eds) (1978) Treatment. *In Diabetes and its management*, 3rd edn, Ch. 7. Blackwell Scientific Publications, Oxford.

Parsons V., Mitchell C., Emond A. & Darby A.J. (1983) The Use of Sodium Fluoride with Calcium Supplements and Vitamin D in the Treatment of Axial Osteoporosis. In Dixon A.St.J., Russell R.G.G. & Stamp T.C.B. (eds), *Osteoporosis a Multidisciplinary Problem*. The Royal Society of Medicine, London. Academic Press, London. Grune and Stratton, New York.

Sönksen, P.H. (1979) Home Monitoring of Blood Glucose by Diabetic Patients. In Ditzel Jørn (ed.) *Proceedings of 3rd Nordic Symposium on Diabetes: Diabetes and Diabetes Treatment III*, pp. 145–56.

Turner R.C. & Williamson D.H. (1982) Control of metabolism and the alterations in diabetes. In O'Riordan J.L.H. (ed.) *Recent Advances in Endocrinology and Metabolism 2*, pp. 73–97. Churchill Livingstone, London.

Index